THE WEB THAT HAS NO WEAVER

Understanding Chinese Medicine

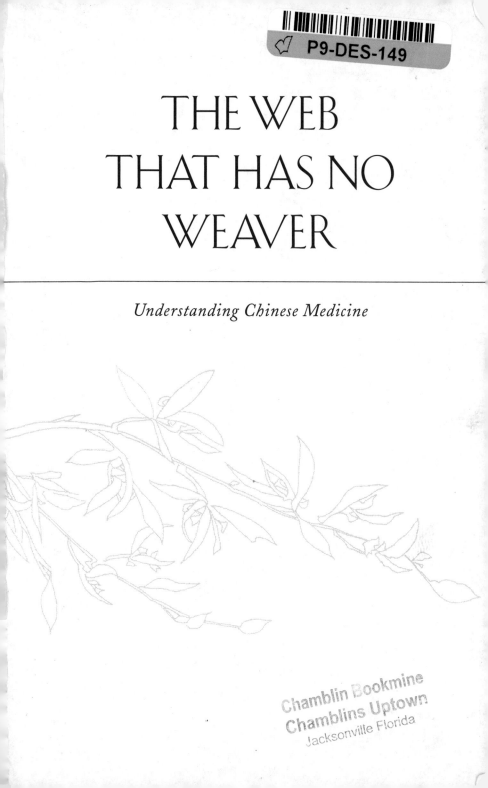

"*The Web That Has No Weaver* opens the great door of understanding to the profoundness of Chinese medicine."

—*People's Daily*, Beijing, China

"*The Web That Has No Weaver* with its manifold merits . . . is a successful introduction to Chinese medicine. We recommend it to our colleagues in China."

—*Chinese Journal of Integrated Traditional and Chinese Medicine*, Beijing, China

"Ted Kaptchuk's book [has] something for practically everyone . . . Kaptchuk, himself an extraordinary combination of elements, is a thinker whose writing is more accessible than that of Joseph Needham or Manfred Porkert with no less scholarship. There is more here to think about, chew over, ponder or reflect upon than you are liable to find elsewhere. . . . This may sound like a rave review: it is."

—*Journal of Traditional Acupuncture*

"This revised version of an essential classic on Traditional Chinese Medicine is a gift for all who share an interest in deep understanding of healing. Ted Kaptchuk is a unique figure in complementary medicine. His combination of scholarship, wisdom, and compassion provides a remarkable window into one of the greatest of all healing traditions."

—Michael Lerner, President, Commonweal, a California
Nonprofit Corporation, author of *Choices in Healing:
Integrating the Best of Conventional and Complementary
Approaches to Cancer*

"Ted Kaptchuk is without question one of the most innovative thinkers in the area of Traditional Chinese Medicine. This new edition is a brilliant synthesis of traditional and scientific knowledge. It is compulsory reading for anyone with a serious interest in this area."

—Professor Edzard Ernst, M.D., Ph.D., Director, Department
of Complementary Medicine, School of Postgraduate
Medicine and Health Sciences, University of Exeter

"In the 20th century, modern China rescued its traditional medicine from oblivion at the cost of removing its soul; in the 21st century, Dr. Kaptchuk has put the ancient discussion of soul back into Chinese medicine. This new edition integrates the seemingly opposing paradigms of ancient Chinese medicine and modern biomedicine and interprets the classical Chinese views on spirit in relation to the medical and existential aspirations of modern humankind."

—Giovanni Maciocia, Honorary Lecturer, Nanjing College of
Traditional Chinese Medicine and author of *The Foundations
of Chinese Medicine*

THE WEB THAT HAS NO WEAVER

Understanding Chinese Medicine

TED J. KAPTCHUK, O.M.D.

McGraw·Hill

New York   Chicago   San Francisco   Lisbon   London   Madrid   Mexico City
Milan   New Delhi   San Juan   Seoul   Singapore   Sydney   Toronto

The McGraw-Hill Companies

Library of Congress Cataloging-in-Publication Data

Kaptchuk, Ted J., 1947–.
 The web that has no weaver : understanding Chinese medicine / Ted
J. Kaptchuk. — 2nd ed.
 p. cm.
 Includes index.
 ISBN 0-8092-2840-8
 1. Medicine, Chinese. 2. Medicine, Chinese—Philosophy.
I. Title.
R601.K36 2000
610'.951—dc21 98-53193
 CIP

*Dedicated to the memory of Ted Gold, my grandparents,
and relatives who died for the Sanctification of the Name*

Copyright © 2000 by Ted J. Kaptchuk. All rights reserved. Printed in the United States of
America. Except as permitted under the United States Copyright Act of 1976, no part of this
publication may be reproduced or distributed in any form or by any means, or stored in a
database or retrieval system, without the prior written permission of the publisher.

15 16 17 18 DOC/DOC 1 9 8 7 6 5 4 3 2 1 0

ISBN 0-8092-2840-8

Cover design by Monica Baziuk

McGraw-Hill books are available at special quantity discounts to use as premiums and sales
promotions, or for use in corporate training programs. For more information, please write to
the Director of Special Sales, Professional Publishing, McGraw-Hill, Two Penn Plaza, New
York, NY 10121-2298. Or contact your local bookstore.

This book is printed on acid-free paper.

CONTENTS

ACKNOWLEDGMENTS

Michael Steinlauf, my oldest friend, who took a series of garbled lectures and made them intelligible. Without Michael's literary help this manuscript might just as well have stayed in Chinese. • Harvey Blume, my oldest comrade, whose poetic and philosophic illuminations are scattered throughout this book. His imprint is especially evident in the remarks on Hegel and Aristotle. • Dan Bensky, my classmate in Macao, who shared my studies and contributed invaluable ideas, writing, and criticism to this manuscript. • Steve J. Bennett, freelance scholar and writer, who helped to clarify the ideas and prose of this manuscript. • Margaret Caudill, my constant medical mentor and collaborator, who provided criticism and stability. • Gretchen Salisbury, for being my editor, and for the enormous work she did to get this book into shape. • Randy Barolet, my teaching colleague, who helped with the writing. • Liz Coffin, June Nusser, and Kendra Crossen for patient editing and rewriting. • Barbara Huntley, who, by her design, transformed an unconventional manuscript into a book. • Satya Ambrose for the illustrations. • Natalia Muina for editorial assistance, and the Jing that helped me to get through the writing of this volume. •

Francesca Loporto for criticism and the gift of Spirit. • Kiiko Matsumoto for scholarly archeology in pre-Tang-dynasty texts. • Andy Gamble, Maria Tadd, and Jon Koritz for help with idea development. • Paul and Andy Epstein for help with writing. • Paul Parker and Mark Epstein for criticism and writing. • Noah Weinberg for help in getting down to basics and lighting fires. • Jonathan Lieff for spiritual and medical advice. • Wendy Pomerantz for editorial assistance. • Fred Klarer and Ken DeWoskin for translation suggestions. • Nancy Trichter for being my literary agent and a source of constant encouragement. • Cody for being Cody. • Lieb Scheiner, E. V. Walter, and Steven Klarer for research assistance. • Marsha Woolf, Joyce Singer, Savitri Clark, Paul Shulman, Richard Michael Zucker, Walter Torda, Chou Man-Xing, Sekyo Nam, Martha Katz, Liu Yun-Hua, Giovanni Maciocia, Ellen Pearlman, Janet Generalli, and Susan Zimelis for support. • The friends, acupuncturists, medical doctors, therapists, healers, and students who attended my lectures in the States, Europe, and Australia and asked the many questions that helped to focus this volume. • My teachers of the traditional medicine of China, who gave so unselfishly, especially Yu Jin-niang, Xie Zhang-cai, Ling Ling-xian, Chen Yi-qing, and Hong Yuan-bain. • My patients, who taught me so much, especially that the effort of writing this volume was more than literary or scholarly. • My adoptive godmother, Lam Pui-yin, whose pureness kept me going physically and spiritually during hard times in medical school. • My parents and sister, whose love is always with me.

FOREWORD

by Margaret A. Caudill

Early in the 1970s, in the wake of a new politically sanctioned exchange of information between China and the United States, there appeared in the press a number of anecdotal descriptions of surgery without anesthesia being performed in China. A technique called acupuncture was used, whereby slender needles pierced the skin at predetermined foci on the body, the patient being fully awake during the procedure but not feeling the scalpel. Over the next several years this ancient technique of acupuncture enjoyed a brief surge of popularity in the United States, where it was touted by some as a new method to induce analgesia, indeed, as the long-awaited panacea from the Orient. This sudden enthusiasm was quickly followed by a backlash within the medical establishment, which, unable to obtain "scientific proof" of claims made by acupuncture proponents, was ready to abandon it and to forbid its practice in the United States. This attempt was unsuccessful, however, and investigations of the possible application of acupuncture to Western medicine have continued. The evidence now indicates that acupuncture can induce analgesia and that its use is associated with measurable physiological changes (see Chapter 4, note 11). Recent medical reviews show that acupuncture is slowly beginning to be integrated into certain areas of Western medicine (*Journal of the American Medical Association* 1998; 280: 1518–1524).

Although acupuncture itself has gained some acceptance, the Western medical and scientific community has never considered seriously the medical tradition and culture from which this technique sprang. As if a full understanding of acupuncture were encompassed by knowing where to stick the needles! This absurdity is compounded by the fact that the idea of isolating a part from its natural environment for investigation is antithetical to the philosophy and culture of the Chinese medical tradition. There may well be inaccuracies, biases, and misrepresentations that have grown up around the acupuncture tradition over the centuries. But any meaningful discussion of acupuncture and its applicability requires more information than has heretofore been presented.

The problem does not lie entirely with the medical and scientific establishment. Almost none of the traditional Chinese medical texts are available in English, and those that are available make little or no attempt to present the cultural medical tradition *in toto*. Even translated works pose the problem of a completely unfamiliar approach to disease and a foreign terminology. Only someone familiar with the Chinese language, naturalist and Taoist philosophy, and with Chinese culture as it has been influenced by these philosophies, would be able to comprehend the Chinese medical tradition.

The chapters to follow begin an important exposition of the ancient art of Chinese medicine in terms that can be understood by a Western audience. The author has deftly avoided, as much as possible, the pitfall of interpreting Chinese theory through Western terminology, thereby leaving the central Chinese concept of medical patterns and disharmonies undisturbed.

A word of caution to those who would judge the images and vocabulary as inconsequential or as the babblings of a primitive society because of their own lack of familiarity with the terms: for thousands of years the Chinese have observed life processes and relationships between man and his environment. From this observation, the art of Chinese medicine has developed vocabulary to describe myriad subtle body patterns, a method of description not available to Western medicine because of its emphasis on disease states. The Chinese approach is a more holistic consideration of health and disease and of the delicate interplay between these opposing forces.

In a time of increased awareness of environment, health, and the personal responsibility of mankind, it seems that an integration of East and West should be mutually beneficial. Dr. Kaptchuk has attempted a most difficult job, to begin bridging the gap by making available this critical and timely exposition to those who wish to understand the art of medicine from a different viewpoint. Indeed, the web may have found its weaver.

Margaret A. Caudill, M.D., Ph.D.

Research Fellow in Medicine, Harvard Medical School, Division of Behavioral Medicine, Beth Israel Hospital, Boston

FOREWORD

by Andrew Weil

The Web That Has No Weaver was my introduction to the theory of Chinese medicine when it first appeared in 1982. In that year I was writing my first book about medicine, *Health and Healing*, in which I surveyed a number of systems of medicine, both conventional and alternative, and discussed their strengths and weaknesses. I found Ted Kaptchuk's book to be the best source of information on the origins, philosophy, and practice of traditional Chinese medicine. Remarkably, almost two decades later, it still is.

In 1982, most Americans were unfamiliar with Chinese medicine, except for some who had tried acupuncture, mostly for temporary relief of pain. Today, Chinese medicine is commonplace in America, with practitioners available throughout the country. Chinese patent medicines are sold widely, and a number of Chinese herbs, like ginseng, astragalus, and dong quai, have become well known. Many American physicians have taken courses in medical acupuncture. Practitioners of traditional Chinese medicine are in demand to join the staffs of integrative medical facilities and healing and wellness centers.

Despite the tremendous popularity of this unique system of medicine in our country, American medical students still receive no formal instruction in it as part of their required studies and most American physicians probably cannot summarize its theoretical structure or explain how it differs from Western medicine.

I find Chinese medicine very appealing because of its strong emphasis on prevention and because of its practical success with conditions that Western medicine is not so good with—inflammatory bowel disease, for example, as well as a range of autoimmune disorders. I recognize also that the emphasis of Chinese practitioners on energy and its balanced flow throughout the body is a stumbling block for Westerners who cannot see beyond the limitations of the paradigm of materialistic science.

As a physician committed to the integration of all safe and effective treatments into a new kind of medicine for the whole person, I think the Chinese perspective on health and illness is invaluable, and I welcome all attempts to make it accessible to Westerners. Ted Kaptchuk did a splendid job of that in the original edition of *The Web That Has No Weaver*. In this second edition he has added much new material, including reviews of recent scientific developments in the study of acupuncture and herbal medicine and a discussion of the possible adverse effects of these therapies. He also presents the traditional psychology of the East and its view of the soul.

Ted Kaptchuk manages to merge the insight of a Taoist sage with the skepticism of a modern, inquiring scientist. I am delighted to see his classic book reappear in a new, expanded edition for the new century. I hope it will continue to help to bring Eastern and Western medicine close together.

Andrew Weil, M.D.
Director, Program in Integrative Medicine
University of Arizona Medical Center

AUTHOR'S NOTES

Certain translated terms I use in this book have connotations for Chinese medicine that are quite different from what is ordinarily expected in English. For example, the Spleen of Chinese medicine is different from the spleen recognized in the West. I have capitalized such English words to account for the special meaning rather than overwhelm the reader with Chinese terminology. Only a few terms for which there are no adequate English equivalents are regularly referred to in romanized Chinese.

Romanization generally follows the Pinyin system used in the People's Republic of China and now accepted throughout the world. (A pronunciation guide appears on xvi.) However, the more conventional spellings are retained for a few familiar terms and names.

Chinese characters are sometimes given in addition to romanized or translated terms, for two reasons. First, Chinese words can often be romanized and translated in so many different ways that ultimately only the character form remains a reliable means of identification. Second, the pronunciation of many characters is identical; for example, the character *shen* that means Spirit is different from the *shen* that means Kidney. Presenting the character serves to make such distinctions clear.

Consideration for those uninitiated into the Chinese language has especially guided the preparation of the notes and the Chinese bibliography. To make the reference notes appear less forbidding, I have cited each Chinese work in short form, with its title in English translation (set in Roman type). In the case of book citations, a bracketed number corresponds to a numbered entry in the Selected Bibliography.

The Chinese sources in the Selected Bibliography are arranged as a kind of catalog of medical literature that may interest readers even if they are unlikely ever to consult a publication in Chinese. They are divided into eight sections: *Nei Jing* and *Nan Jing* and commentaries; other classical sources; reference books; contemporary introductory texts used to train traditional physicians; contemporary writings; miscellaneous sources (including specialty titles); sources on the history of Chinese medicine; and journals. Titles are given first in English translation, then in Chinese (the same is true of the annotated Historical Bibliography in Appendix I).

The reader is encouraged to browse through the rather extensive notes to each chapter, which contain some interesting digressions from the main text and raise some of the complexities inherent in the material.

THE PINYIN PHONETIC ALPHABET

The following table shows pronunciations with approximate English equivalents. In parentheses are the corresponding letters in the Wade-Giles system.

a (a) as in *far*

b (p) as in *be*

c (ts', tz') like *ts* in *its*

ch (ch) as in *church*, strongly aspirated

d (t) as in *door*

e (e) as in *her*

f (f) as in *fit*

g (k) as in *go*

h (h) as in *her*, strongly aspirated

i (i) like the vowel sound in *eat* or the *i* in *sir*

j (c) as in *jeep*

k (k') as in *kite*, strongly aspirated

l (l) as in *last*

m (in) as in *me*

n (n) as in *no*

o (o) like the vowel sound in *paw*

p (p') as in *park*, strongly aspirated

q (ch') like the *ch* in *cheat*

r (j) as in *red* or like the *z* in *azure*

s (s, ss, sz) as in *sister*

sh (sh) as in *shine*

t (t') as in *ton*, strongly aspirated

u (u) as in *too*; also in the French *tu*

v (v) used only to produce foreign words, national minority words, and local dialects

w (w) semi-vowel in syllables beginning with *u* when not preceded by consonants, pronounced as in *want*

x (hs) like *sh* in *sheet*

y semi-vowel in syllables beginning with *i* or *u* when not preceded by consonants, pronounced as in *yes*

z (ts, tz) as in *zone*

zh (ch) like the first consonant in jump

ai like *ie* in *tie*

ao like *ow* in *how*

ei like *ay* in *bay*

ie like *ie* in *experience*

ou like *oe* in *toe*

INTRODUCTION

Many changes have taken place for East Asian medicine in the West since *The Web Than Has No Weaver* was first published. At the time of the first edition, only a handful of obscure and poorly edited acupuncture manuals supplemented one or two academic tomes. Depth and nuance in the discussion of Oriental medicine was mostly absent. No institutions helped guide or shape dialogue and inquiry.

Today, clinical textbooks for all Chinese medical specialties, translations of classical and contemporary Asian source material, and academic works, from anthropology, sinology, sociology, and history, fuel an explosion in knowledge and exploration. Journals of biomedicine, the basic sciences, and Oriental medicine produce a constant stream of studies and finding. Institutions have developed. Professional schools of acupuncture and Oriental medicine confer recognized academic degrees. Universities have become a venue for the critical examination of East Asian medicine. Acupuncture is an ever-widening presence within mainstream health care settings.

Just as Oriental medicine in the West has gone through transformations, so have I. The *Web* was originally written as an effort to communicate what I had recently learned in Asia. I was a novice excited to transmit what I had seen in another world. In the almost twenty years since the first edition, I have continued to learn and study. I have treated many patients and worked in many hospitals. I have come into contact with the many other health care systems. For the last ten years I have had a full-time academic appointment at Harvard Medical School. For four years I worked as a series consultant for a nine-hour British Broadcasting Company (BBC) television series on health care and I was sent to visit various healers on three continents. Currently, I am serving a term on the National Advisory Council of the National Center for Complementary and Alternative Medicine (NCCAM) at the National Institutes of Health (NIH) where I have the opportunity to contribute to the evolving reconfiguration of America's pluralistic medical environment.

Although my home is now in the West, the Asian past has been a constant source of new inspiration. I've pored over sections of classical Chinese medical texts that were often neglected or considered "superstitious" in modern China. Modern ideas have also been a continuous challenge for me. Clinical epidemiology and biostatistics are tools I've managed to acquire, and I am actively involved in scientific research. Medical history and anthropology have also alerted me to the need to be cautious and uncertain. Personal encounters have been just as compelling. Patients have demanded that my practice of Chinese medicine embody authenticity and relevance.

Since the original *Web*, I have written on both Chinese medicine and topics outside its direct scope. I could have left *The Web That Has No Weaver* alone. But the *Web* has been too important to abandon. For many people, it can remain a valuable portal into another way of perceiving the world of health and illness. Instead of forsaking my first book, I have decided to gently update it, allow it to have a natural expansion. I did not want it to become an entirely new book; I wanted it to keep its established identity. In this second edition, I raise and emphasize new questions and underline different connections. My growth is reflected in what has been altered. I have reduced the Chinese transliteration; European languages now seem able to contain more than I once thought possible. This new *Web* has more psychological and existential material derived from historical sources that the first edition overlooked. At the same time, the text is more sensitive to the contemporary debates concerning scientific efficacy in biomedical terms. Every chapter has been given new material and insights. Some sections have had to be rewritten entirely (especially the sections on Qi, Spirit, and the chapter on the patient-physician relationship.) An appendix on Western clinical research has been added. Some material has been dropped because new and more complete resources are now available. Despite such modifications, I have striven to keep the tone, style, and sensibility of the old *Web* intact. In Chapter 1 of the original *Web*, I mention that the book is "another commentary on the commentaries." This second edition is finally a gloss on the first *Web* from the viewpoint of almost twenty years of experience, study, and reflection. It is no longer the writing of a person who has just gotten ashore with the need to tell a fantastic story. While still retaining its distinct orientation, it is now told, I hope, with the feel of a person who is grounded in two distinct cultures. For me, the changes made in the second edition feel like a maturation. I hope that the original Qi of the *Web* has had an opportunity to unfold.

In updating and writing this second edition, I've had to contend with the contradiction between a Talmudic intellect and a Hasidic soul. I have grown acutely aware that East Asian medicine is a huge ocean of texts and interpretations. Any assertion is automatically a complex problematic and an opportunity for contending understandings. My hermeneutic tendency would have liked to pursue the paradoxical knowledge produced by irreducible uncertainty. For this edition, this tendency was overruled (or at least sometimes just moved to a footnote). I want this *Web*, like its predecessor, to continue being an introduction to a coherent and radically distinct approach toward medicine. I want it to ultimately embody hope. Patients need treatment. Practitioners need strategies. Many intellectual problems have been put aside. In the choice between an analytic deconstructionism and provocative narrative, I have adopted the perspective that healing must embody an art with a compelling and even poetic message.

THE WEB
THAT HAS NO
WEAVER

Understanding Chinese Medicine

MEDICINE EAST AND WEST: TWO WAYS OF SEEING, TWO WAYS OF THINKING

and the landscape patterns of nature and humans

East Asian medicine has made a dramatic and unlikely migration. No longer confined to locations such as Shanghai, Seoul, or Singapore, it has become a vibrant component of health care from Sidney to Seattle to Stockholm. Chinese medicine is now international. Acupuncture and Oriental herbalism have become as commonplace and "indigenous" in Boston as in Beijing. This movement of healing techniques, clinical skills, revered literature, traditional knowledge, and distinctive philosophy has been unusually rapid. This swiftness has meant that thoughtful and critical examination can be in short supply.

As a result, many Westerners have strange notions about Chinese medicine. Some of them see it as hocus-pocus—the product of primitive or magical thinking. If a patient is cured by means of herbs or acupuncture, they see only two possible explanations: Either the cure was a placebo effect,[1] or it was an accident, the happy result of hit-or-miss pin-sticking that the practitioner did not understand. They assume that current Western science and medicine have a unique handle on Truth—all else is superstition.

Other Westerners have a more favorable but equally erroneous view of Chinese medicine. Deeply and often justifiably disturbed by many of the products of Western science and culture, they assume that the Chinese system, because it is felt to be more ancient, more spiritual, or more holistic, is also more "true" than Western medicine. This attitude threatens to turn Chinese medicine from a rational body of knowledge into a religious faith system. Both attitudes mystify the subject—one by uncritically undervaluing it, the other by setting it on a pedestal. Both are barriers to understanding.

Actually, Chinese medicine is a coherent and independent system of thought and practice that has been developed over two millennia. Based on ancient texts, it is the result of a continuous process of critical thinking, as well as extensive clinical observation and testing. It represents a thorough formulation and reformulation of material by respected clinicians and theoreticians. It is also, however, rooted in the philosophy, logic, sensibility, and habits of a civilization entirely foreign to our own. It has therefore developed its own perception of health and illness.

Chinese medicine considers important certain aspects of the human body and personality that are not significant to Western medicine. At the same time, Western medicine observes and can describe aspects of the human body that are insignificant or not perceptible to Chinese medicine. For instance, Chinese medical theory does not have the concept of a nervous system. Nevertheless, evidence exists demonstrating Chinese medicine's capacity to treat some neurological disorders.[2] Similarly, Chinese medicine does not perceive an endocrine system, yet it treats what Western medicine calls endocrine disorders.[3] Nor does traditional Chinese medicine recognize *Streptococcus pneumoniae* as a pathological cause of pneumonia, yet before the discovery of antibiotics, its treatments seemed to offer a reasonable and relatively effective response.[4]

Chinese medicine also uses terminology that is strange to the Western ear. For example, the Chinese refer to certain diseases as being generated by "Dampness," "Heat," or "Wind." Modern Western medicine does not recognize Dampness, yet can treat what Chinese medicine describes as Dampness of the Spleen. Modern Western medicine does not speak of fire, but can, from a Chinese perspective, stoke the fire of the Kidney or extinguish excess fire raging out of control in the Lungs. In Western medicine, Wind is not considered a disease factor; yet Western medicine is able to prevent Liver Wind from going to the head, or to extinguish rampaging Wind in the skin. The perceptions of the two traditions reflect two different worlds, but both can affect and often heal human beings regardless of their cultural affiliation.

The difference between the two medicines, however, is greater than that between their descriptive language. The actual logical structure underlying the methodology, the habitual mental operations that guide the physician's clinical insight and critical judgment, differs radically in the two traditions. What Michel Foucault says about medical perception in different historical periods could apply as well to these different cultural traditions: "Not only the names of diseases, not only the grouping of systems were not the same; but the fundamental perceptual codes that were applied to patients' bodies, the field of objects to which observation addressed itself, the surfaces and depths traversed by the doctor's gaze, the whole system of orientation of his gaze also varied."[5]

The two different logical structures have pointed the two medicines in different directions. Biomedicine, a more accurate name for Western medicine, is primarily concerned with isolable disease categories or agents of disease, which it zeroes in on, isolates, and tries to change, control, or destroy. An ontologically circumscribed entity is the privileged ideal of the system. The Western physician starts with a symptom, then searches for the underlying mechanism—a precise *cause* for a specific *disease*.[6] The disease may affect various parts of the body, but it is a relatively well-defined, self-contained phenomenon. Precise diagnosis frames an exact, quantifiable description of a narrow area. The physician's logic is analytic—cutting through the accumulation of bodily phenomena like a surgeon's scalpel to isolate one single entity or cause.

The Chinese physician, in contrast, directs his or her attention to the complete physiological and psychological individual. All relevant information, including the symptom as well as the patient's other general characteristics, is gathered and woven together until it forms what Chinese medicine calls a "pattern of disharmony." This pattern of disharmony describes a situation of "imbalance" in a patient's body. Oriental diagnostic technique does not turn up a specific disease entity or a precise cause, but renders an almost poetic, yet workable, description of a whole person. The question of cause and effect is always secondary to the overall pattern. One does not ask, "What X is causing Y?" but rather, "What is the relationship between X and Y?" The Chinese are interested in discerning the relationships in human activities occurring at the same time. The logic of Chinese medicine is organismic or synthetic, attempting to organize symptoms and signs into understandable configurations. The total configurations, the patterns of disharmony, provide the framework for treatment. The therapy then attempts to bring the configuration into balance, to restore harmony to the individual.

This difference between Western and Eastern perception can be illustrated by portions of clinical studies done in hospitals in China.[7] In a typical study a Western physician, using upper-gastrointestinal x-rays or endoscopy by means of a fiberscope, diagnoses six patients with stomach pain as having peptic ulcer disease. From the Western doctor's perspective, based on the analytic tendency to narrow diagnosis to an underlying entity, all these patients suffer from the same disorder. The physician then sends the patients to a Chinese doctor for examination. The following results are found.

Upon questioning and examining the first patient, the Chinese physician finds pain that increases at touch (by palpation) but diminishes with the application of cold compresses. The patient has a robust constitution, broad shoulders, a reddish complexion, and a full, deep voice. He seems assertive and even aggressive. He seems to be challenging the doctor. He is constipated and has dark yellow urine. His tongue has a greasy yellow coating; his pulse is "full" and "wiry." The Oriental physician characterizes this patient as having the pattern of disharmony called "Damp Heat Affecting the Spleen."

When the Chinese physician examines the second patient, he finds a different set of signs, which indicate another overall pattern. The patient is thin. Her complexion is ashen, though her cheeks are ruddy. She is constantly thirsty, her palms are sweaty, and she has a tendency toward constipation and insomnia. She seems nervous, fidgety, and unable to relax and also complains of feeling pressured. In her life, she is constantly on the go and has been unable to be in a stable relationship. Her tongue is dry and slightly red, with no "moss"; her pulse is "thin" and also a bit "fast." This patient is said to have the pattern of "Deficient Yin Affecting the Stomach," a disharmony very different from that of the first patient. Accordingly, a different treatment would be prescribed.

The third patient reports that massage and heat somewhat alleviate his pain, which is experienced as a minor but persistent discomfort. He is temporarily relieved by eating. The patient dislikes cold weather, has a pale face, and wants to sleep a lot. His urine is clear and his urination frequent. He appears timid, shy, and almost afraid. He seems unable to look the physician in the eye, and his head seems to hang in despair. His tongue is moist and pale, his pulse "empty." The patient's condition is diagnosed as the pattern of "Exhausted fire of the Middle Burner," sometimes called "Deficient Cold Affecting the Spleen."

The fourth patient complains of very severe cramping pain; his movement and affect is ponderous and heavy. Hot-water bottles relieve the pain, but massaging the abdomen makes it worse. The patient has a bright white face and a tendency toward loose stools. He is forty years old and came to the appointment with his mother with whom he still lives. His passion is a world-class stamp collection, which he constantly studies and wants to talk about. His tongue has an especially thick, white, moist coating; his pulse is "tight" and "slippery." These signs lead to a diagnosis of the pattern of "Excess Cold Dampness Affecting the Spleen and Stomach."

The fifth patient experiences much sour belching and has headaches. Her pain is sharp, and, although massaging the abdomen makes it diminish, heat and cold have no effect. She is very moody. Emotional distress, especially anger, seems to precipitate attacks of pain. She feels frustrated and stuck in many of her life activities. During the discussion she says her husband is distant and detached. Strangely enough, the patient's tongue is normal, but her pulse is particularly "wiry." The physician concludes that she is affected by the pattern of "Disharmony of the Liver invading the Spleen."

The sixth patient has an extremely severe stabbing pain in the stomach that sometimes goes around to his back. The pain is much worse after eating and is aggravated by touch. He has had episodes of vomiting blood, and produces blackish stools. The patient is very thin and has a rather dark complexion. His eyes furtively and suspiciously dart around the room, as if to detect a hidden threat. He had been physically abused as a political prisoner. His tongue is a darkish purple and has markedly red eruptions on the sides. His pulse is "choppy." The Chinese physician describes the patient's problem as a "Disharmony of Congealed Blood in the Stomach."

So the Chinese doctor, searching for and organizing signs and symptoms that a Western doctor might never heed, distinguishes six patterns of disharmony where Western medicine perceives only one disease. The patterns of disharmony are similar to what the West calls diseases in that their discovery tells the physician how to pre-scribe treatment. But they are different from diseases because they cannot be isolated from the patient in whom they occur. To West-ern medicine, understanding an illness means uncovering a distinct entity that is separate from the patient's being; to Chinese medicine, understanding means perceiving the relationships among all the patient's signs and symptoms in the context of his or her life. When confronted by a patient with stomach pain, the Western physician must look beyond the screen of symptoms for an underlying pathological mechanism—a peptic ulcer in this case, but it could have been an infection or a tumor or a nervous disorder. A Chinese physician examining the same patient must discern a pattern of disharmony made up of the entire accumulation of symptoms and signs.*

The Chinese method is based on the idea that no single part can be understood except in its relation to the whole. A symptom, therefore, is not traced back to a cause, but is looked at as a part of a totality. If a person has a complaint or symptom, Chinese medicine wants to know how the symptom fits into the patient's entire being and behavior. Illness is situated in the context of a person's life and biography. Understanding that overall pattern, with the symptom as part of it, is the challenge of Chinese medicine. The Chinese system is not less logical than the Western, just less analytical.[8]

⊣ Yɪɴ [阴] ᴀɴᴅ Yᴀɴɢ [阳] Tʜᴇᴏʀʏ

The logic underlying Chinese medical theory—a logic that assumes that a part can be understood only in its relation to the whole—can also be called synthetic or dialectical. In Chinese early naturalist and Taoist thought, this dialectical logic that explains relationships, patterns, and change is called Yin-Yang theory.†

Yin-Yang theory is based on the philosophical construct of two polar complements, called Yin and Yang. These complementary opposites are neither forces nor material entities. Nor are they mythical concepts that transcend rationality. Rather, they are convenient labels used to describe how things function in relation to each other

---

*From a biomedical viewpoint, the Chinese physician is assessing the patient's specific and general physiological and psychological response to a disease entity.

†Although the Chinese identify the relationships between phenomena primarily by the patterns of Yin and Yang, another system of categorization, known as the five Phases, is also used in East Asia. In this system, Wood, fire, Earth, Metal, and Water are seen as a set of emblems by which all things and events in the universe could be organized. (For a detailed discussion of the five Phases in Chinese medicine, see Appendix F.)

and to the universe. They are used to explain the continuous process of natural change. But Yin and Yang are not only a set of correspondences; they also represent a way of thinking. In this system of thought, all things are seen as parts of a whole. No entity can ever be isolated from its relationship to other entities; no thing can exist in and of itself. Fixed essences are abstractions; there are no absolutes. Yin and Yang must, necessarily, contain within themselves the possibility of opposition and change.

The character for Yin originally meant the shady side of a slope. It is associated with such qualities as cold, rest, responsiveness, passivity, darkness, interiority, downwardness, inwardness, decrease, satiation, tranquility, and quiescence. It is the end, completion, and realized fruition.

The original meaning of Yang was the sunny side of a slope. The term implies brightness and is part of one common Chinese expression for the sun. Yang is associated with qualities such as heat, stimulation, movement, activity, excitement, vigor, light, exteriority, upwardness, outwardness, and increase. It is arousal, beginning, and dynamic potential.

Working with these ideas, Chinese thought and Chinese medical tradition have developed five principles of Yin and Yang.[9]

All things have two facets: a Yin aspect and a Yang aspect.

Thus, time can be divided into night and day, place into earth and heaven, season into inactive periods (fall and winter) and active periods (spring and summer), species into female and male, temperature into cold and hot, weight into light and heavy, and so on. Inside and outside, down and up, passive and active, empty and full are all examples of Yin-Yang categories. These qualities are opposites, yet they describe relative aspects of the same phenomena. Yin and Yang qualities exist in relation to each other.

In terms of the body, the front is considered Yin and the back Yang. The upper part of the body is considered more Yang than the lower part; the outer parts of the body (skin, hair, etc.) are more Yang than the inner Organs. In terms of the psyche, willfulness, desire, and assertiveness are Yang; Yin is acceptance, responsiveness, repose, and responsibility. The Yin and Yang are often described metaphorically as Water and fire. Illnesses that are characterized by weakness, slowness, coldness, and underactivity are Yin; illnesses that manifest strength, forceful movements, heat, and overactivity are Yang.

The philosopher Zou Yen (c. 305–240 B.C.E.) describes this idea this way: "Heaven is high, the earth is low, and thus [Heaven and Earth] are fixed. As the high and low are thus made clear, the honorable and humble have their place accordingly. As activity and tranquillity have their constancy, the strong and the weak are thus differentiated. . . . Cold and hot season take their turn. . . . [Heaven] knows the great beginning, and [Earth] acts to bring things to completion. . . . [Heaven] is Yang and [Earth] is Yin."[10]

Any Yin or Yang aspect can be further divided into Yin and Yang.

This means that within each Yin and Yang category, another Yin and Yang category can be distinguished. It is an extension of the logic that divides all phenomena into Yin and Yang aspects, allowing further division within aspects *ad infinitum*. For example, temperature can be divided into cold (Yin) and hot (Yang), but cold can be divided further into icy cold (Yin) and moderately cold (Yang). In the body, the front of the trunk is Yin compared with the back, but the front can be divided further so that the abdomen is Yin in relation to the chest. Within a Yin illness characterized by Coldness there may be aspects of Yang such as sharp, forceful contractions. Within a Yang illness of Heat and hyperactivity there may be weakness and loss of weight, both Yin qualities.

Chuang Tzu (Zhuang Zi), the Taoist philosopher (fl. probably between 400 and 300 B.C.E.), describes the unfolding of Yin and Yang, and the notion of the unity of opposites, in a radical paradoxical way: "There is nothing in the world greater than the tip of a hair that grows in the autumn, while Mount Tai is small. No one lives a longer life than a child who dies in infancy, but Peng Zu (who lived many hundred years) died prematurely."[11]

Yin and Yang mutually create each other.

Although Yin and Yang can be distinguished, they cannot be separated. They depend on each other for definition. And the things in which Yin and Yang are distinguished could not be defined without the existence of Yin and Yang qualities. For instance, one cannot speak of temperature apart from its Yin and Yang aspects, cold and heat. Similarly, one could not speak of height unless there were both tallness and shortness. Such opposite aspects depend on and define each other.

Another example might be the relationship between a couple in which one partner can be (relatively) passive only if the other partner is (relatively) aggressive, and vice versa. Passivity and aggression can be measured only in comparison with each other. The activity (Yang) of the body is nourished by its physical form (Yin), and the physical form is created and maintained by the activity of the body. In illness, overactivity has meaning only in relation to a condition of underactivity, and vice versa.

Lao Tzu (Lao Zi), the reputed founder of Taoism, declares in the *Tao-te Ching* (or *Dao-de Jing*—the Classic of the Tao and Its Virtue):

Being and non-being produce each other;
Difficult and easy complete each other;
Long and short contrast each other;
High and low distinguish each other;
Sound and voice harmonize each other;
Front and back follow each other.[12]

Yin and Yang control each other.

If Yin is excessive, then Yang will be too weak, and vice versa. If the temperature is neither too cold nor too hot, then both cold and hot aspects are mutually controlled and held in check. If it is too cold, then there is not enough heat, and vice versa. Yin and Yang balance each other.

In our example of the couple, the extent to which one partner can be aggressive depends on the extent to which the other is passive, and vice versa. They exert mutual control over each other. An illness of fire may be due to insufficient Water; an illness of Water may be due to insufficient fire.

Lao Tzu alludes to this concept when he says:

He who stands on tiptoe is not steady.
He who strides forward does not go.
He who shows himself is not luminous.
He who justifies himself is not prominent.
He who boasts of himself is not given credit.
He who brags does not endure for long.[13]

Yin and Yang transform into each other.

This principle is a formula for the nature of organic process. It suggests two types of transformations: changes that occur harmoniously, in the normal course of events, and the sudden ruptures and transformations characteristic of extremely disharmonious situations.

Because Yin and Yang create each other in even the most stable relationships, Yin and Yang are always subtly supporting, repairing, and transforming into each other. This constant transformation is the source of all change. It is a give-and-take relationship that is life activity itself. In the dynamics of the body, the nature of transformation can be illustrated by the manner in which inhalation is followed by exhalation, or periods of activity and exertion must be succeeded by nourishment and rest. In human interactions, assertion and responsiveness alternate. In normal life such regular transformations occur smoothly, maintaining a proper, healthy balance of Yin and Yang.

In a relationship in which Yin and Yang are unbalanced for prolonged periods of time or in an extreme manner, the resulting transformations may be quite drastic. Harmony means that the proportions of Yin and Yang are relatively balanced; disharmony means that the proportions are unequal and there is imbalance. A deficiency of one aspect implies an excess of the other. Extreme disharmony means that the deficiency of one aspect cannot continue to support the excess of another aspect. The resulting change may be rebalancing or, if that is not possible, either the transformation into opposites or the cessation of existence.

To return to the couple, let's assume a disharmonious relationship in which one partner is excessively aggressive and the other excessively passive. This situation can have three possible outcomes. They sit down and talk it out, agreeing to a rearrangement of attitudes (i.e., they rebalance their relationship); or one day the passive partner gets fed up and waits for the other with an ax (i.e., a radical transformation of Yin into Yang occurs); or they separate, putting an end to the relationship.

In clinical practice, one of these three kinds of transformation is always possible. For example, when a patient has a pattern with very high fever and much sweating (considered an excess of Yang, or fire), the patient may be in danger of suddenly going into shock (an extreme Yin, or Cold, condition). This is because Yang cannot continue to exist in such extreme relation to Yin without some transformation occurring. Either a gradual transformation, a rebalancing, must take place—medication and healing; or a radical transformation will occur—shock; or Yin and Yang will separate and existence will cease—death.

Lao Tzu describes the transformation process poetically:

> *In order to contract,*
> *It is necessary first to expand.*
> *In order to weaken,*
> *It is necessary first to strengthen.*
> *In order to destroy,*
> *It is necessary first to promote.*
> *In order to grasp,*
> *It is necessary first to give.*[14]

And also:

> *People hate to be orphaned, the lonely ones,*
> * and the unworthy.*
> *And yet kings and lords call themselves*
> * by these names.*
> *Therefore it is often the case that things gain*
> * by losing and lose by gaining.*[15]

Yin-Yang theory is well illustrated by the traditional Chinese Taoist symbol (figure 1). The circle representing the whole is divided into Yin (black) and Yang (white).

The small circles of opposite shading illustrate that within the Yin there is Yang and vice versa. The dynamic curve dividing them indicates that Yin and Yang are continuously merging. Thus Yin and Yang create each other, control each other, and transform into each other.

FIGURE 1 *Traditional Yin-Yang Symbol*

Because of the pervasive influence of Yin-Yang theory on Chinese thought and culture, the Chinese understand and explain events differently than does the West. The idea of causation, central to Western thinking, is almost entirely absent. Aristotle (384–322 B.C.E.), in his *Physics* (one of the basic works of Western philosophy), pens the archetypal formulation of this Western notion: "Men do not think they know a thing till they have grasped the 'why' of it (which is to grasp its primary cause)."[16] For the Chinese, however, phenomena occur independently of an external act of creation, and there is no great need to search for a cause.

> *Tao produced the One.*
> *The One produced the two.*
> *The two produced the three.*
> *And the three produced the ten thousand things.*
> *The ten thousand things carry the Yin and*
> *embrace the Yang and through the blending*
> *of the Qi* they achieve harmony.*[17]

In Chinese thought, events and phenomena unfold through a kind of spontaneous cooperation, an inner dynamic in the nature of things. Wang Cong (c. 27–100 C.E.), the great Taoist scientist, philosopher, and skeptic, describes the inner working of the universe as follows:

> *The way to Heaven is to take no action. Therefore in the spring it does not act to start life, in summer it does not act to help grow, in autumn it does not act to bring maturity, and in winter it does not act to store up. When the . . . Yang comes forth itself, things naturally come to life and grow. When the . . . Yin arises of itself, things naturally mature and are stored up. . . . Originally no result is sought, and yet results are achieved. . . .*
> *Since Heaven takes no action, it does not speak. When the time comes for calamities and strange transformations, the [Qi] produces them spontaneously. . . . When there is [Cold] in the Stomach, it aches. It is not that man causes it. Rather, the [Qi] does it spontaneously. . . .*[18]

Joseph Needham (1900–1994), the great historian of Chinese science, summarizes the Chinese view of causation this way: "Conceptions are not subsumed under one another but placed side by side in a *pattern*, and things influence one another not by acts of mechan-

---

*Qi, often spelled ch'i (or *ki* in Japanese), is discussed in Chapter 2.

ical causation, but by a kind of 'inductance.' . . . The key-word in Chinese thought is *Order* and above all *Pattern*. . . . Things behave in particular ways not necessarily because of prior actions or impulsions of other things, but because their position in the ever-moving cyclical universe was such that they were endowed with intrinsic natures which made that behavior inevitable for them. . . . They were thus parts in existential dependence upon the whole world-organism."[19]

The Chinese assume that the universe is continuously changing. Its movement is the result not of a first cause or creator, but of an inner dynamic of cyclical patterns. Just as the sun maps out four distinct seasons in its yearly round, so all biological organisms go through four seasons in a lifetime: birth, maturation, decline, and death. The constancy of the cosmos is in these patterns of change, which are regular. The cosmos itself is an integral whole, a web of interrelated things and events. Within this web of relationships and change, any entity can be defined only by its function, and has significance only as part of the whole pattern.

This metaphysics that emphasizes the perception of patterns is basic to Chinese thinking. It results in part from Taoism, which altogether lacks the idea of a creator, and whose concern is insight into the web of phenomena, not the weaver. For the Chinese, that web has no weaver, no creator; in the West the final concern is always the creator or cause and the phenomenon is merely its reflection. The Western mind seeks to discover and encounter what is beyond, behind, or the cause of phenomena. In the Chinese view, the truth of things is imminent; in the Western, truth is transcendent. Knowledge, within the Chinese framework, consists in the accurate perception of the inner movement of the web of phenomena. The desire for knowledge is the desire to understand the interrelationships or patterns within that web, and to become attuned to the unfolding dynamic.

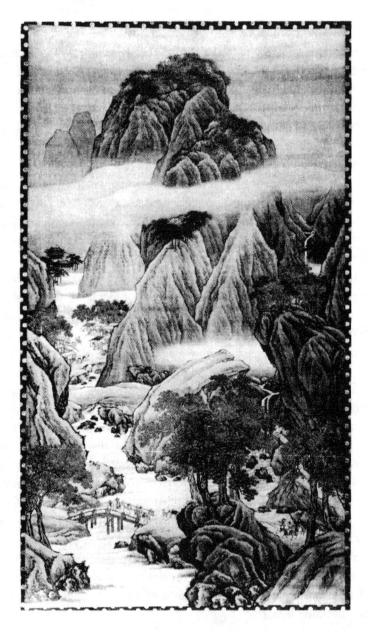

FIGURE 2 **Mountain Landscape** *by Wang Yun (Qing dynasty)*

Courtesy Museum of fine Arts, Boston; purchased in China, received December 1913.

┤ Of Chinese Painters and Chinese Physicians

The arts in China were nourished by the same naturalist and Taoist sensibility that fed Chinese philosophy and medicine. Chinese art attempts to express the ideas of balance, harmony, and change that are contained in Yin-Yang theory. In landscape painting, the harmonious spirit of nature is revealed through the depiction of a scene that depends on proportion and measure to create beauty.

Wang Yun's *Mountain Landscape* (figure 2) is a traditional Chinese landscape painting. In it, the artist has captured the essence of nature as he sees it, in balance and in flux. The painting is like the Taoist symbol (figure 1), containing Yin and Yang in their proper proportions but constantly interacting and transforming into each other.

The scene depicts a vast range of elements, from the towering mountain to the little trickling stream. Nature is shown as a balance of the yielding Yin (foliage, water) and the unyielding Yang (rock, trees). There are the dynamic (water, people) and the quiescent (mountains, houses); the slow (trees) and the fast (mist); the dark and the light; the solid and the liquid. All things contain both Yin and Yang. The water, for instance, is both yielding (Yin) and dynamic (Yang).

The picture is a totality, and each detail takes on meaning only insofar as it participates in the whole. The mountain is immense by virtue of its smaller foothills; the people are small by virtue of the vastness of nature. All things are imbued with interactive qualities and dynamics in their relationships to the things around them.

Through a kind of poetic logic, the Chinese also think of the landscape painting as a microcosm of the universe. In it are contained all the elements of nature, and it serves as a model of the cosmic process. The landscape painter sees in a particular scene a unique configuration of the natural elements. His composition includes those elements, or signs, that are specific to a certain scene, but it also participates in the larger reality. The elements within the microcosm correspond to elements within the macrocosm. For example, winter is death, a budding tree is spring, a lake is all water, a person is humankind. The painting depicts a time and place that through their correspondence with the cosmos become timeless and placeless. As the sinologist François Jullien has noted: "In China, the purpose of painting is to rediscover the elemental and continuous course of the cosmic pulsation through the figurative representation of a landscape. . . . The tension created by the correlation between the lines and the washes, the visible and the invisible, fullness and emptiness, endows the landscape with a power to suggest more than the merely visible and open it to the life of the spirit."[20]

In a similar way, the Chinese think of each person as a cosmos in miniature. A person manifests the same patterns as does the painting or the universe. The Yang or fire aspects of the person are the dynamic and transforming, while the Yin or Water aspects are the more yielding and nourishing. One person projects the heat and quickness of summer fire; another person resembles the quiescence and coolness of winter Cold; a third replicates heaviness and moisture of Dampness; a fourth has the shriveled appearance of a Dry Chinese autumn; and many people display some aspects of the various seasons simultaneously. Harmony and health are the balanced interplay of these tendencies.

In each person, as in every landscape, there are signs that, when balanced, define health or beauty. If the signs are out of balance, the person is ill or the painting does not work. So the Chinese physician looks at a patient the way a painter looks at a landscape—as a particular arrangement of being, behavior, interaction, and life signs in which the essence of the whole can be seen. A person's characteristics, of course, are somewhat different from nature's signs—including color of face, expression of emotions, sensations of comfort or pain, feel of pulse, moral fiber—but they express the texture of the human landscape.

Is Chinese medicine an art? Is it a science? If we mean by science the relatively recent intellectual and technological development in the West, Chinese medicine is not scientific. It is instead a pre-scientific tradition that has survived into the modern age and remains another way of doing things. But it does resemble science in that it is grounded in conscientious observation of phenomena, guided by a rational, logically consistent, and communicable thought process. It has a corpus of knowledge with standards of measurement that allow practitioners systematically to describe, diagnose, and treat illness. Its measurements, however, are not the linear, fixed yardsticks of weight, number, time, and volume used by modern science but rather flexible images of the phenomenal world. Yet Chinese medicine also demands the artistic sensitivity of synthetic logic—always aware that the whole defines the parts and that the pattern may transform the significance of any one measurement within it. What is Yin in one person may be Yang in another. Because it deals with situationally dependent images, Chinese medicine allows and demands a recognition and assessment of quality and context.

This artistic sensitivity allows the physician to stay in touch with subtle refinements of meaning, to discern shades of significance in human and behavioral signs; but, most important, it allows awareness of the process that exists around and between linear measurements. Chinese medicine is not primarily quantitative. It recognizes that each person's pattern has a unique texture; each image has an essential quality.

The Chinese doctor's effort to recognize patterns within the characteristic signs of a particular individual is a creative one. But it is here that the concerns of the artist and the doctor begin to diverge. The artist uses his or her vision and skill to portray an ideal of balance and harmony on a paper scroll. The physician, however, uses his or her perception to recognize *dis*harmony, and must then apply his or her specialized skill to try to restore health—to achieve balance and harmony within a living organism. This balance is a dynamic equilibrium that is appropriate and specifically possible in the particular circumstance and development phase of a person's life. There is no standard or absolute—what is health for one person may be sickness in another. There is no notion of "normal" Yin-Yang—only the unique challenges and possibilities of each human life.

⊣ HALLOWED TRADITION AND MODERN RESEARCH:
IT MAY BE BEAUTIFUL, BUT DOES IT WORK?

Traditional medicine can be considered an art, and it can claim to
be a science. But the important question to ask about a medical practice is: Does it work? Is Chinese medicine just an interesting philosophical curiosity or is it a viable system of healing? Can it treat
what the West defines as real diseases? And can Western science
measure its results and appreciate its value?

Because of the unique history of modern China, traditional
medicine has been the subject of comprehensive study and testing
over the past fifty years.

After the victory of the Chinese Revolution in 1949, the
Chinese decided to take a fresh look at their traditional medical system. Many of China's new leaders were tempted to discard their
prescientific medical inheritance, along with other old-fashioned
practices and remnants of underdevelopment. Their overall desire
was to emulate the developed countries—to industrialize, electrify,
and modernize. Another faction of the leadership, however, saw that,
although China did need to accept modern medicine, there might
also be some practical and theoretical usefulness in the traditional
medicine. At least partially, the issue was whether or not it would
prove efficacious from a modern perspective. To answer that question, the Chinese performed thousands of experiments and clinical
studies during the 1950s. In 1958, for reasons that included scientific
as well as cultural and economic concerns, the Central Committee
decided to give traditional and modern medicine equal respect and
place in China.[21]

The medical reports, which are used to support the official adoption of Chinese medicine, are still produced incessantly, and include
such titles as the following:

Clinical Analysis of 290 Cases of Chronic Glomerular
Nephritis Treated with Traditional Herbs.[22]

Observations of the Efficacy of Subcutaneous Acupuncture in
Treating 121 Cases of Bronchial Asthma.[23]

Study of Treatment of Early Stage Cervical Carcinoma with Traditional Chinese Herbs, Including Analysis of Treatment Effect on Twenty-Four Cases and a Preliminary Investigation of the Treatment Mechanism.[24]

Traditional Chinese Medical Treatment of Angina Pectoris— Report of 112 Cases.[25]

The pages of such studies fill entire libraries, yet it is not their quantity that is important, but rather their conclusions: from the modern Chinese perspective, traditional Chinese medicine can hold its own; it does work clinically.[26]

Even for thoroughly modernized Chinese, Chinese medicine has come to be accepted as an effective healing method. It is now routine for Chinese to think that their traditional methods can alleviate or treat illnesses for which modern medicine is not effective. At other times, the opposite is believed, especially in those cases that require surgery or interventions with high-technology equipment.[27] A partnership has evolved.

For modern Western nations, the scientific judgment as to whether Chinese medicine is an effective therapeutic and should be integrated into "mainstream" medicine has not been as simple or unproblematic. In part, this problem is related to the fact that, until very recently, Chinese medical research has not adopted the modern methodological safeguards of the double-blind randomized controlled trial. Even simple control groups have been missing from most Chinese clinical studies. Recently, in an effort to demonstrate the value of traditional medicine to people outside China, a movement has begun to meet Western research standards. More important, Western researchers, who would consider the Chinese investigations as preliminary evidence, have begun to perform evaluations of Chinese medicine using modern scientific standards. Such outcomes as the National Institutes of Health's Consensus Development Conference on Acupuncture (November 1997), with its positive assessment of the value of acupuncture for some clinical indications and a call for its incorporation into some conventional setting, demonstrate that this recent research has begun to change the status of Chinese medicine's scientific credibility in the West.[28] (For a detailed discussion on the scientific engagement in Western nations with traditional Chinese medicine, see Appendix E.)

Despite its shortcomings, Chinese scientific research is important in understanding how traditional Chinese medicine has come to be understood in modern China. This research also illustrates the provocative assertions Chinese medicine makes for its potential role as a vital component in a future global cosmopolitan medicine. A good example of such Chinese research is the previously mentioned study of ulcer patients. In that study, there were actually sixty-five patients, all of whom were observed by Western-trained physicians while being treated with traditional Chinese methods.[29] Every patient received a complete Western medical examination and was diagnosed as having peptic ulcer disease. The patients were then sent to traditional physicians, whose diagnoses roughly corresponded to the six different patterns described earlier.

The Chinese doctors gave each patient a unique herbal treatment based on his or her particular diagnosis. No Western treatment was administered, nor were any dietary restrictions imposed. The average length of treatment was two months, and modern Western techniques were used to evaluate the treatment's utility. The results were complete recovery in fifty-three patients (81.5 percent), significant improvement in seven patients (10.8 percent), some improvement in two patients (3.1 percent), no change in two patients, and a worsening of the condition in one patient due to complications unrelated to the treatment.

Another example is the angina study listed above. For that study 112 patients with angina pectoris were treated and observed for six months to two and a half years. All the patients were first given complete Western medical examinations and then diagnosed by traditional Chinese methods. In general, one of five distinct patterns was found in each case, and different herbs were prescribed for each pattern. Assessment of the therapy, based on subjective patient findings, was as follows: 34.8 percent of the patients improved markedly, 56.2 percent showed general improvement, and 9 percent remained unchanged. The overall percentage of subjective improvement was 91 percent. There were 91 patients who had abnormal electrocardiograph reports before treatment. Of these, 15.4 percent showed marked improvement after treatment, 23.1 percent showed moderate improvement, 10.9 percent showed an increase to abnormal reports, and 50.6 percent showed no change. The most interesting results, however, were seen when the patients' blood was examined. The serum cholesterol and triglyceride levels had dropped markedly in all cases after treatment. Western medicine considers low levels of these substances beneficial in reducing the threat of artherosclerotic heart disease. These changes occurred without dietary restrictions and without the use of modern drugs to lower the level of blood lipids before or after treatment.[30] Obviously, for a Western scientific audience, the findings of this study and the previous ulcer study would only be considered preliminary data. In order for such results to be maximally persuasive, the outcomes would have needed to be compared to those of concurrent control groups assigned by some randomization procedure that were given an identical-appearing placebo with all subsequent clinical assessments performed without knowledge ("blind") of treatment received. Nonetheless, such evidence is what the modern Chinese generally have accepted as convincing. (For a discussion of the more sophisticated research being performed in the West, see Appendix E.)

Research (both in the East and in the West) has also been done to isolate the effective components of particular Chinese medical treatments in dealing with diseases recognized by the West. For example, experiments have discovered the active ingredients of herbs and have tried to develop efficient nausea treatment using acupuncture. Many studies have attempted to extract from Chinese medicine new, Western-style cures. A sense of the direction of this research can be seen in such recent English-language scientific journal titles:

Qinghaosu (Artemisinin): An Antimalarial Drug from China.[31]

The Effect of Chinese Hepatoprotective Medicines on Experimental Liver Injury in Mice.[32]

Inhibition of Growth of Human Immunodeficiency Virus in Vitro by Crude Extracts of Chinese Medicinal Herbs.[33]

Biologically Active Constituents of Centipeda Minima: Sesquiterpenes of Potential Anti-Allergy Activity.[34]

The Effects of Traditional Antirheumatic Herbal Medicines on Immune Response Cells.[35]

Such studies are aimed at separating out the effective components of Chinese medicine and introducing them into the framework of modern Western medicine. Someday, after much research and development, these components may well appear in Western medicine as practiced in the Occident. Yet, although this knowledge, with its use of traditional herbs and acupuncture, has the veneer of Chinese medicine, the actual application and methodology are clearly Western in orientation. The theory of Yin and Yang and other traditional concepts are left behind. And while valuable techniques may be learned, the extraction of the practice from its theory calls into question the need for the traditional framework.

Fortunately for its future, however, the results of the studies, at least from East Asia so far, generally demonstrate that traditional Chinese medicine does work best when left in the context of Chinese logic.[36] In most cases, pattern weaving based on Yin-Yang theory produced better clinical results than the mechanical application of Chinese remedies within a Western context.[37] The traditional medicine works not only because it has an effective arsenal of therapeutic devices, but also because it may know best how to use them.

Western "style" clinical studies of traditional Chinese medicine, by providing evidence for its practical effectiveness, have helped it win its battle for full recognition in twenty-first-century East Asia. For the Chinese medical claims of efficacy to win acceptance within scientific circles in the West, more rigorous research will certainly be needed (see Appendix E). Undoubtedly, ongoing and future research in Western nations will help clarify Chinese medicine's future in a developing new cosmopolitan medicine.

⊣ ANCIENT BUT STILL ALIVE

Chinese medicine is more than 2,000 years old. Yet over all that time, it has retained an aesthetic and pragmatic relevance for humankind today. Of course, any tradition remains vital only insofar as it allows itself to grow and develop. The Chinese tradition is no different. Based on ancient and revered texts, it has continued to discover itself anew.

The *Huang-di Nei-jing* or Inner Classic of the Yellow Emperor (hereafter referred to as the *Nei Jing*) is the source of all Chinese medical theory, the Chinese equivalent of the Hippocratic corpus. Compiled by unknown authors between 300 and 100 B.C.E., it is the oldest of the Chinese medical texts. The knowledge and theoretical formulations it contains are the basic medical ideas developed and elaborated by later thinkers.

The *Nei Jing* has been called the bible of Chinese medicine, and the rest of Chinese medicine can be compared to rabbinical exegesis or interpretation of doctrine by church fathers. Just as, in the Jewish tradition, later authorities needed to explain theoretical issues raised by the Torah, so Chinese commentators added glosses on the *Nei Jing* that elucidated or even amended its seminal ideas. The Chinese medical tradition thus brings together folk remedies and the therapeutics of China's physician-literati who served the Imperial Court.[38] It synthesized the medicine of one dynasty and another, one place and another, one thinker and another. Every dynasty has produced practitioners equal in stature to Galen, Avicenna, or Paracelsus, and all of them have made important additions and revisions to the tradition.[39]

In China today, the primary textbooks used to train traditional doctors are contemporary interpretations and clarifications of Qing dynasty (1644–1911) commentaries. These books are, in turn, clarifications of Ming dynasty (1368–1644) reworkings, which are also reworkings of earlier material. This process goes all the way back to the Han dynasty (202 B.C.E.–220 C.E.). Such transmission through the dynastic pathway not only preserved and encapsulated the original sources, but also elucidated and reformed them.[40] (See Appendix I: Historical Bibliography.)

It is for this reason that the *Nei Jing*, although it is the source of the tradition, is usually one of the last texts to be studied in contemporary schools of Chinese medicine. The *Nei Jing*, written in archaic language, is often unclear and inconsistent, and can only be understood after much preparation.[41] Without the commentaries and modifications of later eras, the *Nei Jing* would be almost completely unintelligible.[42] So the source requires the tradition to explain it, but both are necessary to guide Chinese theory and practice.

Within Chinese medicine, as in all traditional systems, there is a tension between that which is tacitly recognized as no longer useful and that which continues to be accepted as profound. This book attempts to bring Chinese medicine to a Western audience, and because it does so within the ancient tradition, it is, finally, another commentary on the commentaries.

NOTES

1. For a fuller discussion of the scientific and rhetorical dimension of the placebo accusation see: Ted J. Kaptchuk, "Powerful Placebo: The Dark Side of the Randomized Controlled Trial," *Lancet* 1998; 351: 1722–1725.

2. See, for example, "Treatment with Traditional Chinese Medicine of five Types of Nervous System Disorders," *Shanghai Journal of Traditional Chinese Medicine* (SJTCM), January 1980, pp. 14–16; Y. Shao and B. Shaw, "A Survey of Acupuncture Treatment of Peripheral Nerve Injury," *Journal of Traditional Chinese Medicine*, 1999, 19: 221–226; Y. Sun and X. Liu, "A Review on Traditional Chinese Medicine in Prevention and Treatment of Multiple Sclerosis," *Journal of Traditional Chinese Medicine*, 1999, 19: 65–73; J. Zhang and J. Yi, "Progress in the Treatment of Nerve-Root-Type Cervical Spondylosis with Chinese Herbal Drugs," *Journal of Traditional Chinese Medicine*, 1999, 19: 227–233. For a discussion of evidence from randomized controlled trials performed in the West, see Appendix E.

3. See references to the uses of traditional medicine for treating endocrine disorders in Shanghai Second Medical Hospital, *Handbook of Internal Medicine* [88], pp. 579–650 and Z. Y. Zhou and H. D. Jin, *Clinical Manual of Chinese Herbal Med-*

icine and Acupuncture, New York: Churchill Livingstone, 1997, pp. 172–81. For an example of Chinese research in this area, see X. Gong, "Regulation of Electroacupuncture on the Contents of Endocrine Hormones and Preliminary Exploration for its Mechanism in Rats," *Acupuncture Reasearch*, 1998, 23: 53–62 (Chinese). Also see Appendix E.

4. See three articles on treating lobar pneumonia caused by *Streptococcus pneumoniae* with traditional herbal medicines in *Journal of Traditional Chinese Medicine* (JTCM), February 1959, pp. 31–41. For discussion in the Western literature see, for example, Chaoying Liu and Robert M. Douglas, "Chinese Herbal Medicine in the Treatment of Acute Respiratory Infections: A Review of Radomised and Controlled Clinical Trials," *Medical Journal of Australia*, 1998, 169: 579–582. The review discusses Chinese herbals for pneumonia and bronchiolitis. Also see Appendix E.

5. Michel Foucault, *The Birth of the Clinic* (New York: Vintage Books, 1973), p. 54.

6. Obviously, this statement is an oversimplification necessary to make some distinctions between Eastern and Western medical tendencies. It represents an ideal methodology, not necessarily applicable to all disciplines or all concerns of biomedicine. In fact, biomedicine has multiple perspectives that are selectively utilized.

Reductionism is only one important dimension of biomedical thinking. Its historical trajectory is roughly described by Morgagni's (1761) location of pathology in organs, followed by Bichat's (1800) focus on tissue, leading to Broussais's (1830s) attention to lesion in tissues, to Virchow's (1848) localization in cells, to Koch's (1882) germ theory, all the way to the modern dissection of genes. The scientific quest for mechanical physiochemical agency has led to progressively smaller and smaller analytic units. Yet throughout its history and until the present there have been important corrections to reductionism within biomedicine; organismic tendencies try to counterbalance or prevail over excessive reductionism. Antireductionist tendencies within conventional medicine emphasize homeostasis, predisposition, susceptibility, multi-factorial causation, and psychosocial factors as opposed to isolatable diseases. A few of the many names associated with nonreductionism within orthodox medicine include Claude Bernard, Walter Cannon, L. J. Henderson, Charles Sherrington, Hans Seyle, George Engels, and Arthur Kleinman.

In addition, in clinic, biomedicine can be multidisciplinary and holistic. For example, a chronic pain unit or an oncology unit may include multiple disciplines from pathology and anesthesiology to psychiatry and social work to music therapy and physical therapy. Increasingly, such units may add meditation, relaxation therapy, or yoga. The recent tendency to add practitioners of Oriental medicine to such treatment teams has made the distinction between East and West even more complex. (For example, a survey of 172 chronic pain clinics in the U.K. found 84 percent had adopted acupuncture as a treatment modality. C. H. M.

Woollam and A. O. Jackson, "Acupuncture in the Management of Chronic Pain," *Anesthesia* 1998; 53: 589–603.)

The focus of this inquiry is East Asian medicine, and the author apologizes that to illustrate and contrast for clarification purposes, biomedicine is sometimes portrayed in an oversimplified manner. For a more nuanced discussion on the *a priori* assumption of biomedicine see: Margaret Lock and Deborah Gordon (eds.), *Biomedicine Examined* (Boston: Kluwer Academic, 1988); E. K. Ledermann, *Philosophy and Medicine* (Hants, U. K.: Gower House, 1986); and Stuart F. Spicker, *Organism, Medicine, and Metaphysics* (Boston: D. Reidel, 1978). For a historical discussion on this issue see John V. Pickstone, "Ways of Knowing: Towards a Historical Sociology of Science, Technology and Medicine," *British Journal of History of Science* 1993; 26: 433–458. Generally speaking, unlike modern biology with its theory of evolution and genetics, the concrete practice of biomedicine lacks any general overarching theory. Biomedicine's practical unity comes from the availability of a system of mutiple explanatory schema such as infectious diseases, nutritional diseases, autoimmune diseases, and molecular-genetic diseases. See: Paul Thagard, *How Scientists Explain Disease*, Princeton: Princeton University Press, 1999. Psychogenic disease often represents a waste-basket category. Some of the unity of biomedicine also comes from its recent adoption of "rules of evidence" for clinical interventions (see Appendix E). For a discussion of the term "biomedicine" itself see Ted J. Kaptchuk, "In the Name of Medicine," *Annals of Internal Medicine*, 1998: 128: 246.

7. See "Clinical Observations of Traditional Chinese Medical Approaches to 65 Cases of Ulcers," (JTCM), June 1959, pp. 30–33. See also "Typing of Peptic Ulcer Disease According to Traditional Chinese Medicine and Preliminary Exploration of Its Pathological Basis," (JTCM), February 1980, pp. 17–21. The research report "Analysis of Effectiveness of Traditional Chinese Medicine in Treating 126 Cases of Gastrointestinal Ulcers" in JTCM, February 1960, distinguishes twelve distinct traditional medical patterns in its study group. See note 29.

8. Manfred Porkert states this idea this way: "We should always keep in mind that Western science is not more rational than Chinese science, merely more analytical" (Porkert, *The Theoretical Foundations of Chinese Medicine*, p. 46).

9. I have translated these five principles from the discussion appearing in Shanghai Institute, *Foundations of Traditional Chinese Medicine* [53], pp. 22–25. It should be noted that the presentation of material in this volume follows the sequence and general content of this standard textbook. For an intriguing account of how Yin-Yang theory was transformed by Marxism and modernist China see Elizabeth Hsu, "YinYang and Mao's Dialectics in Traditional Chinese Medicine," *Asiatische Studien*, 1998, 52: 419–443.

10. Quoted in Wing-tsit Chan, *A Source Book in Chinese Philosophy*, p. 248.

11. Ibid., p. 186. Some minor changes in romanization have been made in this quotation.
12. From chap. 2 of the *Tao-te Ching*. Ibid., p. 140. There is considerable scholarly debate over who should be assigned the title or nickname Lao Tzu. Some scholars place Lao Tzu in the seventh century B.C.E., some in the sixth as an elder contemporary of Confucius, and some in the fourth as the teacher of Chuang Tzu. Still other scholars say Lao Tzu is merely a legendary figure. Even if he was a historical personage, it may be that the *Tao-te Ching* in its present form was compiled by several authors after his time. In any case, the *Tao-te Ching* is the classical formulation of Taoist philosophy.
13. From chap. 24 of the *Tao-te Ching*. Ibid., p. 152.
14. From chap. 36 of the *Tao-te Ching*. Ibid., p. 157.
15. From chap. 42 of the *Tao-te Ching*. Ibid., p. 161. During the Warring States period (475–221 B.C.E.) Chinese kings referred to themselves as solitary or lonely ones.
16. *Physics* 194.18–20. In R. McKeon, *The Basic Works of Aristotle*, p. 240.
17. From chap. 42 of the *Tao-te Ching*, in Chan, *Chinese Philosophy*, p. 160.
18. From the Balanced Inquiries by Wang Cong (Wang Ch'ung). Ibid., pp. 298–299.
19. J. Needham, *Science and Civilization in China*, vol. 2, pp. 280–281. Judith Farquhar makes the same point in the following way:

> *When the "ontological ground" of effects is a state of constant transformation, where there is no European metaphysic requiring fixity of essence or discreteness of material form as a criterion of "reality," it is patterns in and of time and space, rather than material structures and mechanical functions, that must be perceived. And for this profoundly temporal project, applied in medicine, yinyang is a clarifying model.* [Knowing Practice: The Clinical Encounter of Chinese Medicine, *1994, p. 218*]

Again it must be said that the emphasis of this chapter is the contrast of Far East and West, and in order to make distinctions, some simplification is necessary. The synthetic proclivity of Chinese thought is the main tendency but not its exclusive method. Needham writes:

> *Chinese scientific thought saw related phenomena as synchronous or emblematically paired rather than caused or causing. . . . But it would, I think, be most unfortunate if one were to assume that there were never any elements of temporal causal succession in their world-outlook. . . . Simultaneous appearance of widely separated events was surely, for the ancient Chinese, the manifestation of an underlying cosmic pattern. . . . But we never maintained that this exhausted the Chinese way of looking at Nature, and it is possible to find many passages and descriptions of natural events which indicate conceptions of causes and effects in time.* [Annals of Science 32 (1975): 491]

20. François Jullien, *The Propensity of Things*. The first part of the quote is on page 94; the second part is on page 174. For a discussion of the importance of medical the-

ory in the Chinese theory of art see John Hay, "The Human Body as a Micro-cosmic Source of Macrocosmic Values in Calligraphy." In: S. Bush and C. Murck (eds.) *Theories of the Arts in China* (Princeton, N.J.: Princeton University Press, 1983).

21. For a discussion of the political, economic, and social influences (i.e., extramedical forces) at work in establishing traditional Chinese medicine on an equal footing with modern medicine, see "The Ideology of Medical Revivalism in Modern China" by Ralph C. Croizier in *Asian Medical Systems*, ed. by Charles Leslie (Berkeley: University of California Press, 1976). Also see David M. Lampton, *Health, Conflict and the Chinese Political System* (Ann Arbor: Center for Chinese Studies, University of Michigan, 1974). For a discussion of the relationship of modern and traditional medicine in the recent pre-Communist period with implicit or explicit continuities into the present, see Bridie J. Andrews, "The Making of Modern Chinese Medicine 1895–1937" (Ph.D. diss. Cambridge University, 1996); AnElissa Lucas, *Chinese Medical Modernization: Comparative Policy Continuities, 1930s–1980s.* (New York: Praeger, 1982); Ralph C. Croizier, *Traditional Medicine in Modern China: Science, Nationalism, and the Tensions of Cultural Change* (Cambridge: Harvard University Press, 1968); Mary Brown Bullock, *An American Transplant: The Rockefeller Foundation and Peking Union Medical College* (Berkeley: University of California Press, 1980); S. W. Hillier and J. A. Jewell, *Health Care and Traditional Medicine in China 1800–1982* (London: Routledge and Keagan Paul, 1983); Carol Benedict, *Bubonic Plague in Nineteenth-Century China* (Stanford: Stanford University Press, 1996); M. P. Sutphew, "Not What, but Where: Bubonic Plague and the Reception of Germ Theories in Hong Kong and Calcutta, 1894–1897. *Journal of the History of Medicine* 1997; 52:81–113. Peter Buck, *American Science and Modern China.* (Cambridge: Cambridge University Press, 1980). For discussion of parallel issues in Japan, see Emiko Ohnuki-Tierney, *Illness and Culture in Contemporary Japan* (Cambridge: Cambridge University Press, 1984); Margaret M. Lock, *East Asian Medicine in Urban Japan* (Berkeley: University of California Press, 1980). For a recent discussion on the state of traditional medicine in China, see Xiang Zheng and Sheila Hillier, "The Reforms of the Chinese Health Care System: County Level Changes: The Jiangsi Study, in *Social Science and Medicine* 1995; 41: 1057–1064. Therese Hesketh and Wei Xing Zhu, "Traditional Chinese Medicine: One Country, Two Systems," *British Medical Journal* 1997; 315: 115–117. For additional textured insights into recent changes in the medical system of modern China, see Gail Henderson, "Increased Inequality in Health Care in China," in *Chinese Society on the Eve of Tiananmen: The Impact of Reform.* Deborah Davis and Ezra F. Vogel, eds., Cambridge, MA: Council on East Asian Studies, Harvard University, 1990; Judith Farquhar, "Market Magic: Getting Rich and Getting Personal in Medicine After Mao," *American Ethnologist* 1996; 23: 239–257.

22. *Chinese Journal of Internal Medicine* (CJIM), January 1965.

23. Ibid., October 1963.
24. See JTCM, June 1965.
25. *Chinese Medical Journal* (English edition), Beijing, May 1977.
26. To get a further idea of the scope of these titles, it is worth glancing at John E. Fogarty International Center for Advanced Study in the Health Sciences, *A Bibliography of Chinese Sources on Medicine and Public Health in the People's Republic of China: 1960–1970* (Washington, D.C.: U.S. Dept. of HEW, NIH, 1973). Many of the titles listed concern studies on traditional Chinese medicine. For a more recent discussion of clinical research in China, see J. L. Tang, S. Y. Zhang, and E. Ernst, "Review of Randomised Control Trials of Traditional Chinese Medicine," *British Medical Journal*, 1999, 319: 160–161. Also see Appendix E for extensive discussion of this issue.
27. For all the research on the traditional medicine in China by Western-style scientists and medical workers, a survey of the extensive literature uncovers little or no generalized discussion of which illnesses call for one medical approach rather than the other. The thrust is to examine the efficacy of the traditional medicine and not to compare it with Western medicine. My observation in clinical situations in China and in reading the literature points to a rough tendency to use Western medicine in acute and emergency situations and Chinese medicine in chronic situations. Often, however, the choice is left to patients, and also commonly both systems are used simultaneously. From my own experience, Western medicine is often more effective when it has a definite and clear idea of the disease etiology (e.g., bacterial infections). When a precise etiology evades Western medicine (e.g., in cases of chronic low back pain), Chinese medicine seems more effective. Also, it seems that Chinese medicine is preferable for functional disorders, benign self-limiting problems, psychosomatic complaints, psychological stress, and intractable and catastrophic conditions that resist resolution with biomedicine. Chinese medicine is also valuable in helping people adopt and cope with incurable conditions and serious emotional conflict. It is often adopted for illness prevention and health maintenance. Western medicine has a clear edge in organic disorders that have delineated pathophysiology with available successful interventions. Generalizations sometimes can be heard in discussion with doctors in China; for example, for chronic bronchial asthma or arthritis, Chinese medicine is often said to be better, while in bacterial infections and in cases needing surgery, Western medicine is better. But with a stubborn persistence these generalizations are unable to predict any particular patient's response to treatment. Many times I have seen clinical cases in which Western medicine worked better in treating arthritis or Chinese medicine eliminated the need for an operation or cleared up a persistent infection.

Western medical scientists often suspect that much of Chinese medicine's effectiveness is due to the power of the placebo effect. While to some extent (as in any medicine) this is likely to be true, it should be noted that in China, Western medicine is more likely to enjoy this advantage. To Chinese patients, Western medicine has prestige and an aura of the mysterious and foreign, whereas their own country's medicine is more ordinary and common.

28. For a discussion of the NIH Consensus Conference, see National Institutes of Health Consensus Conference. "Acupuncture," *Journal of the American Medical Association* 1998; 280: 1518–1524. C. Marwick, "Acceptance of Some Acupuncture Applications," *Journal of the American Medical Association*, 1997; 278: 1725–1727; National Institutes of Health, *NIH Consencus Development Conference on Acupuncture*, (Bethesda, MD: NIH 1997). (Also see Appendix E.) For shifts in acupuncture's acceptance in health delivery settings see K. R. Pelletier, A. Marie, M. Krasner, W. L. Haskell, "Current Trends in the Integration and Reimbursement of Complementary and Alternative Medicine by Managed Care, Insurance Carriers, and Hospital Providers," in *American Journal of Health Promotion*, 1997; 12: 112–123. For discussion of the availability of Chinese medicine or acupuncture in European nations, see George Lewith and David Aldridge (eds.), *Complementary Medicine and the European Community* (Essex, U.K.: C. W. Daniel, 1991); Usuala Sharma, *Complementary Medicine Today: Practitioners and Patients* (London: Tavistock/Routledge, 1992).

29. See "Clinical Observations of Traditional Chinese Medical Approach to 65 Cases of Ulcers," JTCM, June 1959, pp. 30–33. For a more recent English-language example of a double-blind controlled trial, see Z. H. Zhou, Y. H. Hu, D. H. Pi et al., "Clinical and Experimental Observations on Treatment of Peptic Ulcer with Wie Yan An (Easing Peptic Ulcer) Capsule," in *Journal of Traditional Chinese Medicine* 1991; 11: 34–39. Also, for a summary of English-language research into acupuncture treatment of gastrointestinal complaints, see Y. Li, G. Tougas, S. G. Chiverton and R. H. Hunt, "The Effect of Acupuncture on Gastrointestinal Function and Disorders," in *American Journal of Gastroenterology* 1992; 87: 1372–1381 and D. L. Diehl, "Acupuncture for Gastrointestinal and Hepatobiliary Disorders," *Journal of Alternative and Complementary* Medicine, 1999, 5: 27–45.

30. For examples of more recent rigorous investigations of Chinese medicine and heart disease, see H. Zhang, M. J. Liang, H. L. Ye, "Clinical Study on the Effects of Bu Yang Huan Wu Decoction on Coronary Heart Disease," in *Chinese Journal of Integrated Traditional and Western Medicine* (Chinese language) 1995; 15: 213–215; G. R. Lu, Y. C. Zhao, "The Use of Xue Fu Zhu Yu Decoction in the Treatment of 84 Cases of Coronary Heart Condition," in *Chinese Journal of Integrated Traditional and Western Medicine* (Chinese language) 1995; 15: 44–45. It has been noted that many Chinese herbs dramatically reduce blood cholesterol even though the traditional system does not recognize cholesterol. For an interesting discussion combining Western and Chinese methodologies, see "Eight Methods of Lowering Lipidemia by Traditional Chinese Medicine," SJTCM, November 1979. Also see, R. Gao and L. Li, "Clinical Observation on 300 Cases of Angina Pectoris Treated

by the Spleen-Stomach Regulatory Method," *Journal of Traditional Chinese Medicine*, 1998, 18: 87–90; D. Zhong, "TCM Differential Treatment of Angina Pectoris," *Journal of Traditional Chinese Medicine*, 1999, 19: 234–237.

31. Daniel L. Klayman, "*Qinghaosu* (Artemisinin): An Antimalarial Drug from China," in *Science* 1985; 228: 1049–1055. Research in the West has emphasized identification of the active ingredients of a single herb using chemical and bioassay procedures. For a discussion of this approach and how it ignores Chinese theories of herb interaction and the possible mutual relationship between the constituents of complex herbal mixtures, see E. L. Way and C. F. Chen, "Modern Clinical Applications Related to Chinese Traditional Theories of Drug Interactions," *Perspectives in Biology and Medicine*, 1999, 42: 512–525.

32. Jie Liu, Yaping Lu, Curtis D. Klaasen. "The Effect of Chinese Hepatoprotective Medicines on Experimental Liver Injury in Mice," in *Journal of Ethnopharmacology* 1994; 42: 183–191.

33. R. Shihman Chang, H. W. Yeung, "Inhibition of Growth of Human Immunodeficiency Virus in Vitro by Crude Extracts of Chinese Medicinal Herbs," in *Antiviral Research* 1988; 9: 163–175.

34. Jin-Bin Wu, Yui-To Chun, Yutaka Ebizuka, Ushio Sankawa, "Biologically Active Constituents of Centipeda Minima: Sesquiterpenes of Potential Anti-Allergy Activity," in *Chemical Pharmacology Bulletin* 1991; 12: 3272–3275.

35. Deh-Ming Chang, Wei-Yen Chang, San-Yuan Kuo, Mu-Lan Chang, "The Effects of Traditional Antirheumatic Herbal Medicines on Immune Response Cells," in *Journal of Rheumatology* 1997; 24: 436–441.

36. See Qin Bo-wei's discussion in the chapter on Suitability of Using Traditional Chinese Medical Theory and Methods to Treat Western Diagnosed Disease in his famous *Medical Lecture Notes of Qian Zhai* [64], pp. 168–192. An excellent translation of this volume has been done by Charles Chase, *A Qin Bowei Anthology: Clinical Essays by Master Physician Qin Bowei*. C. Chase and Z. T. Liang (trans.) Brookline, MA: Paradigm Publications, 1997. Obviously, this research needs to be replicated in the West.

37. A common opinion in modern China is that acupuncture, as opposed to herbal medicine, works almost as well in a high proportion of cases even when isolated and disentangled from the traditional Chinese medical view. This has allowed it to be easily incorporated into modern medicine in China and is one factor that makes it more easily transmitted to the West. This ability to isolate from the traditional theory probably is related to the fact that acupuncture seems to induce the body toward homeostasis, so an incorrect selection of points (from the traditional view) does little harm and only somewhat reduces the treatment's positive effect. The herbs seem to have more harmful effects if improperly used (because their actions seem to be through complex biochemistry), and the traditional theory prevents such misuse. Also, the precise use of herbs seems to maximize the positive

effect of the treatment more than the precise use of the acupuncture point. A discussion of the single-directional effects of herbs as compared with the homeostatic effects of acupuncture is presented by Wei Jia in his theoretical essay "On the Applicability of Moxibustion in Heat Patterns," JTCM, November 1980, p. 48. An opposite approach to acupuncture, suggesting the continued need for a traditional framework, underlies Yang Ming-yuan's *Concise Acupuncture* (*Jian-ming Zhen-jiu Xue*) (Harbin: Heilongjiang People's Press, 1981). The successful series of randomized controlled trials using a single acupuncture point (P6) to treat nausea and vomiting is an example of acupuncture being applied independent of its traditional theory. See Andrew Vickers, "Can Acupuncture Antiemesis Have Specific Effects on Health? A Systematic Review of Acupuncture Antiemesis Trials," in *Journal of the Royal Society of Medicine.* 1996; 89: 303–311. (Also see Appendix E.)

38. In general one ought to distinguish traditional Chinese medicine, which is the subject of this volume, from Chinese folk medicine. Folk medicine is largely empirical, involving relatively simple remedies applied by nonprofessional, informally educated practitioners. The traditional medicine, however, is, as Ralph Croizier defines it, "a theoretically articulated body of ideas about disease causation and treatment contained in a written tradition and practiced by men whose knowledge of that tradition causes their society to recognize them as medical specialists." "Traditional Medicine as a Basis for Chinese Medical Practices" by Ralph Croizier in *Medicine and Public Health in the People's Republic of China*, ed. by J. R. Quinn (Washington, D.C.: John E. Fogarty International Center, U.S. Dept. of HEW, NIH, 1973), p. 5.

In fact, the literate medicine of China may not have been available to most Chinese people throughout history. Paul Unschuld estimates that "the history of high medicine in China was never the medicine of ninety percent of the population." (Paul U. Unschuld, "Discussion on David McQueen's Paper," *Social Science and Medicine* 1978; 12: 75–78, p. 78.) In the rural areas of China, literacy was extremely rare and health care was primarily in the hands of various magico-religious practitioners or folk herbalists. Even in the cities, during every epoch this was true. Spence comments:

> *Magicians and exorcists, midwives, herbalists, apothecaries and Taoist adepts, self-taught practitioners, eminent Confucian scholars who turned to medicine out of intellectual interest or financial necessity, families of physicians jealously guarding inherited family lore, skillful practitioners with nationally known names, court specialists—all of these "practiced" during the Ching dynasty, and none can be ignored in a comprehensive study of medical systems.*
> (Jonathan Spence, *"Commentary on Historical Perspectives and Ching Medical Systems,"* Medicine in Chinese Cultures: Comparative Studies of Health Care in China and Other Societies, *Arthur Kleinman [ed.] p. 81)*

Similarly, in the Song dynasty: "For every illness, the diagnosis and remedies varied widely according to the different schools of medicine and sick people for their part did not hesitate to try out different treatments at the same time." (J. Gernet, *Daily Life in China on the Eve of the Mongol Invasion, 1250–1276.* Palo Alto: Stanford University Press, 1970, p. 170.) Even Confucius speaks of health care as being the domain of both physicians (*yi*) and sorcerers (*wu*). A full discussion of the pluralistic medical environment of historical China would have to additionally include shamans, soothsayers, geomancers, fortune-tellers, eye-and-ear specialists, surgical specialists, itinerant drug peddlers and various religious practitioners. An examination of Sun Si-miao's Tang dynasty writings even shows the active presence in China of Ayuravedic, Persian, and Tibetan practices. (Sun Si-miao, Supplemental Wing to the Thousand Ducat Prescriptions [*Qian-jin Yi-fang*]. Beijing: People's Press, 1982 [682 c.e.]. In fact:

within a well-defined historical period the entity we call [Chinese medicine] turns out not to be a single system at all, but a whole complex of interacting systems of health care. Some of these are openly hostile towards one another, while others have relations that are hierarchical or even complementary. Some are linked with the elite culture which underpins the legitimacy of the Chinese state; some are perceived by that elite culture as deviant and dangerous; some are more or less neutral. Some claim to be based on authoritative written texts, while others are purely oral. Some are at least ostensibly public, while others set great store by secret traditions. Some are fit occupations for gentlemen, while some are mere trades. Some exclude women, while in others women are dominant. And in a country as vast as China, practice may differ from region to region as markedly as does the spoken dialect. (C. Cullen, "Patients and Healers in Late Imperial China: Evidence from the Jinpingmei," History of Science *1993; 31: 99–150, p. 100–101).*

For a discussion and examples of medical pluralism and non-literate traditions in modern China see such studies as Elizabeth Hsu, *The Transmission of Chinese Medicine*, 1999; Volker Scheid, *Plurity and Synthesis in Contemporary Chinese Medicine*, 1997; Judith Farquhar, "Market Magic: Getting Rich and Getting Personal in Medicine after Mao," *American Ethnologist*, 1996; 23: 239–257; S. Harrell, "Pluralism, Performance and Meaning in Taiwanese Healing: A Case Study," *Culture, Medicine and Psychiatry* 1991; 15: 45–68; J. M. Potter, "Wind, Water, Bones and Souls: The Religious World of Cantonese Peasants," *Journal of Oriental Studies* 1970; 8: 131–153; A. Kleinman and J. L. Gale, "Patients Treated by Physicians and Folk Healers: A Comparative Outcome in Taiwan," *Culture, Medicine and Psychiatry* 1982; 6: 405–423; Judith Farquhar, "Medicine and the Changes Are One: An Essay on Divination Healing with Commentary," *Chinese Science*, 1996; 3: 107–134. This volume primarily describes the state-sanctioned modern variant of the literate version of traditional Chinese Medicine. In fact, this tradition is itself influenced by earlier shamanic imagery (see e. g., Kuriyama Shigehisa, "Concepts of Disease in East Asia," in *Cambridge World History of Human Disease*, Cambridge University Press, 1993). Any absolute boundary demarcation between the multiplicity of healing options available in China can become problematic. (See footnote 42 below.)

39. While the point of the discussion is that Chinese medicine is progressive in a qualitative sense, it should be noted that this is true also in quantitative ways. Joseph Needham makes the point, perhaps even too emphatically, in *The Grand Titration: Science and Society in East and West* (p. 277): "It would be quite a mistake to imagine that Chinese culture never generated this conception [of a progressive development of knowledge], for one can find textual evidence in every period showing that in spite of their veneration for the sages, Chinese scholars and scientific men believed that there had been progress beyond the knowledge of their distant ancestor. . . ." Needham goes on to plot a curve on a graph demonstrating the tremendous increase in the number of entries in pharmacopoeias through the centuries. Also see note 6 for Chapter 4 for a discussion of the increased number of acupuncture points recognized in various historical periods. For a discussion of the conceptual transformation of Chinese medical perspectives, see Ted J. Kaptchuk, "Oriental Medicine: Culture, History and Transformation," in East Asian Medical Studies Society, *Fundamentals of Chinese Medicine* (Brookline, MA: Paradigm, 1985); Paul U. Unschuld, *Medicine in China: A History of Ideas*, 1985.

40. It should also be remembered that the historical lineage is also "a Chinese historiographical tradition that has so idealized its classical origins and the continuity of its transmitted medical wisdom that it successfully conceals much of the strangeness of its own past. [China's medical traditions] . . . were shaped by decentralized authority; by forgetting as well as by learning; and by the eclectic use of the past knowledge as bricolage, preserved or adapted or reassembled at will." Charlotte Furth, *A Flourishing Yin: Gender in China's Medical History, 960–1665*, p. 16. The examination of the creation of "history" in an entirely different context in Eric Hobsbawn and Terence Ranger (eds.), *The Invention of Tradition* (Cambridge: Cambridge University Press, 1983), might also be helpful in this discussion.

Also, it can easily be overlooked that East Asian medicine necessarily is undergoing a dramatic transformation as it migrates to the Western world. This transplantation is only possible if Oriental medicine creatively adapts to its new environment and unavoidably develops a new sensibility and historiography. Important discussions of this process include: Linda B. Barnes, "The Psychologizing of Chinese Practices in the United States," *Culture, Medicine and Psychiatry*, 1998; 22: 413–443; H. A. Baer, C. Jen, L. M. Tanassi, C. Tsia and H. Wahbeh,

"The Drive for Professionalization in Acupuncture: A Preliminary View from the San Francisco Bay Area," *Social Science and Medicine* 1998; 46: 533–537.

41. Many translators prefer not to deal with this problem. Translating ancient Chinese scientific texts into comprehensible language is an extraordinarily difficult task. First, determining that the text in hand is actually what it is purported to be is a laborious job for the scholar. Through the millennia, original texts have gone through series of emendations and alterations so that what actually comes down to us must be thoroughly compared with other editions and traced in the literary documents left by each dynasty.

Second, and much more troublesome, is the problem of creating an accurate vocabulary for translating Chinese technical terms. Chinese is a pictographic language, and once it passed its formative stages, people simply did not invent a new character to express a narrow technical concept, as is done with an alphabetic language when a new word is needed. Old characters were simply given new meanings—which must be ferreted out by translators separated from the original material by a vast gulf of time and space. To translate Chinese medical texts directly, using the everyday meanings of such characters, would result in inscrutable gibberish. At the other extreme, to arbitrarily introduce Western technical terms would be to turn the Chinese text into a projection of the Western mind. Unfortunately, most translations of the *Nei Jing* in whole or in part reflect little sensitivity to either of these considerations and should be read with considerable caution.

42. The compilation of various "disparate texts [into the *Nei Jing*] has brought about repetitions, uncertainties, contradictions even, which a full commentary cannot always manage to clarify or reconcile." Huard and Wong, *Chinese Medicine*, p. 39. For a discussion of the lineage of various discourses in the *Nei Jing*, see Yamata Keiji, "The Formation of *Huang-Ti Nei-Ching*," *Acta Asiatica*, 1979; 36: 67–89. For an analysis of the history of the *Nei Jing* text and a presentation of the state of medical knowledge at the time of its creation, see David J. Keegan, "'*The Huang-Ti Nei-Ching*': The Structure of the Compilation; the Significance of the Structure" (Ph.D. diss. University of California, 1988).

A provocative and relevant sense of how commitment to canonical text can replace theoretical or practical consistency in an entirely different intellectual tradition can be found in Moshe Halbertal's discussion of textual interpretation in Judaism. (*People of the Book: Canon, Meaning and Authority.* Cambridge: Harvard University Press, 1997.) Because by definition, a sacred text can have no contradiction and is perfect, the tradition must read text in the best possible light. The degree of canonicity of a text corresponds to its authority and the "charity" it receives in its interpretation. For a historic medical tradition in the modern era this can pose a peculiar tension: on the one hand it claims a "golden" and "sacred" point of departure and on the other hand it must value "thousands of years" of experience and presumed refinement.

Similar complexity and commitment to sacred text can be found in the Hippocratic tradition of medicine. Reading the collection of some seventy Greek medical writings of about 400 B.C.E. attributed to Hippocrates, one is struck by a similarity in structure. The doctrine of humors is used in terminology and outlook but nowhere does a systematic or clear presentation appear. Contradictory ideas are frequent, but at the same time there is a sense of a rational perspective not bound by fixed rules but based on empirical observation. Only later do codifiers provide systematization and consistency.

Also, both Hippocrates and the *Nei Jing* represent the same monumental break from earlier supernatural and magical healing systems. Hippocrates explicitly rejects magico-religious notions of disease and speaks of illness as a knowable, natural phenomenon subject to investigation and observation:

> *My own view is that those who first attributed a sacred character to this malady were like the magicians, purifiers, charlatans and quacks of our own day. . . . This disease styled sacred comes from the same causes as others, from the things that come from the changing restlessness of winds. These things are divine. So that there is no need to put the disease in a special class and to consider it more divine than the others; they are all divine and all human. Each has a nature and power of its own; none is hopeless or incapable of treatment. . . . So the physician [can give] . . . useful treatment, without having recourse to purifications and magic.* [The Sacred Disease, *Jones, (trans.)*, Hippocrates, *vol. 2, p. 139, p. 183.*]

The *Nei Jing* speaks in the same terms: "In treating illness, it is necessary to examine the entire context, scrutinize the symptoms, observe the emotions and attitudes. If one insists on the presence of ghosts and spirits one cannot speak of therapeutics." (Inner Classic of the Yellow Emperor: Simple Questions [1], sec. 3, chap. 11, p. 78. Later cited as *Su Wen*. This is the first half of the *Nei Jing*.)

Elsewhere in the *Nei Jing* the Yellow Emperor asks:

> *What if there has been no encounter with a Pernicious Influence nor any emotional disturbance and suddenly one falls ill? Is this not the result of the supernatural?*

And Qi Bo (his minister and teacher) replies:

> *This also has its reason. A Pernicious Influence lies dormant and waits to manifest; the will has its loathings and yearnings; the Blood and Qi are thrown into turbulence and the two Qis clash. The origin is subtle, neither visible nor audible, and it only seems to be the supernatural. [Classic of the Spiritual Axis [2], sec. 9, chap. 58, p. 397. Later cited as Ling Shu. This is the second half of the Nei Jing.]*

While these rational notions clearly dominated both medical traditions, the problem of grave diseases unaffected by human endeavor, and of fate in general, could not be banished altogether—just moved to the periphery. The Imperial Medical Academy (tai-yi-shu) of the Tang dynasty (618–907 C.E.) had an incantation-taboo department, and one of the thirteen departments of the Yuan dynasty (1271–1368 C.E.) Academy was spirit-healing. Likewise, the Greek physicians often relied on the temples of Asclepius as a friendly ally, just as a chaplain is sometimes called into the intensive care unit in a modern hospital.

For a discussion of pre–*Nei Jing* magico-religious Chinese medicine see, for example, Donald Harper, "The Conception of Illness in Early Chinese Medicine, as Documented in Newly Discovered 3rd and 2nd Century B.C. Manuscripts," *Sudhoffs Archives* 1990; 74: 210–235 and Paul U. Unschuld, *Medicine in China: A History of Ideas.*

2

THE FUNDAMENTAL TEXTURES: QI, BLOOD, ESSENCE, SPIRIT, AND FLUIDS

or the basic ingredients of human life

The highly developed constructs of chemistry, biochemistry, anatomy, and physiology that form the groundwork for modern biomedicine are of little importance to traditional East Asian medicine. What concerns it is organizing signs and symptoms to arrive at an accurate perception of "what is going on." Chinese medicine therefore has a very limited theory of the human organism itself. Where biomedicine, seeking a pathological mechanism behind the veil of symptoms, needs a theory that also goes beyond the meeting of patient and doctor to an auxiliary body of knowledge, Chinese medicine rarely looks further than the patient. There is no expectation of an underlying pathological mechanism behind the appearance. Any theory is necessary only to guide the physician's perceptions.

Because this is a book on fundamental perspectives and principles, it is mainly about how the Oriental physician looks at human beings and perceives a clinical landscape. The word *diagnosis* may be close to what is being described, but if this word is used in this book it is meant improvisationally. Any classificatory category is not meant as a discrete entity; rather it is a temporary synthesis that is to be pragmatically tested in the therapeutic intervention. What concerns the Chinese physician is gaining a flexible perspective on the dynamic texture of a person's life. For the Chinese clinician, the first goal, at least after making the initial therapeutic alliance, is to organize signs and symptoms into an emblematic image. Any description of imbalance allows the physician to reflexively consider a suitable clinical response. Any label, or diagnosis, is understood to be a set of words that allows discourse between patient and physician, between physicians and society in general. It is not meant to be mistaken for the ineffable flux that makes a person a unique being.

The essential ideas of Chinese medicine are not elaborate; they are not even strictly the province of the physician. Most of them are the views about health and disease that are shared by the ordinary members of Chinese society. These ideas include axioms, modes of perception, and organization schema.

The "truth" of many of these ideas exists in the deep cultural orientation and root intuitions of a unique civilization. Any attempt to "prove" these organizing principles may be a non sequitur and futile. They represent a world view that is prior to argument and proof. They may just be another point of departure for approaching the phenomenal world.[1] These ideas are cultural and speculative constructs that provide framework and direction.

There are few secrets of Oriental wisdom buried in this book. When presented outside the context of Chinese civilization, or of practical diagnosis and therapeutics, these ideas can seem fragmented and without great significance. The practical "truth" of these ideas lies in the way the physician can use them to treat real people with real complaints. They are valuable because they comprise a medical paradigm that makes possible the substantive discussion of "what is going on," thereby allowing the physician to understand people and discern patterns of disharmony. The ideas also guide the use of therapeutics.

Because this is a book on fundamental principles and perspectives, it is mainly about "diagnosis." (Its counterpart in the West would be about chemistry and biology, or anatomy and physiology.) This chapter begins with a discussion of the all-important Chinese notion of Qi and resonance and revisits the Chinese understanding of causality and the macroscosm-microcosm landscape. It then proceeds to describe the fundamental textures of human life and their relationships. The fundamental textures are the basic human subcategories of the universal substratum that the Chinese call Qi. Finally, this chapter will introduce ideas and vocabulary that will lead, later on, into a fuller exposition of the human landscape and what is going on within it.

It is important to remember that Chinese medical theory does not move in a linear way from proposition to proposition. Instead, learning Chinese medicine is like going from simple drawings to fine paintings. The whole is always present; the Yin and Yang can only be refined, never abandoned.

⊣ QI AND RESONANCE

The notion of Qi is as fundamental to Chinese culture and medical thought as Yin and Yang.[2] Like these polar complementary opposites, no one English word or phrase can adequately capture Qi's meaning. One can say that, for the Chinese, everything in the universe, inorganic and organic, is composed of and defined by its Qi. Mountains, plants, and human emotions all have Qi. Qi is not so much a force added to lifeless matter but the state of being of any phenomena. For the Chinese, Qi is the pulsation of the cosmos itself.

Qi is not some primordial, immutable material, nor is it merely vital energy, although the word is occasionally so translated.[3] Chinese thought does not easily distinguish between matter and energy. We might think that Qi is somewhere in between, a kind of matter on the verge of becoming energy, or energy at the point of materializing. But it is far beyond this simple attempt to bridge the chasm of a Western dichotomy. In a single syllable, the word *Qi* proclaims one of the deepest root intuitions of Chinese civilization.

Qi is the thread connecting all being. Qi is the common denominator of all things—from mineral to human. Qi allows any phenomenon to maintain its cohesiveness, grow, and transform into other forms. Metamorphosis is possible because Qi takes myriad forms. Qi is the potential and actualization of transformation. The universe moves—ceaselessly manifests and engenders because of Qi. Qi is the fundamental quality of being and becoming.

Without Qi, there would be no Yin and Yang. Qi is the universe's underlying plastic texture that explains change, the inexhaustible ink of the world. Qi takes countless forms. Qi allows things to become other things. But Qi is more than cause. Qi is the cause, process, and outcome of all activity in the cosmos. Qi is the ceaseless throbbing, the substratum of the cosmos.

In the classical physics and the common parlance of the modern West, change is produced by one object exerting a force on another: change is from external movement. Matter is inert; external force propels change. There is a basic dichotomy. (Obviously, modern notions of physics have begun to modify these notions, but for modern medicine and everyday reality, these notions persist.) As we have mentioned earlier, for the Chinese, causation is primarily an inner transformation. Qi does not "cause" change; Qi is present before, during, and after any metamorphosis. The change has to do with the manifestation of what is already inherent in the earlier state. Things transform because Qi takes on different forms. Qi is the propensity or inclinations of things. "At the most embryonic stage, the tendency toward the fullness of actualization is already latent."[4]

While change is primarily internal, forms of being can influence other forms of being. Things "evoke" change in other things. For the Chinese, this kind of "causing" or "inductance," however, is not because of an external compulsion. Things influence other things because they "connect" or "elicit" what is already a "disposition" in things. This ability for one thing to influence another is called in

Chinese *gan ying*, which is usually translated "resonance."[5] If Qi is the link, resonance is the method.

The Qi of the sun, rain, and soil resonate with the Qi of the seed to bring forth a plant that already contains the germ of the plant and qualities that the sun, rain, and soil touch. Anger can be an aggressive awareness of another person; self-reflection can foster the "same" Qi of awareness to manifest as a benevolent concern for the other. The Qi of illness can be transformed into healthy Qi by a medicine that resonates between the two particular states. Illness contains the seed of health. Resonance is the process "by which a thing, when stimulated, spontaneously responds according to the natural guidelines of the particular phases of vital energy engendered in itself and active in the situation."[6] The Qi does not "cause" change; the Qi is present before, during, and after the transformation. One Qi elicits the propensity of another Qi that shares a similar kind of "frequency." Things "energize" each other. Through resonance, one Qi evokes another.

Resonance allows the universe (or any of its parts) to influence a human being. In fact, the macrocosm-microcosm relationship discussed earlier is possible because of resonance. The universe can affect a human being because a person already contains latent forms of the cosmic Qi. Otherwise, a person would be impervious to outside influences. Causality is relationships of resonance and resemblance. Connection, contact, and compulsion is the intimacy of similar Qi. The *Nei Jing* eloquently explains:

> *Heaven is round and Earth is square; the roundness of the head and squareness of the Earth resonate accordingly. Heaven has the sun and moon, humans have two eyes; Earth has nine provinces, humans have nine orifices; Heaven has thunder and lightning, humans have sound and speech; Heaven has wind and rain, humans have joy and anger. . . . Heaven has five musical sounds, humans have five Yin Organs. . . . Heaven has winter and summer, humans have cold and hot; Heaven has Yin and Yang and*

humans have husband and wife. . . . Earth has twelve rivers,
humans have twelve Meridians. . . . Heaven has morning and
evening, humans go to sleep and awake. . . . Earth has times of no
crops, so humans can be childless. In these ways, Heaven and
Earth resonate with humans.[7]

The Chinese believe that the human "cosmos in miniature" is a
statement of relationship and "fact." For the Chinese, the landscape
metaphor of the last chapter is more than a descriptive device. It is
a statement of resonance and interpenetration. Components of the
universe, the Qi of herbs (plants, animal parts, and stones), acupuncture points (junctions of the human rivers), lifestyle activities
(movement and rest, food, and relationships), or living environment
(seasons, weather, or even air conditioning) share a resonating frequency that already exists in a person. A medicine or a conscious
shift in a person's behavior can resonate with the condition within a
person (e.g., a pattern of a disharmony) and induce a person toward
health. Also, the different layers of human life, as disparate as the
corporeal, psychological, ecological, and moral mutually interact for
the same reason: their various forms of Qi resonate. Qi is the cosmic breath that unites disparate forms.

⊣ Qi [气]

The all-pervasive global sense of Qi tends to confound discussion.
It includes all Yin and Yang. It is hard to get beyond the fundamental intuition and be more specific. In Chinese medicine, beside
this all-inclusive generic meaning, Qi can also have a more narrow
and specific sense. Qi, in its more practical and clinical sense, means
the particular dynamic of engendering, movement, tension, and acti-
vation. (Other textures or energies of the global aspect of Qi, such
as repose, quiescence, and self-reflection, are described with different names.) In this focused sense, Qi is considered in its Yang aspect

alone. (In the generic sense, Qi is both Yin and Yang.) On a physical level, this specific clinical sense of Qi has to do with strength, effort, and capacity for work. On a psychological level, this Qi concerns desire, awareness of possibilities, considerations of options, resolution, and motivation. The narrower sense of Qi has a sense of future orientation, potential manifestation, and creative vision.

Both senses of Qi exist in the medical literature. The all-encompassing larger one allows the label *Qi* to be attached to anything, while the narrower sense has mainly to do with its creative dynamic aspect. In the discussion in this book, when the word *Qi* is used (unless otherwise stated) it is being used in the narrow sense as it pertains to clinical Chinese medicine.

Origins of Qi

The Qi that is directly involved with a person's life has three sources. The first of these is Original Qi (*yuan-qi*), also called Prenatal Qi, which is transmitted by parents to their children at conception. This Qi is partly responsible for an individual's inherited constitution. The second source is Grain Qi (*gu-qi*), which is derived from the digestion of food. The third is Natural Air Qi (*kong-qi*), which is extracted by the Lungs from the air we breathe.

These three forms of Qi intermingle to produce the Qi that permeates the entire person. There is "no place that does not have it, and no place it does not penetrate."[8]

Functions of Qi

Qi, once formed, can be divided into many different specific types of Qi, which have specific functions. In fact, any activity could be a "type" of Qi. One sinologist has identified thirty-two distinct categories in the literature of the past 2,500 years, and has posed a useful analogy between Qi and electrical energy. Just as Westerners recognize electricity as a general phenomenon displayed in specific forms (high and low voltage, high and low amperage), the Chinese recognize Qi as a general phenomenon with many variant aspects and functions.[9]

Within the person, Qi has at least five major functions.[10] Through these activities, Qi is responsible for the integrity of any entity and for the changes that entity undergoes.

Qi is the source of all movement and accompanies all movement.

This function includes movement in its broadest sense: gross physical activity (walking, dancing), involuntary movement (breathing, heartbeat), willed action (eating, speaking), mental action (thinking, rejoicing, dreaming), and development, growth, and life process (birth, maturation, and aging) are all movements that depend on the Qi.

Qi is *not* the cause of movement, because Qi is inseparable from movement. For example, Qi is the source of growth in the body, but also grows with the body. For the Chinese, Qi is the process that makes possible integrative descriptions of human changes. Diagnostic methods exist for determining its strength and motion, and there are specific treatments for supplementing its deficiency, draining its excess, and regulating its flow.

In the body, Qi is in constant motion and has four primary directions: ascending, descending, entering, and leaving. The *Nei Jing* states: "Without entering and leaving there is no development, without ascending and descending no transformation, absorption, and storing."[11] Normal physiological activity is Qi moving harmoniously in these various directions. If there is insufficient Qi, if the Qi is obstructed or moves in "rebellion" or moves "recklessly," or if any of the Qi directions lose their "regulation," disharmony will result. *without dynamism of Qi, There is no life present.*

Qi protects the body.

It resists the entry into the body of pathological environmental agents, called External Pernicious Influences (discussed in Chap-

eg. Spleen Qi "is" the process of digestion!

ter 5), and combats them if they do manage to penetrate. The *Nei Jing* says: "If Pernicious Influences abide, the Qi must be deficient."[12]

Qi is the source of harmonious transformation.

When food is ingested it is transformed into other states of being such as Blood, Qi itself, tears, sweat, thought, and aspirations. These changes depend on the transformative function of Qi.

Qi ensures stability and governs retention.

While Qi is mainly described as moving, the stability and integrity of human life—the persistence of activity—requires the dynamic tension of Qi. Qi maintains structure. Standing still or watching for a long time requires the force of a kind of "structural" Qi. Qi also helps things from falling. Qi "keeps everything in"—it holds Organs in their proper place, keeps the Blood in the Blood pathways, and prevents excessive loss of the various bodily fluids, such as sweat and saliva. Qi also steadies volitional commitments.

Qi warms the body.

Maintenance of normal heat in the body as a whole, or in any part of the body (e.g., the limbs) depends on the warming function of the Qi.

Types of Qi

Each of the five functions of Qi is apparent in all the specific types of Qi, of which there are many. Five of them, however, are especially important. These types of Qi are associated with particular actions or particular parts of the body, and most Chinese medical discussions of Qi center on one of the five primary types.

Organ Qi *(zang-fu-zhi-qi)* The major functions of any Organ are referred to in terms of that Organ's Qi. Every Organ is conceived of as having its own Qi, whose activity is characterized by the Organ to which it is attached. When the Chinese speak of Heart Qi or

Lung Qi, the texture of Qi is the same, but its activity when related to the Heart is different from its activity when related to the Lungs; and the Heart and Lungs operate differently depending on the nature of their Qi. (Details of the particular Organ Qis are discussed in Chapter 3.)

Meridian Qi (*jing-luo-zhi-qi*) Meridians are a unique and crucial part of Chinese medical theory. They are the channels or pathways through which Qi flows among the Organs and various bodily parts, adjusting and harmonizing their activity. Qi flowing in this comprehensive network is called Meridian Qi (See Chapter 4).

Nutritive Qi (*ying-qi*) This is the Qi most intimately associated with the Blood. It manifests itself in the Blood and moves with the Blood through the Blood Vessels. Its activity helps transform the purest nutrients derived from food into Blood. Nutritive Qi is an essential factor in bodily nourishment.

Protective Qi (*wei-qi*) This is the Qi responsible for resisting and combating External Pernicious Influences when they invade the body. Considered the most Yang manifestation of Qi in the body, Protective Qi is "fierce and bold."[13] It moves within the chest and abdominal cavities and travels between the skin and muscles. This Qi regulates the sweat glands and pores and moistens and protects the skin and hair.

Qi of the Chest or Ancestral Qi (*zong-qi*) This Qi gathers in the chest, where it forms a "sea of Qi."[14] The *Nei Jing* states that this Qi "collects in the chest, goes out the throat, connects with the Heart and Vessels, and moves respiration."[15] Its main function is to aid and regulate the rhythmic movement of respiration and heartbeat, and so it is intimately connected with the Lungs and Heart. The relative strength and evenness of respiration, of the voice, the heartbeat, and the movement of Blood are all related to the Qi of the Chest.[16]

Disharmonies of Qi

There are two major patterns of disharmony associated with Qi. Such patterns are generally called Qi disharmonies. The details and intricacies of Qi and other disharmonies will be discussed in later chapters.

Deficient Qi (*qi-xu*) This is the general designation for patterns of disharmony in the human being, in which the Qi is insufficient to perform any of the five Qi functions. If Deficient Qi affects the whole person, symptoms might include lethargy and exhaustion. Deficient Qi can be one or more of the following feelings: "not being able to do things," "not being able to want to do things," or "not wanting to be able to do things." Deficient Qi may also describe a particular Organ unable to perform its functions. For example, in the pattern of Deficient Kidney Qi, the Kidneys may be incapable of harmoniously regulating water, and the individual may develop such symptoms as incontinence or edema. Deficient Qi can also apply to any of the various types of Qi. Deficient Protective Qi, for instance, may lead to frequent colds.

Collapsed Qi (*qi-xian*) A subcategory of Deficient Qi, this implies that the Qi is so insufficient that it can no longer hold Organs in place. When there is Collapsed Qi, such disorders as prolapse of the uterus or piles or loss of motivation or commitment may occur.

Stagnant Qi (*qi-zhi*) This is the second broad category of Qi disharmonies. In this disharmony, the normal movement of Qi is impaired—the Qi does not flow through the body in a smooth and orderly fashion. Stagnant Qi in the limbs and Meridians may be the origin of pain and aches in the body. Stagnant Qi can also lead to impairment of an Organ. Stagnant Qi in the Liver may result in abdominal distention, moodiness, or a sense of frustration.

Rebellious Qi (*qi-ni*) This is a particular form of Stagnant Qi. It implies that the Qi is going in the wrong direction. For example, Chinese medicine says that Stomach Qi should go downward; if it rebels and goes upward, there may be vomiting and nausea or explosive forms of mania.

All the fundamental textures can be defined as either mostly Yin or mostly Yang. They embody the five Yin-Yang principles, and so contain both Yin and Yang aspects, but one aspect is dominant. All patterns of disharmony can be considered either Yin conditions or Yang conditions.

Within the group of fundamental textures, Qi is a Yang texture. Deficient Qi is a Yin condition, a condition of depletion, in which a person exhibits the underactivity characteristic of Yin. Relative to Deficient Qi, Stagnant Qi is a Yang condition, a condition of surfeit, associated with the Yang characteristics of excessiveness.

⊣ BLOOD [*xue* 血]

As discussed already, in the generic sense, the fundamental quality of human life, like the cosmos itself, is an all-pervasive Qi. In the narrow sense, Qi is the quality of life that is dynamic and transforming. Blood is the responsive, accepting, effortless, soft, and nurturing complement of the clinical Qi. Qi and Blood are the Yin and Yang of ordinary life activity.

Qi activates, Blood relaxes. Qi quickens, Blood softens. Qi is tense and tight; Blood is smooth and languid. Qi embodies effort, Blood is effortlessness. Qi is becoming. Blood is being. Qi moves forward in time; Blood circulates in repetitive cycles. Qi is the potential; Blood is the actualized. Qi is creative and fosters newness; Blood is the already achieved and recognizes what has already been created. Qi is visionary; Blood is memory. Qi is Yang, Blood is Yin.

Obviously, the Blood of Chinese medical terminology is not the same as what the West calls blood. Although it is sometimes identifiable with the red fluid of biomedicine, its characteristics and functions are not so identifiable.[17]

A major activity of the Blood is to circulate continuously through the body, nourishing, maintaining, and to some extent moistening its various parts. Blood moves primarily through the Blood Vessels, but also through the Meridians (see Appendix F). Chinese medicine does not make a clear distinction between Blood Vessels and Meridians. The Chinese rarely concern themselves about precise inner physical locations—the Stomach Qi "goes upward," or the Blood "circulates," but it is seldom entirely clear what internal paths they travel or where, precisely, they go. The physical pathway is less important than the function. This tendency not to fix sites for things is contrary to the Western approach, but it is inevitable with Chinese medical theorizing, which emphasizes process over fixed entities.

Origins of Blood

Blood originates through the transformation of food. After the Stomach receives and "ripens" the food, the Spleen distills from it an extremely fine and purified essence. The Spleen Qi then transports this essence upward to the Lungs. During the upward movement, Nutritive Qi begins to turn the essence into Blood. The change is completed when the essence reaches the Lungs, where the now-transformed food combines with the portion of air described as "clear." This combination finally produces Blood. The Blood is then propelled through the body by the Heart Qi in coordination with the Qi of the Chest.

Relationships of Blood

Three Organs in the body have special relationships with the Blood: the Heart, Liver, and Spleen. Blood depends on the Heart for its harmonious, smooth, and continuous circulation throughout the body. It is therefore said that "the Heart rules the Blood." The body needs less Blood when it is inactive, and then "the Liver then stores the Blood." finally, the Blood depends on the retentive properties of Spleen Qi to keep it within the Blood Vessels and, therefore, "the Spleen governs the Blood."

Blood and Qi, though generally distinct from each other, have a mutually dependent and indissoluble relationship. Qi creates and moves the Blood and also holds it in place. Blood in turn nourishes the Organs that produce and regulate the Qi. Their relationship of tension and ease, desire and acceptance exemplifies the principles of Yin (Blood) and Yang (Qi). A traditional saying summarizes this relationship in two principles: "Qi is the commander of the Blood . . . Blood is the mother of Qi."[18]

Disharmonies of Blood

The two major categories of Blood disharmony are Deficient Blood (*xue-xu*) and Congealed Blood (*xue-yu*). A pattern of Deficient Blood exists when the entire body, or a particular Organ or other part of the body, is insufficiently nourished by the Blood. If this condition affects the entire body, signs such as a pale and lusterless face, dizziness, tight muscles, restlessness, and dry skin may appear. On a psychological level, Blood is about effortless acknowledgement of accomplishment. Insufficient Blood may be accompanied by poor self-esteem, lack of a sense of self-worth, or poor memory. When a particular Organ is affected, there will be different signs. Deficient Blood of the Heart, for example, may lead to palpitations, insomnia, or shyness.

Congealed Blood means the Blood is not flowing smoothly, has become obstructed, and accumulates in a manner contradictory and opposite to its nature. What should be effortless and soothing becomes its opposite. "Just being," turns upon itself and becomes an intolerable, impossible, or threatening situation. This condition is often characterized by sharp, stabbing pains and/or tumors, cysts, or swelling of the Organs. On a psychological level, the inability to feel safe, excessive vigilance, suspiciousness, paranoid ideation, and delusions can also be associated with Congealed Blood.

⊣ Essence [*jing* 精]

Essence, the translation of the Chinese word *Jing*, is the texture that is specific to organic life. It is the stuff that makes living beings unique and distinct from inorganic things. Essence is a kind of deep, "soft," "juicy" potential inherent in living beings which forms and fills the life cycle as it unfolds. In the usual Chinese manner that defies simple categories, it is the potential, guidance, and actuality that shapes birth, development, maturation, decline, and death. Essence has a forward direction in time, but it concerns a form of time that is almost imperceptible and inexorable. It is barely noticeable in an everyday sense. It is time that goes through a person—only recognizable when we look back and see big chunks of the life cycle. Essence's transformation is noticed most easily in reflection and contemplation. At the age of seventy it is easy to notice the unfolding that has happened since age twenty or thirty. Essence moves slowly, but with a slowness that seems not to move at all. Essence is automatic, autonomous, and inevitable. Although Essence is "soft," paradoxically Essence's inexorability has a nonstoppable and relentless power.

Origins of Essence

Essence has two sources, which are also its characteristic aspects. Prenatal Essence (*xian-tian-zhi-jing*), also translated as Congenital Essence, is inherited from the parents. In fact, the fusion of this parental Essence is conception. Each person's Prenatal Essence is unique and will determine his or her particular growth patterns. The quantity and quality of the Prenatal Essence is fixed at birth and, together with Original Qi, determines an individual's basic makeup and constitution.

Postnatal Essence (*hou-tian-zhi-jing*) is the second source and aspect of Essence. It is derived from the purified parts of ingested food and continuous physical, emotional, and mental stimulation from a person's environment. The Postnatal Essence allows for modification of Prenatal Essence. Together, they compose the overall Essence of the person.

Functions of Essence

An individual's development is accompanied by corresponding changes in his or her Essence. The *Nei Jing* speaks of women's development in seven-year stages:

> At seven years the Kidney [Essence][19] is ascendant: The teeth change and the hair grows. At fourteen years the Dew of Heaven [Essence] arrives: The Conception Meridian flows, the Penetrating Extra Meridian is full, the menses come regularly, and the woman can conceive. At twenty-one years the Kidney [Essence] plateaus: The wisdom teeth come in and growth is at its peak. At twenty-eight years the tendons and bones are strong, the hair is at its growing peak, and the body is strong; at thirty-five years the Yang Brightness Meridian weakens, the face begins to darken, and hair falls out. At forty-two the three Yang Meridians are weak above [in the face], the face is dark, and the hair begins to turn white. At forty-nine the Conception Meridian is Deficient, the Penetrating Extra Meridian is exhausted, the Water of Heaven is dried up; the Earth Road [the menses] is not open, so weakness and infertility set in.[20]

A similar process of eight-year transitions is described for men:

> At eight years the Kidney [Essence] is full: The hair is grown, and the teeth change. At sixteen years the Kidney [Essence] is abundant: The Water of Heaven [Essence] arrives, the Jing Qi is

able to flow, the Yin and Yang are in harmony, and the man is fertile. At twenty-four the Kidney [Essence] plateaus: The tendons and bones are strong, the wisdom teeth come in, and growth is at its peak. At thirty-two the tendons and bones are at their strongest and the flesh is full and strong. At forty the Kidney [Essence] is weakened, the hair falls out, and the teeth are loose. At forty-eight the Yang Qi is exhausted above, the face darkens, and the hair whitens. At fifty-six the Liver [Essence] is weak, the tendons cannot move, the Dew of Heaven is used up, there is little semen, the Kidney is weak, and the appearance and body are at their end. At sixty-four the hair and teeth are gone.[21]

Thus, Essence is the quality or texture that imbues an organism with the possibility of development, from conception to death. Essence is also responsible for the development of the deepest awareness and wisdom.

Disharmonies of Essence might involve improper maturation, sexual dysfunction, inability to reproduce, ungraceful aging, or the incapacity to be self-reflective as a person matures.

Qi and Essence both have to do with movement. Qi (in the narrow sense) has to do with the dynamic movement of ordinary time. Qi flows with the "external" aspects of movement; Jing—dark, moist, warm—is the inner essence of growth and decline. An individual's Qi and Essence are mutually dependent. Qi emerges out of Essence, since Prenatal Essence is the root of life. But Qi helps transform food into Postnatal Essence, thereby maintaining and expanding that life. In relation to each other, Essence is Yin and Qi is Yang.

When compared with Blood, however, Essence is the more active, or Yang, phenomenon. Blood is associated with the everyday cyclical process of maintenance, nourishment, and repair. Essence is tied to ongoing, long-range development. Blood may be conceived as remaining static in time, presiding over repetitive cycles; Essence is the fluid that moves forward through time and history—the basis of reproduction, growth, ripening, and withering. Therefore, in relation to Blood, Essence is Yang; in relation to Essence, Blood is Yin.

⊣ SPIRIT [*shen* 神]

Spirit is the translation for the Chinese word *Shen*. Spirit is the fundamental texture that is unique to human life. In the same way that Essence (*Jing*) distinguishes organic life from inorganic material, Spirit separates human life from animal life. While the Chinese believe animals share instinctive drives, reactivity, and various "emotions" with humans (see Chapter 5), only humans are thought to have Spirit.

Spirit is the domain of human life that defies the limitations of time and space. It is the human capacity for relationships that are not restricted by physical or temporal contact. For example, for the Chinese, Spirit allows a person to worship an ancestor or revere Confucius. Spirit recognizes and pursues ultimate goals such as "self-transformation," "being the 'knight' (*jun-zi*) of the Way," "the arduous effort of will not to will," "seeking the Tao," and "the ceaseless cultivation of virtue." Western equivalents might include being deeply connected to revelations on Mt. Sinai or by the Sea of Galilee and seeking to live the life of a tsaddick or saint.

But Spirit has no necessary link with a particular religion or even religiosity. In a more secular vein, Spirit may have to do with efforts at cleaning rivers so future generations can enjoy them or appreciating the beauty of an ancient vase. Spirit allows the dedication and commitment of the physician, police officer, or plumber. Spirit is involved in the most prosaic aspects of life. Spirit allows for such simple but life-affirming activities as consuming personal hobbies, honoring cultural or national traditions, the expansiveness of leisure travel, or feeling "connected" when puttering around the house. Spirit is felt whenever human consciousness forges compelling bonds and special relationships. Spirit is invoked by imagination, will, intention, awe, enchantment, and wonder.

Spirit depends on more than mind-consciousness. Spirit is self-awareness that fosters the human experience of authenticity and personal meaning. Spirit allows self-reflection, art, morality, purpose, and values. It depends on self-relationship.

Spirit is not some "spiritual" goodness in people; it can produce both virtue and its absence, beauty and its opposite. Spirit is the process of self-examination, not its outcome. (For religion, as opposed to medicine, Spirit may be an outcome defined by a pre-scribed tradition.) In medicine, Spirit allows a person to tread his or her self-chosen and self-directed path.[22] China's oldest herbal text (150 B.C.E.) treats Spirit when it prescribes herbs that will support a person to self-consciously shape his or her own destiny (*ming*).[23] Spirit is the capacity that allows self-reflection on volitional inten-tions, creativity, meaning, and moral cultivation. It is the capacity of the human being to be "an initiator, a participant, and a guardian of the universe."[24] It is also what allows for humans to insert or interject their "authentic self" into their mundane lives and be par-ticipants in shaping their fate.

The Five Spirits

The medical tradition generally considers Spirit to be divisible into five smaller Spirits. Each of these small Spirits has a primary respon-sibility for a particular virtue.[25] Occasionally, some of the discussion concerning Spirit presented here can appear "religious" (and indeed it borrows from a shared vocabulary with Asian religious traditions). But it should be emphasized that this is not a section on East Asian religious beliefs or spirituality. This discussion of Spirit and virtue is about capacities and responsibilities inherent in the human con-dition that are recognizable across cultures and can be absolutely independent of religious belief, preferences, or inclinations. The focus is how Chinese medicine (as a "secular" healing art) has tra-ditionally sought to conceptualize and integrate the nonphysical aspects of a person's life into its discussion of illness and health.

EARTH

***Consciousness of Potentials, or* Yi** *Yi* is sometimes translated as thought, consciousness, or intention, and, in this book, it is trans-lated by the cumbersome but more accurate phrase "Consciousness of Potentials." Operationally, it is the Spirit that is responsible for considering, deliberating, and deciding on what is likely, possible, or conceivable. It is responsible for discerning various directions and perspectives. The Consciousness of Potentials is ultimately responsible for allurement, vision, motivation, and creativity.

The Consciousness of Potentials (*Yi*) is responsible for the virtue of faithfulness, loyalty, or sincerity (*xin*) and has the task of enabling and supporting new manifestations to come into being. Because the Yi is insightful, it can understand others and be generous and extremely aware of the needs of other people and situations. It can see both what can and what needs to be done.

If Yi lacks intactness, instead of creative possibilities a person will experience worry, confusion, exaggerated sympathy, "sticky" or "stifling" loyalty, or uncontrolled and even self-destructive generosity. At other times, a weak Yi will manifest with boredom, monotony, or indifference. Yi can be said to be the Qi aspect of the Spirit.

Non-Corporeal Soul, or **Hun**   The *Hun* is even more difficult to translate than *Yi*. In fact, *Hun* is a common word in many East Asian languages and appears with extreme frequency in the medical literature, but its precise meaning is linked with specific cultural notions of Spirit that make an exact equivalence or translation elusive. In the parlance of East Asian culture, Hun is considered that part of the person that is "not attached to the physical body" and supposedly continues to exist after the cessation of physical life. It is what remains after death that still bears the name of the once-breathing person, hence the translation "Non-Corporeal Soul." (In the various religious traditions of the East, the Non-Corporeal Soul is the crucial issue addressed in any rites for the dead.[26])

China's medical and philosophic systems deal with the matrix of phenomena that belong to the Non-Corporeal Soul as it pertains to the "earthly" realm. (A Chinese doctor does not treat the afterlife of a person, which would be a usurpation of the role of clergy.) In the living world, the Hun has to do with the "good deeds" performed in this life that potentially can abide after death. One could say that the Hun is the "good name" or "acts of kindness" that continue after a person's demise.

A Chinese doctor can help the Non-Corporeal Soul of a person be steady, clear, and sensitive in this life. An intact Hun produces acts of kindness or benevolence toward others and self. In fact, human kindness (*ren*) is the specific virtue of the Hun. If the Hun is not intact, a person can be unkind toward others (e.g., overly angry and belligerent) or unkind to himself or herself (e.g., unable to feel self-worth or be self-deprecating). The disturbed Non-Corporeal Soul can easily foster envy, jealousy, and inappropriate hatred.*

The Non-Corporeal Soul's responsibility for human kindness and benevolence has an intimate relationship to a person's capacity to feel and endure pain and suffering. In fact, awareness of suffering is often considered to be the insight that propels the Non-Corporeal Soul's cultivation of human kindness. On an existential level, this means that the Non-Corporeal Soul understands another person's or a person's own suffering as a call for heightened compassion. Because of the Hun, pain awakens empathy. Suffering is the fundamental awareness that fosters benevolence toward others or self. Without this capacity, a person is numb (*bu ren*) and incapable of experiencing the depth of another person's humanity or his or her own. On a physical level, the Non-Corporeal Soul (through its rela-

---

*Historical medical texts see herbs, acupuncture, and the therapeutic relationship as possible modalities that can help heal the Non-Corporeal Soul. Whether the Hun is "real" or not is an unimportant question for the physician. This author feels that the Hun is a Chinese cultural construct that is helpful in discussing aspects of human behavior and in searching medical texts for potentially useful treatments. Essentially, the Non-Corporeal Soul is the vocabulary for describing ordinary people's daily struggles around such critical issues as uncontrollable anger, absence of self-esteem, inability to forgive, resentment, and jealousy. The reality or nonreality of the Hun should never interfere with the physician's job of "treating" a person's body and soul. Also, it should be mentioned that if the physician imposes on the patient any of his or her own religious or moral beliefs, an abuse of power in the therapeutic relationship is occurring.

tionship with Blood, see Chapter 3) allows for the sensation of pain and at the same time reduces the "wanting things to be other than they are." The Non-Corporeal Soul increases tolerance and acceptance of the pain sensation, which paradoxically automatically reduces pain's noxiousness and intolerableness. The more room for pain, the less it hurts. For the Non-Corporeal Soul, pain and suffering are not something to flee, but a catalyst for the authentication of humanity and the generation of human kindness.[27] The Non-Corporeal Soul is considered the Blood aspect of Spirit.

Will, or Zhi

On its simplest and most superficial level, Will has to do with resolution and the basic volition and intentions of a person. It has the quality of force, self-determination, and arduous effort. This first level of the the will is the Yang Will.

The deeper Will—the Yin Will—is more difficult to describe. The Yin Will is paradoxical: it is a kind of "will that cannot be willed." The Yin Will is mostly a direction, a willfulness that moves to an end that cannot be known until it is already reached. The Yin Will goes through a person and is noticeable only when a person turns around and can reflect over a time and say, "Oh yes! There was a Will that worked independent of my own knowing volition." Li Shi-zhen, the great Ming-dynasty physician, described it as being "lengthy" and enduring.[28] The Yin Will is noticed as an abiding and persistent presence detectable only after what was willed has already manifested. It is the profound sense of "it was always there," or "it was always meant to be." The Yin Will has the sense of the unknown, fate, or destiny. The Yin Will embodies the inexorable and irreducible mystery of life.

The Will is responsible for the virtue of Wisdom (*zhi*). Wisdom is not certainty or knowledge. One cannot decide to obtain this Wisdom; it comes on its own. It accumulates like our years. Wisdom is a knowing that has to do with learning to have a relationship with what is unknown and unknowable. Wisdom infuses; it does not proclaim. Wisdom has some of the qualities of fear in that it has a relationship to the unknown; but, unlike fear, it possesses a deep trust that the unknown eventually reveals an inevitable destiny.* Facing death with equanimity and grace (whether from a religious or a secular perspective) has to do with the Wisdom a person gathers in a lifetime.

A weak Yang Will means profound passivity and being devoid of assertiveness. A deficiency of the Yin Will may produce such signs as the absence of tranquility or deep restlessness. A diminished Yin Will may also cause the Yang Will to become reckless and unrestrained. In this situation a person tries to will what cannot be willed. Signs can include being incongruent with the life cycle (e.g., acting like a teenager when one is eighty years old, or trying to be wise when one is twenty) or wanting the Essence (*Jing*) to be different (e.g., wanting to be born Japanese when one is born Italian). Inordinate existential fear can result from Will disturbances. The Yang Will's fear is paralyzing; the Yin Will's fear is agitating and seeks to run. The Yang and Yin Will are not quite balanced. The Yang Will is about the primordial assertions, fundamental decisions, and the most arduous efforts undertaken during a person's life. The Yin Will is trust and knowing that Wisdom and destiny inevitably are revealed. Ultimately, the Yang Will cannot push beyond the constraints imposed by the Yin Will; the Yin Will is supreme. Fate is the final arbiter. The Will is considered the Essence (*Jing*) aspect of Spirit.

Spirit, or **Shen** Here the vocabulary can be confusing. *Spirit* is the Chinese word for the combination of all five spirits; it is also the name of one of these five Spirits in particular. This small Spirit is said

---

*The closest Western word for the Chinese sense of Wisdom is probably faith. This faith does not imply a parochial religious identity, but speaks to a sense of trust and being able to embrace the unknown.

to reside in the Heart (see Chapter 3) and composes, so to speak, one-fifth of the larger Spirit. (The character for *Shen* is a homonym for both the generic Spirit and the Heart's small Spirit.) The small Heart Spirit has the responsibility of making sure that the big Spirit connects properly with the world of time and space. This Spirit makes sure that the inner "timeless" aspect of a person does not lose the ability to connect to the actual ongoing world of real people in real places. This Spirit is the most visible of the Spirits. It has to do with connecting with people, saying the right words, calculations of appropriateness, looking a person in the eyes, and responding to a question with an answer that makes sense. The Heart Spirit has to do with communication and being able to "click" with people and situations.

The virtue of the Heart Spirit is *li*, which can be translated as ceremony, ritual, or propriety. Propriety ensures that correct behavior fosters timely and appropriate interactions and relationships. The Heart Spirit governs the essential East Asian concern for "face." If the Heart Spirit is intact, a person behaves in a socially correct manner and acts with a proper demeanor and style. The right things happen at the right time. If the Heart Spirit is disturbed, a person can have awkward social relationships, behave in a socially incorrect manner, be shy and easily blush, not be able to look a person in the eyes, or, in extreme cases, be obviously disoriented and delusional, as might happen in a serious mental illness.

Animal Soul, or Po Po is a very distinct Chinese notion. In Chinese religious thought, unlike Non-Corporeal Soul (*Hun*), Po ceases to exist when a person physically dies. (Therefore, some have translated *Po* as "corporeal soul.") Po is the portion of a person's Spirit that is absolutely dependent on the person's physical life. When breathing ceases, the Po disintegrates. The Po is about momentary reactions; unlike the other Spirits (with the possible exception of the Heart Spirit), it is utterly tied to time and space. Po is the reactivity or animation of a person, hence the alternative translation Animal Soul.

In the medical tradition, the Animal Soul is often said to be equivalent to the seven emotions (see Chapter 5). The Po is the unthinking and compelling passion that propels life. The Animal Soul can be reckless and unthinking. The Animal Soul is the Chinese way of acknowledging that part of the nonmaterial aspect of a person is just plain knee-jerk reactions that are utterly linked to transitory feelings. An intact Po has short-term power and assertiveness; a weakened Po is lifeless and lethargic. The Po's activity is reactive and momentary.

The Animal Soul's virtue has two dimensions. In one sense, it has to do with being impartial and not being easily swayed. This virtue is called justice (*yi*). From this perspective, an intact Animal Soul can be deliberate and fair. When it is disturbed, a person can be emotionless or haughty or, the opposite, be wildly reactive or hysterical, and seem like an enraged animal.

From another perspective, the virtue of the Animal Soul is described as preciousness (*bao*). In this vein, the Po is said to capture the perfection and completeness of a single moment or a short time span. This aspect of Po grasps the overflowing fullness of a momentary flash of inspiration or the profound awe and eternity in a single work of great art. When the Po is disrupted, in this sense, a person has difficulty appreciating the completion and sublimity of something that has passed away, ceased existing, or died. Grief lingers and is never resolved. A person always feels loss or incompletion. Po is the fluid aspect of Spirit.

Two final notes on the Spirit are in order. First, it is worth mentioning the surprising similarity of the Chinese notion of Spirit as portrayed here and Ian Hacking's philosophic-historical analysis of the notion of soul: "[which is not meant] to suggest something eternal, but to invoke character, reflective choice, self-understanding, values that include honesty to others, and oneself, and several types of freedom and responsibility. . . . I do not think of the soul as unitary, as an essence, as one single thing, or even as a thing at all. It does not denote an unchanging core of personal identity. One person, one soul, may have many facets and speak with many tongues.

... To think of the soul is not to imply that there is one essence, one spiritual point, from which all voices issue. In my way of thinking the soul is a more modest concept than that. It stands for the strange mix of aspects of a person that may be, at some time, imaged as inner."[29] Second, it is worth stating, at least in the medical tradition, Spirit is always considered to be embodied and have no independence from a human life.[30] The Chinese physician resists, both intellectually and clinically, a separation of human life into components or dichotomies; mind and body, mental and physical, soul and body, moral virtues and autonomic activities are linked. Obviously, in some clinical situations one aspect has priority over another. One needs to stop acute bleeding or an asthma attack. At other times, issues of the soul take precedence. But during the course of the patient-physician encounter, the physician will necessarily consider and engage the multidimensional and integrated nature of a person's life.

⊣ FLUIDS [*jin-ye* 津液]

Fluids are bodily liquids other than Blood—including sweat, saliva, gastric juices, and urine. The term *jin* refers to lighter and clearer fluids, while *ye* connotes fluids with a heavier, thicker nature.

The function of the Fluids is to moisten and partly to nourish the hair, skin, membranes, orifices, flesh, muscles, Inner Organs, joints, brain, marrow, and bones. Although the Fluids are considered a fundamental texture, they are perceived as being less refined, less essential, or less "deep" than Qi, Blood, Essence, and Spirit. The time frame for Fluid activity tends to be of a very short duration—minutes, hours, or days.

The Fluids are derived from ingested food and drink and are absorbed and regulated by the Qi of various Organs, particularly the Kidneys. Therefore, the Fluids depend on the Qi, and the Qi, to some extent, depends on the Fluids to moisten and nourish the Organs that regulate Qi.

Blood and Fluids are part of a continuum of liquids in the body. Their basic natures are much the same, but they differ in the degree of their ability to nourish. The Blood is "deeper," more potent, and touches important cycles of time. In Chinese theory, the cleanest or clearest part of the Fluids enters the developing Blood and unites with purified food as part of the process that creates Blood. This relationship between Fluids and Blood is seen clinically when a severe acute hemorrhage causes insufficient Fluids or, conversely, when chronic damage to the Fluids causes Deficient Blood.

Fluids, as liquids, are Yin Substances. Disharmonies of Fluids generally include dryness—of the lips, skin, eyes, etc. Most Fluid disharmonies, however, blend into the more general category of Yin or Water disharmonies, which will be discussed later.[31]

These five fundamental textures of the human being are the basics of the Chinese system. But any aspect of Chinese medical knowledge is meaningful only in relation to the signs, symptoms, and patterns displayed by people. The concrete natures of Qi, Blood, Essence, Spirit, and Fluids will become clearer in the myriad patterns of their disharmonies.

NOTES

1. Judith Farquhar describes these issues in the following way: the "difference between a world of fixed objects and a world of transforming effects accounts for many of the difficulties encountered by moderns who attempt to understand Chinese medicine. Assumptions about the nature of being cannot be 'proved'; no evidence can support or refute them. Like the solid inertial world of modern natural science traditions, the processual and transformative world of Chinese medicine seems to exist prior to all argument, observation, and intervention. Perhaps with a certain discomfort, Western readers must acknowledge that 'their' abstractions about such things make as much sense as 'ours.'" Judith Farquhar, *Knowing Practice: The Clinical Encounter of Chinese Medicine*, p. 26.

2. The concept of Qi has a complex history. Given the key position the concept of Qi holds in explaining the process of change in Chinese scientific, medical, and spiritual thought, one is tempted to assume that it is one of the oldest and most central concepts in the Chinese world view. A look at the history of both the character and the concept show otherwise.

The oldest inscriptions in Chinese, the bones used in Shang-dynasty oracles, are concerned with understanding the process of change in such uncertain areas as agriculture and illness. Nowhere in the more than 200,000 known extant oracle bones can one find the character *Qi* or anything that might be its close antecedent or relative. Throughout the oracle bone inscriptions we see that, in Shang culture, change was brought about by the actions of spirits rather than naturalistic forces.

The character *Qi* is originally composed of an element that signifies vapors that rise to form clouds and another element that means grain. The character may mean vapors arising from cooked food or simply steam. At this level of the character's history, Qi is a simple notion. Qi is what makes the lid of boiling water rattle.

In the course of its development Chinese thought began to look for the origins of change in sources other than the spirits. For a time, change, especially illness, was understood to come from the winds of the eight directions, each of which was responsible for causing particular diseases at particular seasons and each of which was personified as a deity. Although this model of change brought about by wind is a step toward a world of naturalistic causality and away from a world of supernatural causality, it still has a strong component of the latter. It is probably, however, a major step in the development of the concept of Qi that later comes to permeate all of Chinese thought.

By the time of Confucius (551–479 B.C.E.), the word *Qi* appears in the literature, but it is rare, and its meaning is confined to purely human qualities. The *Analects*, the record of Confucius's teaching, uses the word less than a handful of times, each distinctly related to some aspect of human behavior such as appetite, tone of voice, breath, and physical stamina. In none of these does it refer to anything beyond a specific physical quality of human life. At this stage of its history, Qi still shows its origin as a common, ordinary term.

The several centuries following Confucius were a critical time of change in Chinese culture. One of the key concepts to emerge at this time was Qi. Mencius (371–289 B.C.E.), the follower of Confucius, refers to Qi almost a score of times, and each time it is a concept of major philosophical import. Chuang Tzu (Zhang Zi), between 399 and 295 B.C.E., author of a major Taoist text, refers even more frequently to Qi. In this text we can see one of the earliest and clearest uses of Qi to refer to a natural force, something that, although an attribute of human beings, is also a power that makes things happen in the world. We see this conceptualization of Qi (although it is still connected to wind) as a moving power in the universe in a famous passage from Chuang Tzu.

> *The great cloud belches out breath (Qi) and its name is wind. So long as it does not come forth nothing happens, but when it does, the ten thousand hollows begin crying wildly. . . .Blowing on the ten thousand things in a different way, so each can be itself.* (Chuang Tzu *Burton Watson (trans.), New York: Columbia University Press, 1964, p. 31–32).*

Here Qi is a conceptual model for explaining and understanding the process of change in the observable world. The Shang world of a supernatural spirit causality, which had developed into the world of semisupernatural wind causality, has now become a world of natural causality. The Qi model explains the process of change and development in a naturalistic way, conducive to the expansion of philosophic and scientific thought and inquiry.

By the late third century B.C.E., Qi had become a concept used throughout Chinese thought. This conceptualization/experiential model is used to explain the qualities of plants and animals, the use of herbs, and the influence of climate, weather, and geographic location of people. From its use to explain the process of disease comes psychological insights into character and personality types. Eventually, through philosophers such as Wang Yang-ming (1472–1529 C.E.), Qi becomes an essential quality that enables all change, because no matter how they seem to differ, all things share the same Qi. It also becomes a moral and spiritual quality allowing for the oneness of all being.

Perhaps the best single statement concerning Qi that summarizes the sense that Chinese history has conferred on the concept appears in Tu Wei-ming's writings:

> *All modalities of being, from a rock to heaven, are integral parts of a continuum (ta hua). Since nothing is outside of this continuum, the chain of being is never broken. A linkage will always be found between any given pair of things in the universe. . . . The continuous presence of Qi in all modalities of being makes everything flow together as the unfolding of a single process. Nothing, not even an almighty creator, is external to this process.*

For a more detailed discussion of the history of Qi, see Shigehisa, Kuriyama, *Varieties of Haptic Experience: A Comparative Study of Greek and Chinese Pulse Diagnosis* (Ph.D. dissertation, Harvard University, 1986). For a general discussion on Qi, see Nathan Sivin, "Chinese Alchemy and the Manipulation of Time," *Isis*, no. 239 (1976): 513–525; S. Bennet, "Chinese Science: Theory and Practice," *Philosophy East and West* 28, no. 4 (1978): 439–453; Nathan Sivin, *Traditional Medicine in Contemporary China*, 1987.

3. Qi has frequently been identified with the Western concept of vital energy. Westerners are by no means the only ones to make this connection. To characterize Qi as energy is to invoke a world view the Chinese never had, a world view in which matter and energy are different things. While it is true that modern scientific

theory no longer holds that matter and energy are separate entities, in most senses the words have come to connote distinct and separate entities. To the Chinese, matter was never inert; it always had dynamic and teleological properties. As Western concepts of physics have caused some to think of Qi as energy, nineteenth-century Western concepts of vitalism caused Qi to be identified, especially in medicine, as some form of vital force that distinguishes living things. Historically, however, Qi has been as much an attribute of a rock or river as of a person or animal. To call Qi energy or life force is probably as erroneous as it is to call it matter. See Ted J. Kaptchuk, "Historical Context of the Concept of Vitalism in Complementary and Alternative Medicine," in M. S. Micozzi (ed.), *Fundamentals of Complementary and Alternative Medicine* (New York: Churchill Livingstone, 1996).

Tui Wei-ming has noted "that the unusual difficulty in making Qi intelligible in modern Western philosophy suggests that the underlying Chinese metaphysical assumption is significantly different from the Cartesian dichotomy between spirit and matter. . . . (Furthermore) the continuous presence in Chinese philosophy of the idea of Qi as a way of conceptualizing the base structure and function of the cosmos, despite the availability of symbolic resources to make an analytical distinction between spirit and matter, signifies a conscious refusal to abandon a mode of thought that synthesizes spirit and matter as an undifferentiated whole. The loss of analytical clarity is compensated by the reward of imaginative richness. The fruitful ambiguity of Qi allows philosophers to explore realms of being which are inconceivable to people constricted by Cartesian dichotomy. . . . Qi, in short, seems inadequate to provide a philosophical background for the development of empirical science as understood in a positivistic sence. What it does provide, however, is a metaphorical mode of knowing, an epistemological attempt to address the multidimensional nature of reality by comparison, allusion and suggestion." *Confucian Thought*, 1985, p. 37–38.

4. François Jullien, *The Propensity of Things*, p. 223.

5. The most important English-language discussion of resonance appears in Joseph Needham, *Science and Civilization in China*, vol. 2. Another important English-language source is Charles LeBlanc, *Huan Nan Tzu: Philosophic Synthesis in Early Han Thought* (Hong Kong: Hong Kong University Press, 1985).

6. Harold D. Roth, "Psychology and Self-Cultivation in Early Taoist Thought," in *Harvard Journal of Asiatic Studies*, 1991:51: 599–650, p. 640. For a discussion of resonance specific to Chinese medicine, see Judith Farquhar, *Knowing Practice*, 1994, pp. 36, 218–220.

7. Classic of the Spiritual Axis with Vernacular Explanation [2], sec. 10, chap. 71, p. 471. This text, hereafter referred to as the *Ling Shu*, is the second half of the *Nei Jing*. Tu Wei-ming has stressed that "the notion of humanity as forming one body

with the universe has been so widely accepted by the Chinese, in popular as well as elite culture, that it can very well be characterized as a general Chinese world view." *Confucian Thought*, 1985, p.43.

8. Shanghai Institute, *Foundations* [53], p. 38.

9. See discussion in Porkert, *Theoretical Foundations*, pp. 166–196.

10. Based on discussions appearing in Shanghai Institute, *Foundations* [53], pp. 23–24.

11. *Su Wen* [1], sec. 19, chap. 68, pp. 399–400.

12. Ibid., sec. 9, chap. 33, p. 197.

13. Ibid., sec. 12, chap. 43, p. 245.

14. *Ling Shu* [2], sec. 11, chap. 75, p. 519.

15. Ibid., sec. 10, chap. 71, p. 468.

16. The Qi of the Chest, unlike the other kinds of Qi, has only two of the three constituents of Normal Qi. It lacks Original Qi.

17. The identification of red fluid with Blood is clearly stated thus: "The Middle Burner receives Qi [here meaning pure essences of food], obtaining a sap that is transformed into a red color and is called Blood" (*Ling Shu*, sec. 6, chap. 30, p. 267). Blood is a fluid, but it also has aspects of Qi and is especially involved in activating the sense Organs. "Blood and Qi are different in name but are of the same category" (*Ling Shu*, sec. 4, chap. 18, p. 198).

18. Shanghai Institute, *Foundations* [53], p. 42. The quotation derives from Tang Zong-hai's Discussion of Blood Patterns (1885) [20], p. 17. Tang, however, uses the word *protector* (*shou*) instead of *mother*. At this point Tang is very reminiscent of Gong Ting-xian's discussion of Qi and Blood in Preserving Vitality in Life (*Shou-shi Bao-yuan*). In fact, the first half of the saying ("the Qi is the commander of the Blood") is taken from Gong's text (Taipei: Whirlwind Press, 1974), sec. 1, chap. 20, p. 24. Gong's book originally appeared in 1615 C.E.

19. At this point in the *Nei Jing*, the word *Qi* is often used to mean Jing (Essence).

20. *Su Wen*, sec. 1, chap. 1, pp. 4–5.

21. Ibid., sec. 1, chap. 1, pp. 5–6.

22. It might be that the closest analogous concept that Western thought has to the Chinese notion of "cultivation of destiny" is related to the Western notion of "free will." Both the "cultivation of desity" and "free will" convey a notion of inner directed self-transformation. But free will implies important cultural differences. As Eng-Kung Yeh has noted: "The word freedom is seldom used in the Confucian classics or current literature. In the Chinese mind, freedom, both from external pressures and internal psychological restraints, has been entirely a matter of cultivation of the individual's moral character according to his social roles." "The Chinese Mind and Human Freedom," in *International Journal of Social Psychiatry*, 1978; 18: p. 133. Godwin Chu comments in a similar vein: "The traditional Chinese self . . . appears to be relatively more oriented toward the significant others,

rather than toward the individual self." "The Changing Concept of Self in Contemporary China," in Anthony J. Marsella et al. (eds.), *Culture and Self: Asian and Western Perspectives* (New York: Tavistock, 1985), p. 258.

23. Pharmacopoeia Classic of the Divine Husbandman with Investigations (*Shen-nong Ben-cao Jiao-Zheng*). Wang Zhu-mo (ed.), Jilin: Science and Technology Press, 1988, p. 33. My translation of *ming* as "destiny" is an example of the difficulty of making transmissions of medical meaning through various languages and how translation is necessarily interpretation. The only English translation of the *Shen-nong Ben-cao* is Yang Shou-zhong's *The Divine Farmer's Materia Medica*, Boulder, CO: Blue Poppy Press, 1998. Wang translates *ming* as "life". I have chosen to use the "destiny" meaning of *ming* for two reasons. First, the *Shen-nong* has an extensive discussion of the various Spirits and virtues in places that correspond to the location of the discussion on *ming*. Second, the place in the text where *ming* is explicitly raised contrasts *ming* to *xing* and *bing*. In the text, *xing* (temperament or disposition) is also always considered "life" and it makes no sense to contrast life with life. For me, the structure of the discussion clearly implies that *ming*, *xing*, and *bing* ("disease") are three different levels of the totality of life experience. My contrasting reading of the *Shen-nong* continues in many places from Wang's valuable translation. For example, Wang translates *zhi* as wit, while I translate it as Wisdom (see later discussion in Chapter 2).

24. Tu Wei-ming, "Pain and Suffering in Confucian Self-Cultivation," in *Philosophy East and West*, 1984; 34: 379–388, p. 385.

25. The *Nei Jing* discusses the Spirit in many different places; in fact, it is a major focus of the text. Self-consistency, however, in these discussions (as with most issues) is not characteristic of the text, and multiple traditions clearly are expressed. The most systematic discussion of the Spirit is probably *Ling Shu*, Chapter 8 (which will be often cited in Chapter 3). This section has been the basis of most major discussion in later historical periods. Also it should be emphasized that the discussion of Spirit and smaller Spirits appears in the earliest Chinese written traditions, e.g., Burton Watson (trans.), *The Tso Chuan: Selections from China's Oldest Narrative History*, New York: Columbia University Press, 1989, and most of the Taoist and Confucian writings. The most *systematic* early correlation of the virtues and the Spirits as they are formally developed in the medical tradition appears in Liu Shao's Records of Personages (*Ren-wu Zhi*), written around 200 C.E. (Unfortunately, no English translation exists.) Few of the later systematic classical discussions of the virtues have been translated into English. The most important exception is Tjian Tjue Som's translation of the Tang classic, *The Comprehensive Discussion of the White Tiger Hall (Po Hu Pung)* (Leiden, E. J. Brill, 1952). The classic English-language presentation on the different Spirits as they affect the Chinese scientific and medical tradition is Joseph Needham, *Science and Civilisation in China*, vol. 2, pp. 71–113. Needham's presentation shows the importance of the

classical herbal literature in understanding the Chinese view of Spirit. An excellent English discussion on the link between virtue, character cultivation, and the medical tradition is Scott Davis, "The Cosmobiological Balance of the Emotional and Spiritual Worlds: Phenomenological Structuralism in Traditional Chinese Medical Thought," *Culture, Medicine and Psychiatry* 1996; 20: 83–123. Also see A. C. Graham, *Yin-Yang and the Nature of Correlative Thinking* (Singapore: Institute of East Asian Philosophies, National University of Singapore, 1989); Zhaojiang Guo, "Chinese Confucian Culture and the Medical Ethical Tradition," in *Journal of Medical Ethics*, 1995; 21: 239–246. The Chinese concepts of the soul and Spirit are complex and reflect multiple religious, scholarly, and popular traditions that can be contradictory. For an insightful English discussion on this issue, see Ying-Shih Yü, "'O Soul, Come Back!' A Study in the Changing Conceptions of the Soul, Afterlife in Pre-Buddhist China," in *Harvard Journal of Asiatic Studies*, 1987; 47: 363–395; and Stevan Harrell, "The Concept of Soul in Chinese Folk Religion," in *Journal of Asian Studies*, 1979; 38: 519–528. Walter Liebenthal, "The Immortality of the Soul in Chinese Thought," *Monumenta Nipponica*, 1952; 8: 327–397; Edwin D. Harvey, *The Mind of China*, New Haven: Yale University Press, 1933; Kristofer Schipper, *The Taoist Body*, Karen C. Duval (trans.) Berkeley: Unversity of California Press, 1993. It has been suggested that the plurality of souls in Chinese thought itself may be due to the overlap of diverse religious perspectives. See Myron L. Cohen, "Souls and Salvation: Conflicting Themes in Chinese Popular Religion," in James L. Watson and Evelyn S. Rawski (eds.), *Death Ritual in Late Imperial and Modern China*, 1988.

26. See James L. Watson and Evelyn S. Rawski (eds.), *Death Ritual in Late Imperial and Modern China*, 1988; Michael Loewe, *Chinese Ideas of Life and Death: Faith, Myth and Reason in the Han Period* (202 B.C.–A.D. 220) (London: George Allen & Unwin, 1982); P. Steven Sangren, *History and Magical Power in a Chinese Community*, Stanford: Stanford University Press, 1987.

27. For an especially insightful English discussion on the question of suffering and the Non-Corporeal Soul, see Wei-ming Tu, "Pain and Suffering in Confucian Self-Cultivation," in *Philosophy East and West* 1984; 34: 379–387.

28. Li Shi-zhen, The Great Pharmacopoeia, vol. 1 (*Ben-cao Gang-mu*), Beijing: People's Press, 1985 [original edition, 1578 C.E.], p. 1020. This discussion concerns *Rehmannia glutinosa*. For a modern Western discussion of the "will" that bears a resemblance to this Chinese notion, see Leslie H. Farber, *The Ways of the Will: Essays Toward a Psychology and Psychopathology of Will*, New York: Basic Books, 1966. Similar notions of will and destiny can easily be found in Western theological or philosophic writings. For example, Martin Buber writes that "to the extent to which the soul achieves unification it becomes aware of direction, becomes aware of itself as sent in quest of it. . . . [This direction] is revealed to the human person's retrospection, his cognizance of himself in the course of the life he has

lived. . . . [This direction] is the presentiment implanted in each of us, but of what is meant and purposed for him and for him alone." (*Good and Evil*, New York: Charles Scribner's Sons, 1952, pp. 127, 132.)

29. Ian Hacking, *Rewriting the Soul: Multiple Personality and Sciences of Memory*, Princeton: Princeton University Press, 1995, p. 6.

30. Note that this discussion of Spirit is derived from the medical tradition, which is not necessarily congruent with some of the Taoist and other esoteric traditions in China.

   Needham writes concerning this entire question: "In accord with the character of all Chinese thought, the human organism was an organism, neither purely spiritual in nature nor purely material. It was not a *machina* with a single *deus* in it, which could go off and survive somewhere else; and for any recognizable continuance of identity its parts were not separable. . . . Taoist immortality inescapably involved elements of materiality, and it had to be a continuance within this world . . . since no other, purely 'spiritual,' was conceivable. . . . The line drawn between spirit and matter in all characteristic Chinese thinking was extremely vague." Joseph Needham, *Science and Civilization in China*, vol. 5, part 2 (Cambridge: At the University Press, 1974), p. 92. For an example of the imprecision in finding a boundary between religion and medicine, see Livia Kohn, "Medicine and Immortality in T'ang China," *Journal of the American Oriental Society* 1988; 108: 465–469.

31. The best English study of Fluids as it develops historically, theoretically, and clinically can be found in Steven Clavey's *Fluid Physiology and Pathology in Traditional Chinese Medicine* (Melbourne, Australia: Churchill Livingstone, 1995). This volume is a good example of how a simple concept in this book is actually a complex and multifaceted inquiry.

3

THE ORGANS OF THE BODY: THE HARMONIOUS LANDSCAPE

and on anatomy and its absence

Another major feature of the human landscape is the Organs. Chinese medical theory recognizes a number of important Organs, which work in unison with each other and with the fundamental textures. This network of Organs and textures sustains the human activities of storing and spreading, preserving and transforming, absorbing and eliminating, ascending and descending, activating and quieting. When all these activities take place harmoniously, the person is healthy and in balance.

This concept of health is very simple. The Chinese cannot measure health as is customarily done in the West. Health is not a composite of quantifiable entities, such as chemical levels in the blood and urine. In the West, health is analyzable independent of illness; it is an elaborate edifice upon which a practice of medicine is built. Health for the Chinese, however, is a simple sense of equilibrium. The image is balanced. The important Taoist notion—that the Tao (or Dao, the balanced and harmonious Way) that can be talked about and described is not the Tao—pervades medicine. Harmony is a simple assertion. It is enough to say, for instance, "The Lungs in harmony administer respiration." No elaboration is needed.

The detail and precision of Chinese medicine lie instead in its perception of *disharmony,* in its ability to recognize in signs and symptoms a pattern that becomes the basis for treatment. This theory of health is an attempt to make sense out of the practice of treating illness. For instance, in the process of finding a treatment for the symptom of edema (excessive accumulation of fluid in tissues), the Chinese formulated their theory of harmonious movement of Fluids in the body. They did not study healthy people first; they probably moved from perceiving and treating a *dis*harmony to the understanding of harmony.

The tendency of Chinese thought is to seek out dynamic functional activity rather than to look for the fixed somatic structures that perform the activities. Because of this, the Chinese have no system of anatomy comparable to that of the West. Thus, for example, the Organ known as the Liver is for the Chinese very different from the Western liver. The Chinese Liver is defined first by the activities associated with it, the Western liver by its physical structure. This divergence of conceptual approach makes it possible for Chinese medicine to identify Organs not recognized in the West—such as the Triple Burner—and for it not to recognize organs and glands clearly identified by Western medicine—such as the pancreas and the adrenal glands.

It is impossible to read into the Chinese system the classifications of the West. One Western authority on Chinese medicine states, erroneously: "The endocrine glands were not known to the ancient Chinese and were therefore not considered. . . . I think the thyroid should be classified as belonging to the heart in the system of classification under twelve organs (likewise . . . the adrenal belongs to the kidney)."[1] This sort of attempt to impose simple parallelism on the two systems is inappropriate and leads to misunderstanding.

The Chinese system must first be approached and dealt with on its own terms.

Chinese medicine is a coherent system of thought that does not require validation by the West as an intellectual construct. Intellectually, the way to approach Chinese concepts is to see whether they are internally logical and consistent, not to disguise them as Western concepts or dismiss them because they do not conform to Western notions. And the system *is* internally consistent—it is an organization of all the observable manifestations of human life into an integrated set of functions and relationships. Understanding of these functions and relationships enables the practitioner to identify and treat a disharmony in them.

As a clinical construct, the Chinese concepts can be evaluated more easily. Western techniques can be used to study whether the practice derived from the theory really works. This has been done, and the results have begun to show that Chinese medicine can be effective in Western terms, as noted in Chapter 1. (See Appendix E for a more meticulous discussion on scientific research.) But the treatment is usually often achieved through the use of a non-Western theoretical framework. Chinese medicine can, for instance, treat the disharmonies that Western medicine would associate with a thyroid condition. The Western doctor would treat the thyroid itself, in most cases either biochemically or surgically. The Chinese physician, however, might effect a cure through treatment of the Heart or, depending on the total configuration of signs, through treatment of the Liver, Spleen, Kidneys, or some combination of these Organs.[2] The two paradigms embrace a person differently; there is not a simple correspondence.

China's lack of a refined anatomical theory like the West's does not mean its system is quaint or primitive, it means only that there exist alternate systems of thought, one Eastern, one Western. In the West, even the early Greeks developed sophisticated anatomies based on the dissection of humans and apes.[3] These anatomies were often incorrect, but they grew out of the same emphasis on finding fixed entities that motivates modern medicine. The description of Organs that follows, however, is "not a Chinese version of anatomy, but its very antithesis."[4]

In the Chinese system, the Organs are discussed always with reference to their functions and to their relationships with the fundamental textures, other Organs, and other parts of the body. Indeed, it is only through these relationships that an organ can be defined. The Organs are bundles or intersecting matrixes of resonating human activity. The relationships discussed herein are those that the Chinese medical tradition considers most important in the clinical perception of patterns.

Chinese medicine recognizes five Yin Organs (*wu-zang*) and six Yang Organs (*liu-fu*). The Yin Organs are the Heart, Lungs, Spleen, Liver, and Kidneys. The Pericardium is sometimes considered a sixth Yin Organ.[5] The function of the Yin Organs is to produce, transform, regulate, and store the fundamental textures—Qi, Blood, Essence, Spirit, and Fluids.

The six Yang Organs are the Gall Bladder, Stomach, Small Intestine, Large Intestine, Bladder, and Triple Burner. The Yang Organs receive, break down, and absorb that part of the food that will be transformed into fundamental textures, and transport and excrete the unused portion.

The Yin Organs are thought of as being deeper inside the body, and are therefore Yin in relation to the Yang Organs, which are more external. The Yin Organs are generally more important in medical theory and practice.

There are also six miscellaneous or Curious Organs (*qi-heng-zhi-fu*) mentioned in the classical literature. They are the Brain, Marrow, Bone, Blood Vessels, Uterus, and Gall Bladder.[6] The Gall Bladder is considered both a Yang Organ and a Curious Organ—Yang because it is involved in the breakdown of impure food; curious because it alone among the Yang Organs contains a pure substance: bile. (The Curious Organs are discussed further in Appendix F.)

⊣ YIN ORGANS [*wu-zang* 五 脏]

Spleen [*pi* 脾]

The Spleen is most closely associated with Qi. It also has an intimate relationship to Blood. Enabling phenomena to be transmuted from one state of being to another is its central dynamic.

"The Spleen rules transformation and transportation."[7] The Spleen is the crucial link in the process by which food is transformed into Qi and Blood. For the Chinese, it is the primary organ of digestion. The Spleen extracts the pure nutritive essences of ingested food and fluids and transforms them into what will become Qi and Blood. Because the Spleen is the source of sufficient Blood and Qi in the body, it is traditionally referred to as the "foundation of postnatal existence" (*hou-tian-zhi-ben*).[8] The Spleen or Spleen Qi is also responsible for sending Grain Qi, derived from food and "pure essences" that will become Blood, upward to the Lungs, where finally the synthesis of Blood and Qi takes place. The Spleen directs "ascending" movement. It is also involved in the movement and transformation of Water in the body. A modern text summarizes these aspects of the Spleen by saying that it "rules the raising of the pure."[9]

If the transmutative and transporting functions of the Spleen are harmonious, the Qi and Blood can be abundant and the digestive powers strong. If the Spleen is in disharmony, then the whole body, or some part of it, may develop Deficient Qi or Deficient Blood. If digestion is affected, such symptoms as abdominal distention or pain, diarrhea, or appetite disorders may appear.

"The Spleen stores the Consciousness of Potentials (Yi)."[10] Through this activity, the Spleen has an additional link to Qi. In its consciousness of potentials dimension, the Spleen is responsible for considerations of options, pondering, possibilities, and making final decisions. It is the source of motivation and creativity. If the Spleen is healthy, a person has clear thoughts, can make decisions, and has the insight to faithfully support the needs of other people and situations. A harmonious Spleen enthusiastically engages the world. If the Spleen is unbalanced, a person can worry easily, have difficulty making decisions, be mentally unclear and confused, be excessively helpful, or just feel bored and uninterested.

"The Spleen governs the Blood."[11] Not only does the Spleen help to create the Blood, it also governs the Blood in the sense that it keeps the Blood flowing in its proper paths. In general, the Qi commands the blood, and the particular aspect of Qi that holds the Blood in place is the Spleen Qi. If the Spleen Qi is weak, the Spleen's governing function loses its harmony, and the Blood can escape its pathways and "move recklessly." This leads to symptoms such as vomiting blood, blood in the stool, blood under the skin, menorrhagia, or uterine bleeding. Many chronic bleeding diseases are treated through the Spleen.

CLINICAL SKETCH* *A man comes to an Oriental physician and complains of chronic problems with digestion including loose stools, abdominal discomfort, and inability to control his appetite. He's slightly overweight and is unable to care for himself outside of the realm of food. He obsesses about eating and ruminates about menus. He obviously enjoys the physician's sympathy. A series of treatments to regulate the Spleen, using herbs such as atractylodes and tangerine peel and acupuncture points such as Spleen 2* (Da-du, *Great Metropolis), and Bladder 49 (*Yishe, The Consciousness of Potentials' Abode) *seem to help considerably. An inquiry concerning other ways to nourish himself and a few lifestyle suggestions tied to the timing of taking the herbs seem to contribute to the success of the exchange.*

"The Spleen rules the muscles, flesh,"[12] and the four limbs.[13] Not only is the Spleen the origin of Qi and Blood, but the Spleen also transports these substances to the muscles and flesh. The dynamic movement of the muscles, flesh, and, consequently, the four limbs, depends on the power of the Spleen Qi. Muscle tone or the appearance of the limbs often indicates the relative strength or weakness of the Spleen.

---

*This illustration and the ones that follow throughout the book are intended only as sketches to clarify the working of East Asian medicine. They are not necessarily meant to prove or to explain theoretical details.

"The Spleen opens into the mouth."[14] "The Spleen's brilliance is manifested in the lips."[15] The mouth and lips are closely related to the Spleen. The Spleen's Qi empowers the mouth to detect and distinguish the five tastes,[16] and brings Blood to the lips so they will be red and moist. If the Spleen is weak, the mouth will be insensitive to taste and the lips will be pale.

Liver [*gan* 肝]

The Liver is most closely connected with the Blood and at the same time tempers and "softens" the Qi. The Liver is exquisitely sensitive to boundaries and demarcations and maintains the smoothness and harmony of movement throughout the body. The *Nei Jing* metaphorically calls the Liver "the general of an army"[17] because it ultimately embodies a refined assertiveness that is timely, skillful, and strategic and forcefulness yet remains mobile and flexible.

"The Liver stores the Blood."[18] The Liver's Blood is responsible for softening the Qi and ensuring that the Qi's dynamic strength is not too tense, restless, and awkward. The Liver's Blood is the essential balance for the Qi, especially the Spleen's Qi and the Liver's own Qi. The Liver's Blood is responsible for the repetitive cycles of human life. A woman's menstrual cycle depends on the Liver's Blood, and disharmonious Liver Blood can make an irregular or painful menstruation.

The Liver's Blood's ability to temper the Qi has been characterized as "The Liver rules flowing and spreading (shu-xie)."[19] A modern Chinese text uses the word *sprinkle* to describe its gentle touch.[20] The *Nei Jing* says "The Liver is the foundation of curtailing extremes."[21] One classic herbal formula to restore the Liver's Blood effect on Qi is named "The Free and Easy Wanderer Pill" (also translated as "Rambling Powder").[22] The Liver fosters a relaxed, easygoing internal environment—an even disposition. Creating this ambience can be thought of as the function of the Liver, as well as a basic need of the Liver itself.

The Liver's Blood, by first tempering the Liver's Qi and then the entire body's Qi, ensures the smooth movement of Qi. And all activity that depends on Qi depends also on the Liver. Any impairment of Liver function can influence the circulation of Qi and Blood, leading to either Stagnant Qi or Congealed Blood. The Liver Qi often becomes stuck and blocked in its own pathways and will then manifest symptoms such as pain or distention in the flanks, swollen or painful breasts and genitals, gas distention, or lower abdominal pain. If the stagnation affects the psyche, a sense of frustration, being hampered, or edginess can easily develop.

The Liver's soothing aspect can be especially valuable for digestion. The Liver's Blood tempers the Liver's Qi and fosters cycles of movement. The Spleen Qi is more linear and transformative in a single creative direction. The Spleen Qi needs the gentle touch of the Liver. If the Liver loses its pliable nature, it can "invade" and cause disruption of the Spleen. This may be accompanied by such digestive problems as abdominal pain, nausea, belching, intestinal rumbling, or diarrhea.*

"The Liver stores the Non-Corporeal Soul (Hun)."[23] Because the Non-Corporeal Soul is responsible for human kindness or benevolence, it is sensitive to the boundaries that make for the recognition of self and others. A modern text speaks of the Liver as "a Yin Organ that has an 'edge': it is Yin but uses the Yang."[24] The acknowledgment of the humanity, whether in others or in oneself, depends on the receptivity of the Hun. When the Hun "takes too much ground," a person can easily be angry, belligerent, or stubborn or "fly off the handle." When the Hun is insufficiently assertive, it can lead to a lack of self-worth or self-esteem. The *Nei Jing* implies this dual aspect of the Hun when it says Liver Blood excess leads to anger and its deficiency leads to a sense of absence.[25]

The Non-Corporeal Soul (Hun) and Blood also concerns the capacity to be sensitive to pain. While Stuck Qi often causes pain, Blood has more to do with how a person reacts to pain. The ability to stay "soft" while experiencing pain, to not tense up, to give pain "more room," depends on the Liver's Blood and Hun. Blood allows

---

*An additional digestive aspect of the Liver is that it controls bile secretion. See the section on the Gall Bladder in this chapter.

pain to be more bearable and less debilitating. Without this capacity, a person can be numb or insensitive to either his or her own physical or spiritual suffering or that of others.

CLINICAL SKETCH *A woman visits a Chinese physician with the complaint of painful and irregular menses. During the intake, it is both obvious that the woman is extremely kind and that a lack of self-esteem has been a major problem in her work and relationships. Herbs such as angelica sinensis, rehmannia, ligusticum, and peony, which nourish the Liver's Blood, regulate the menses and strengthen the Hun, and acupuncture points such as Liver 3 (Tai Chong, Great Pouring), Spleen 10 (Xue-hai, Sea of Blood), Bladder 47 (Hun-men, Non-Corporeal Soul Gate), after a number of treatments, alleviate the condition. Discussion with the woman concerning how her compassion does not extend to herself also seemed helpful.*

"The Liver rules the tendons and is manifest in the nails."[26] The proper movement of all the tendons in the body is closely related to the Liver. To Chinese medicine, "tendons" is a broader category than it is in Western anatomy, for it includes ligaments and, to some extent, muscles.[27] If the Liver's Blood is insufficient and incapable of nourishing the tendons, symptoms such as spasms, tightness, numbness of the limbs, and difficulty in bending or stretching may result. Liver disharmonies may also cause the nails to be thin, brittle, and pale. When the Liver's Blood is plentiful, however, the tendons are supple and the nails appear pink and moist.

"The Liver opens into the eyes."[28] All of the Yin and Yang Organs contribute the purest part of their energy to the eyes; the Liver, however, has a special relationship to the function of the eyes. The *Nei Jing* says, "When the Liver is harmonized, the eyes can distinguish the five colors,"[29] and "When the Liver receives Blood, the eyes can see."[30] Therefore, many disorders of the eyes and of vision are taken to be Liver-related.

Kidneys [shen 肾]

"The Kidneys store the Essence (Jing)"[31] and rule birth, development, and maturation. Essence is the texture most closely associated with life itself; it is the source of life and its unfolding. It is the texture that gives organic life its specific character. It is the stuff of growth and development. Essence is the potential for differentiation into life's Yin and Yang. Essence, in one form or another, is the primordial seed of the life process, the life process itself, and life's final fruit.

The entire body and all the Organs of the body need Essence in order to thrive. The Kidneys, because they store Essence, bestow this potential for life activity. They have, therefore, a special relationship with the other Organs in that they hold the underlying texture of each Organ's existence and are the foundation of each Organ's Yin and Yang. In other words, the Yin and Yang, or life activity, of each Organ ultimately depends on the Yin and Yang of the Kidneys. Thus, the Kidneys are the "root of life." As the medical tradition states, "The Kidneys are the mansion of Fire and Water, the residence of Yin and Yang . . . the channel of death and life."[32]

All the Organs can be characterized as either Yin or Yang. But within each Organ there is both a supportive, nourishing Yin aspect and a dynamic active Yang aspect. For example, the Liver's storing of Blood is Yin, while its spreading of Qi is Yang. As the primordial organic texture, Essence can be thought of as coming "before" Yin and Yang; but because of its "soft," unhurried, and unfolding nature, it is Yin as well. It is characteristic of the dialectical movement of classical Chinese thought that Jing *can* be both before Yin and Yang and be Yin as well, and that within that Yin there is another Yin and Yang differentiation.

The Kidneys, like all organs, have both Yin and Yang aspects. Their storing activity is Yin, but some of their other activities are Yang. The Yin of the Kidneys, depending on context, is called either Jing or Water (if Jing is before Yin and Yang). The Yang of the Kidneys has a special name. It is called *Ming-men huo*, or Life Gate Fire.[33]

The Kidneys are also called the "root of life" because Essence is the source of reproduction, development, and maturation. Conception is made possible by the power of Essence; growth to maturity is the blossoming of Essence; and the decline into old age reflects the physical decline of Essence. As time passes, the Essence decreases in its physical vitality. Because the Kidneys store Essence, all these processes are governed by the Kidneys. Therefore, reproductive problems such as sterility or impotence and developmental disorders like retarded growth or lack of sexual maturation are seen as dysfunctions of the Kidneys' storing of Essence. Aging is considered a normal process—when it proceeds gracefully it is not seen as an illness or a problem. If aging is premature, or if it lacks the dignity of a sense of completion, it may be the result of Kidney Essence irregularities.

"The Kidneys rule Water."[34] All Organs participate in the metabolism of Water, but the Kidneys are the foundation upon which this entire process of Water movement and transformation is built.

The words *Water* and *Fluids* are often used interchangeably, but sometimes one or the other is preferred. *Water* has a more general connotation than *Fluids*. While *Fluids* refers to Water in its particular aspects (perspiration, urine, etc.), Water refers to all the moisture in the body. Water is also thought of as the opposing principle to Fire, the Yin to Fire's Yang. Since Water and Fire are two of the basic forces at work both in the body and in the universe, Water is the broader, more metaphorical term.

The Kidneys rule Water through their Yang aspect, the Life Gate Fire. This Fire, or Heat, transforms Water into a "mist," a necessary first step before Fluids can ascend or circulate. All the circulation of Water in the body depends on the vaporizing power of the Kidneys. The Spleen also vaporizes pure Fluids as it raises the pure essences of food and Fluids, but its vaporization power—its Fire—is ultimately dependent on the Kidney Fire, which acts as a kind of "pilot light."

CLINICAL SKETCH *A patient is diagnosed by a Western physician as suffering from right-sided heart failure. The patient's chief complaint is serious edema of the*

*entire body (anasarca). An Oriental physician gives the man a complete exami-
nation and decides that he has the pattern of Deficient Kidney Fire, unable to rule
Water. The physician prescribes very warming herbs, including aconite, and the
use of moxibustion (burning substances such as mugwort to stimulate acupuncture
points) at such points as Kidney 7* (Fu-liu, Returning Current) *and Conception
Vessel 4* (Guan-yuan, Hinge Source). *After a course of treatment, the patient's
symptoms are visibly alleviated. Examination by a Western physician confirms
great improvement in the heart. A partial explanation of these results in Western
terms could be that modern pharmacological studies have demonstrated that
aconite is a potent cardiotonic. Chinese medicine, however, describes it as a warmer
of the Kidney.*[35]

"The Kidneys store the Will."[36] The Kidneys are associated with
both aspects of the Will. The Yang Will, the forceful assertions that
shape the course of decades, belongs here. The big shifts, decisive
efforts, and fundamental commitments that allow a person to take
responsibility for his or her life are the creation of the Yang Will's
volition. The Yang Will is the most dynamic assertive aspect of a person, the ultimate Fire.

The Yin Will is the other side of Will. It is the deeper encounter
with the inexorable and ultimate destiny that already exists hidden
in the undifferentiated seed. It is the recognition that the deepest
force requires no effort. The Yin Will is elusive, almost intangible.
It is noticed in stillness. It has a quality of irreducible mystery. The
Yin Will is about the inevitable, about a direction we each move
toward that can be seen only when we turn around and look at how
we have developed through time. It is about fate and destiny. It is
about the unknown and death.

Recognition of the Yin Will allows for the creation of the virtue
of Wisdom. This Wisdom is not about knowing things. In fact, it
is more about being deeply connected to the unknown. Wisdom is
a recognition of that fact that life is an intertwining of known and
unknown. We know that death is involved; but we also know that
the unknown is involved. Wisdom is a recognition of a deep knowing that infuses life. The Yang Will ultimately must accept the Yin

Will in order that the Essence bear the fruit of Wisdom. Resolution must acknowledge the inevitable; certitude must bow before the unknown. Age often weakens the physical aspect of Essence, but maturity is the necessary ingredient for the spiritual dimension of Essence to unfold. Essence reflects itself in Wisdom gained through a reflective life.

Obviously, an Oriental physician cannot and should not give a person Wisdom. Every person needs to find his or her own (perhaps with the help of religious figures, family, friends, teachers, poets, or philosophers). The Oriental physician can, however, strengthen the Kidney's Will. When the Will is not intact, a person can have uncontrollable fear or a dread of death, existential anxiety, or inability to feel the gracefulness of becoming older. Fear and Wisdom share a similar energetic—both are an encounter of the unknown. Fear, however, cannot embrace the unknown with trust; fear cannot recognize the inevitability of the unknown. Wisdom, on the other hand, acknowledges the profound truth and tranquility of the unknown. When an East Asian physician successfully helps nourish the Essence, a patient will receive support to reclaim some of his or her own Wisdom. When Essence flourishes, Wisdom can abide.

"The Kidneys rule the bones."[37] "The Kidneys produce the marrow."[38] These two functions are an aspect of control by the Kidney Essence of birth, development, and maturation. The Kidneys store the Essence, and it is said that the Essence produces marrow. The marrow, in turn, is responsible for creating and supporting bones. Therefore, the bones' development and repair depend on the nourishment of the Kidney Essence. In a child, insufficient Kidney Essence may result in soft bones or incomplete closure of the bones of the skull. In an adult, insufficient Kidney Essence can produce weak legs and knees, brittle bones, or stiffness of the spine.

The teeth are considered the surplus of the bones, and so they too are ruled by the Kidneys. When a child's teeth develop poorly or fall out, or an adult's teeth are a constant problem, a Chinese physician will suspect an insufficient Kidney Essence.

"The Kidneys open into the ear."[39] The Kidneys manifest in the head hair.[40] There is a close relationship between the Kidneys and the ears. As the *Nei Jing* says, "The Kidney Qi goes through the ear; if the Kidney is harmonized, the ear can hear the five tones."[41] Many hearing problems are treated through the Kidneys. The poor hearing common in the elderly, for example, is a consequence of weakened Kidney Essence.

The relative moistness and vitality of head hair are also related to the Kidney Essence. The head hair also depends on the Blood for nourishment, which is why the tradition calls head hair "the surplus of the Blood."[42]

"The Kidneys rule the grasping of Qi."[43] While the Lungs administer respiration, normal breathing also requires assistance from the Kidneys. The Kidneys enable the Natural Air Qi to penetrate deeply, completing the inhalation process by what is called "grasping the Qi." Kidneys are thus the "root of Qi," while the Lungs are the "foundation of Qi." Proper breathing thus depends on the Kidneys; and Kidney disharmonies may result in respiratory problems, especially chronic asthma or being deeply locked in grief and fear.

Heart [xin 心]

"The Heart stores the Spirit (Shen)."[44] The Heart guarantees connection and stores the small Spirit component of the person's entire Spirit. The Heart Spirit ensures that whatever consciousness, intention, volition, thought, reflection, and self-awareness exist within the large composite Spirit intersects and "clicks" with the world of time and space. The Heart is responsible for appropriate behavior, timely interactions, and being suitable to the context. Being respectful, helpful, thoughtful, or emotional is only virtuous when the Heart Spirit ensures that the moment is right. The Heart's little Spirit makes sure that the big composite Spirit of a person is on target.

The Heart Spirit guides the larger Spirit into the world of manifestation. Intending to take an elderly person shopping is helpful before going shopping, not afterward. The Heart Spirit ensures the timing. Wearing a bathing suit with a towel around one's neck at poolside is fine, but not before a gathering of businesspeople with whom you are negotiating a financial transaction. Figuring out the details of a money deal before going to sleep is probably also poor timing. The Heart Spirit ensures picking suitable places for particular actions.

When the Heart Spirit is disturbed, one has symptoms such as insomnia, situational anxiety, and inappropriate or even bizarre behavior. Discomfort with situations and people often has to do with the Heart, as do the somatic correlates of anxiety, such as sweating, blushing, being flustered, and palpitations. When the Heart Spirit is intact, one connects with propriety and tact.

"The Heart opens into the tongue."[45] "The Heart's brilliance manifests in the face."[46] The tradition also says that "the tongue is the sprout of the Heart."[47] The ability to choose words precisely, to convey meaning well, and to connect in dialogue belongs to the Heart Spirit's relation with the tongue. Expressing warmth and appropriate engagement through facial expression is another Heart function. On a more physical level, the connection between the Heart and tongue means that pathological changes of the tongue such as ulceration and inflammation can often be treated by acupuncture or herbal therapy directed at the Heart. Stuttering is also linked to the Heart.

"The Heart rules the Blood and Blood Vessels."[48] The Heart regulates the flow of Blood. When the Heart Qi (partly related to the heartbeat) and Heart Blood (which are mutually dependent on each other) are abundant and normal, then the pulse will be even and regular.

The Heart Blood is critical for treating insomnia because it is said to "embrace" the Heart Spirit and allow it to peacefully disconnect with the world. Also, short-term memory—"where are the car keys"—depends on the Heart Blood's ability to effortlessly remember and connect gently to time and place. (One cannot remember something with Qi; one has to "let go" with the Blood before the memory flows back.)

The Heart Organ moves in a time frame that is of very short duration; it is situational and contextual. This contrasts with the Kidneys whose trajetory marks the developmental stages in life and the Spleen and Liver whose time frame is shorter than the Kidneys' but longer than the Heart's.

Pericardium [xin-bao 心包]

The Pericardium is the outer protective shield of the Heart. For clinical purposes it is considered a sixth Yin Organ. But in general theory, the Pericardium is not distinguished from the Heart, except by being the first line of defense against External Pernicious Influences attacking the Heart. In acupuncture it has a separate Meridian. The role of the Pericardium is developed in Appendix A.

CLINICAL SKETCH *A man is suffering from insomnia. He goes to a Western doctor, who finds nothing wrong but offers a referal to a behavioral sleep clinic. Later, the patient decides to try an Oriental physician. An examination confirms the doctor's suspicion that the Heart is not storing the Spirit properly, and a series of treatments is prescribed. The doctor will use acupuncture points such as Heart 7* (Shen-men, *Spirit Door) and herbs such as the fruit of* Euphoria longana, *which alleviate the condition, as they strengthen that aspect of the Heart that stores the Spirit. These treatments have no sedating side effects, and, from a Western viewpoint, they appear to strengthen the nervous system.*[49]

Lungs [fei 肺]

The Lungs concern the momentary and ephemeral. Healthy Lungs allow for a single moment or any singular episode of time to become complete. Traditionally, the Lungs are called the "tender organ"[50] because they are easily affected by fleeting events, whether it is respiration, an acute cold or flu,[51] short-lived emotions, or acknowledging and accepting both the completeness and impermanence of a precious enounter or cherished life.

"The Lungs store the Animal Soul (Po)."[52] The Animal Soul is the animation, emotional reactivity, and pressing urges of human life. It can be erratic and untamed. It lacks the deliberation of reason. Without a healthy Animal Soul (Po) a person can be either emotionless or hysterical. An intact Po is flexible and reactive but quickly regains composure and sees the entire situation. Of all the emotions (see Chapter 5), the Po is especially sensitive to mourning and grief and disturbances in gaining a sense of completion. The Lungs experience loss and longing easily. Disturbed Lungs can produce unresolved grief and a failure to see the delicate integrity of the temporal world. In another sense, when the Po is intact, it produces the virtue of impartial justice and the sense of perfect, nonreplicable beauty. The Po also has the ability to receive flashes of inspiration, which can be the source of understanding and intuition when taken into other Organs.

"The Lungs rule Qi."[53] The aspect of Qi meant here is respiration and other short-term aspects of the Qi. The Lungs are the arena in which the Qi (meaning air, Natural Air Qi) outside the body meets the Qi inside the body. The Lungs take in Natural Air Qi, propelling it downward. This is inhalation. The Lungs are then said to "disseminate" and "make things go round," and expel "impure" air (exhalation). When the Lungs are healthy, the Natural Air Qi enters and leaves smoothly, and respiration is even and regular. When an imbalance or obstruction interferes with the Lungs, symptoms such as cough, dyspnea, or asthma may result. For any Lung disorder to remain chronic, it must link with another organ.

The Lungs are closely allied with the Qi of the Chest. Because the Qi of the Chest is involved with the movement of all the Qi and Blood in the body, a disharmony of the Lungs can produce Deficient Qi anywhere in the body. These Qi disruptions tend to be of a shorter duration, such as recovering after a hard day's work.

"The Lungs move and adjust the Water Channel."[54] The Lungs have a role in the movement and transformation of water in the body. The Lungs move the water in two directions. By "descending and liquefying" (*su-jiang*), the Lungs move water to the Kidneys. By "disseminating" (*xuan*), the Lungs circulate and scatter water vapor throughout the body, particularly through the skin and pores. (Chinese medicine postulates that water in liquid form descends, while in vapor form it circulates or ascends.) The movement of water by the Lungs is summarized thus: "The Lungs are the upper origin of water."[55]

Disharmonies of the Lungs' Water-descending function are likely to result in problems of urination or in edema, particularly edema in the upper part of the body. Disturbances involving the disseminating function may produce respiratory problems.

The entire system of water and Fluid movement may now be summarized as follows in what is one of the most "concrete" physiological discussions one finds in Chinese medicine. Fluids are received by the Stomach, which begins a process of separation, by which the unusable portions of food are sent to the intestines as waste and the pure Water is extracted. This process is continued by the Spleen, which then sends the pure Fluids in a vaporized state upward to the Lungs. The Lungs circulate the clear part of the Fluids throughout the body, but liquefy whatever has become impure through use and send it downward to the Kidneys. In the Kidneys, the impure part is further separated into relatively "clean" and "turbid" parts. The clear part is transformed into a mist and sent upward to the Lungs, where it rejoins the cycle. The final impure portion goes into the Bladder, where it is stored and subsequently excreted.[56]

"The Lungs rule the exterior of the body."[57] "The brilliance of the Lungs is manifested in the body hair."[58] The word *exterior*, in relation to the Lungs, is a standard usage referring to the skin, sweat glands, and body hair.[59] In other words, the Lungs regulate the secretion of sweat, the moistening of the skin, and resistance to External Pernicious Influences (See Chapter 5). These functions also depend on the Protective Qi, which in turn depends on the Lungs' disseminating ability. This particular relationship is considered another example of the Lungs ruling Qi. If the Lung Qi is weak, there may be too much or too little sweat, and the resistance of the Protective Qi will be poor.

"The brilliance of the Lungs is manifested in the body hair" means that the quality of the body hair may indicate the condition of the Lung Qi.

CLINICAL SKETCH *A person whose Lungs or Lung Qi are not functioning well may constantly get colds. Every time something is going around, he or she catches it. An Oriental physician may determine that the Protective Qi of such a person is weak. A series of herbal treatments, such as one called the Jade Screen, which includes* astragalus, *and the use of acupuncture points such as Lung 9 (* Tai-yuan, Great Abyss) *and Bladder 38 (*Gao-huang-shu, *Vital's Hollow), should improve the situation, as they strengthen both the Lung and the Protective Qi.*[60]

"The Lungs open into the nose."[61] The nose is the "thorough-fare for respiration" and is intimately connected to the function of the Lungs. The throat is said to be the "door" of the Lungs and the "home" of the vocal cords, so both the throat and the vocal cords are also related to the Lungs. Many common nose and throat disorders are therefore treated through the Lungs.

⊣ YANG ORGANS [*liu-fu* 六 腑]

The main function of the Yang Organs is to receive food, absorb the usable portions, and transmit and excrete waste. The Yang Organs are less directly involved with the fundamental textures than are the Yin Organs and are generally described less psychologically. They are also considered more exterior than the Yin Organs. The word *exterior* (*biao*) has more to do with the ultimate life significance of an organ than with its physical location. Thus, the important Yin Organs are thought to be more interior than the less important Yang Organs.

Each Yang Organ is coupled with a Yin Organ in what is called an interior-exterior relationship. (See Table 1.)

TABLE 1   *Coupled Yin and Yang Organs*

YIN ORGAN	YANG ORGAN
Spleen	Stomach
Liver	Gall Bladder
Kidneys	Bladder
Heart	Small Intestine
Lungs	Large Intestine
(Pericardium)	Triple Burner

This means that their Qi's interpenetrate and can mutually resonate and that the Meridian pathways (discussed in Chapter 4) are connected. Sometimes this connection has clinical significance and at other times it mainly completes a hypothetical symmetry (See Appendix B.)

Stomach [*wei* 胃]

The Stomach is responsible for "receiving" and "ripening" ingested food and fluids. It is therefore called "the sea of food and fluid."[62] Food begins its decomposition in the Stomach. The "pure" part is then sent to the Spleen, which transforms it into the raw material for Qi and Blood. The "turbid" part is sent to the Small Intestine for further digestion. The Stomach and Spleen activities are closely related. While the Spleen rules "ascending," the Stomach rules "descending"; that is, it makes things move downward. Thus, the directions of their Qi activity complement each other. If the Stomach's receiving and descending functions are impaired, symptoms such as nausea, stomachache, distention, belching, or vomiting may ensue.

Gall Bladder [*dan* 胆]

The Gall Bladder stores and secretes bile. Bile is a bitter yellow fluid continuously produced by the surplus Blood and Qi of the Liver. The Gall Bladder sends bile downward, where it pours into the Intestines and aids the digestive process.

The Liver that produces bile and the Gall Bladder that secretes it are very dependent on each other. Any disruption of the Liver's flowing and spreading activity will affect the Gall Bladder's bile secretion. Disharmonies of the Gall Bladder will affect the Liver, possibly resulting in such symptoms as vomiting bitter fluid.

The *Nei Jing* says that the Gall Bladder rules courage and decisiveness.[63] Behavior characterized by anger and rash decisions may be due to an excess of Gall Bladder Qi. Timidity and fear of particular places and things (such as a dark room or bugs) may be a sign of Gall Bladder disharmony and weakness.*

Bladder [*pang-guang* 膀胱]

The function of the Bladder is to receive and excrete the urine. Urine is produced in the Kidneys, out of the final portion of the turbid fluids transmitted from the Lungs, Small Intestine, and Large Intestine. Disharmonies of the Bladder may lead to urinary problems such as incontinence, burning urination, or difficulty in urinating. The coupling of the Bladder and the Kidneys reflects a clinical importance based on their complementary functions.

Small Intestine [*xiao-chang* 小肠]

The Small Intestine rules the separation of the "pure" from the "turbid." It receives what the Stomach has not completely decomposed and continues the process of separation and absorption. The "clear"

---

*Deeper existential fear belongs in the Kidneys.

part is extracted by the Small Intestine and sent to the Spleen, and the "turbid" part continues downward to the Large Intestine. Some impure ingested fluid is also sent directly to the Kidneys and Bladder. Disharmonies involving the Small Intestine may produce abdominal pain, intestinal rumblings, diarrhea, or constipation.

Large Intestine [da-chang 大肠]

The Large Intestine continues to move the turbid parts of the food and fluids downward, while at the same time absorbing water from this waste material. At the end of this process, the feces are formed and eliminated under the control of the Large Intestine. If the Large Intestine loses its harmony, abdominal pain, intestinal rumblings, diarrhea, or constipation may result.

Triple Burner [san-jiao 三焦]

The Chinese word for this Organ can be translated as Triple Burner, Triple Warmer, or Triple Heater. Literally, it means "three that burn" or "three that scorch." The Triple Burner is the sixth Yang Organ, although its exact Organ nature is not clear from the classical texts. Ambiguity and dispute surround this Organ.[64]

The majority of Chinese physicians agree that the Triple Burner "has a name but no shape."[65] It may best be understood as the functional relationship between various Organs that regulate Water. These are mainly the Lungs, Spleen, and Kidneys, but they also include the Small Intestine and the Bladder. The Triple Burner does not exist as an entity outside of these other Organs, but rather it is the pathway that makes these Organs a complete system.

In Chinese medical thought, Fire is necessary to control Water. The name Triple Burner implies Fire, and the *Nei Jing* emphasizes the Triple Burner's control of the body's Water. In the *Nei Jing*, the Triple Burner is called the "Official of the Bursting Water Dam" and is referred to as "where the Water Channel arises."[66] The *Nei Jing* implies, so tradition has it, that those aspects of the Spleen, Kidney,

Stomach, Large Intestine, Small Intestine, and Bladder that are involved in Water movement are all regulated by the Qi of the Triple Burner.

The *Nei Jing* says further that "the Upper Burner is a mist."[67] A mist is pervasive, and traditionally this would correspond to the vaporized Water in the Lungs that is later disseminated throughout the body. "The Middle Burner is a foam."[68] This is traditionally interpreted as referring to the digestive churnings of the Stomach and Spleen. "The lower Burner is a swamp."[69] It is in charge of excreting impure substances. The reference here is primarily to the Kidneys, Large and Small Intestines, and the Bladder.

There is also general agreement on another definition of the Triple Burner. This concept considers the Triple Burner a demarcation of three areas of the body. The Upper Burner is the head and chest, including the Heart and Lungs. The Middle Burner is the area below the chest but above the navel, and includes the Spleen and Stomach. The Lower Burner corresponds to the abdominal area below the navel and especially encompasses the Liver and Kidney. (The location of the Liver is related to its Meridian pathway in the lower groin.)[70]

The Organs of the body, defined as they are by their psychophysiological functions and relationships, are another part of the human web. They cannot be discussed out of context. The Chinese notions about Organs (or about anything else) are not meant to be hard pieces of a theory that can be proved or disproved. They are part of an organizing network to be used when convenient. The Chinese would be indifferent to proof in our accustomed scientific sense. In the Song dynasty (960–1279 C.E.) introduction to the Systematic Classic of Acupuncture (282 C.E.), the Imperial Medical Scholars are explicitly aware that the Meridians and much of the rest of the system are not to be found when one dissects and physically investigates. They are not troubled. They say it does not matter. The verification is the classics, the wisdom of the ancients, and the fact that it is an important conceptual tool and resources.[71]

In the West, since the scientific revolution, a theory must rest on a provable physical substratum of repeatable events and measurable facts. Each fact holds up the next level. William Harvey helped usher in this scientific revolution when on April 17, 1616, in a public lecture, he overthrew the classic Greek notion of blood movement and replaced it with the modern concept of circulation. The entire Greek medical edifice began to crumble. Early speculations and imaginative constructs were found to be insufficient. Hard and substantial facts were to be the basis of the new knowledge. Qualities had to be reduced to quantities, images to lines, speculation to experimentation. The Chinese theories, however, resemble those of Greek antiquity. This type of fact is a speculative interpretation. For the Chinese, it is a sensory image, a poetic exploration of what is going on. The value of the Chinese theories is in aiding the organization of observation, discerning patterns, capturing interconnectedness and qualities of being. Can one prove a poetic image? It can be shared. It can be used. One can decide if it's worth listening to. . . .

NOTES

1. F. Mann, *The Meridians of Acupuncture* (London: Heinemann Medical Books, 1964), p. 57.
2. See the discussion of thyroid problems and their relationship to traditional Chinese patterns of disharmony in Chengdu Institute, *Internal Medicine and Pediatrics* [40], pp. 538–544. For further examples see "Introduction to Experience of Using Chinese Herbal Medicine in Hyperthyroidism," JTCM, March 1960, pp. 22–30 and D. W. Guo, "Effect of Longdan Jiedu Decoction for the Treatment of Subacute Thyroiditis: Report of 40 cases," JTCM, 1998; 39: 158–162.
3. While it is unlikely that Hippocrates of Cos (460–377 B.C.E.) performed dissection, many schools did. Erasistratus of Julis (c. 304 B.C.E.) was noted for his anatomical studies and rigorous seeking of causal explanations of diseases. For example, he described the valves of the heart, distinguished sensory and motor nerves, and accurately described the movement of food in the body. The other noted early anatomist was Herophilus of Chalcedon, who may have performed

vivisection on criminals, but whose interest was not in finding causal explanations. Aristotle's anatomy was quite advanced, and Galen of Pergamum (c. 129–200 C.E.) made a very sophisticated anatomy and physiology the cornerstone of his medicine. For a description of Greek anatomy, see "The History of Anatomy in Antiquity" in *Ancient Medicine: Selected Papers of Ludwig Edelstein*, ed. by Temkin and Temkin (Baltimore: Johns Hopkins Press, 1967), pp. 247–303; and Charles Singer, *A Short History of Anatomy and Physiology from the Greeks to Harvey* (New York: Dover, 1957), pp. 9–62.

In China, internal anatomy is generally irrelevant to clinical practice. The *Nei Jing* mentions dissection (*Ling Shu*, sec. 3, chap. 12, p. 156) and has records of anatomical investigation (e.g., *Ling Shu*, sec. 6, chap. 31, p. 270), but these descriptions are incidental and crude. China also had Confucian religious and ethical prohibitions against dissection, which were first written in legal code form in 653 C.E. Despite the general lack of interest and the religious barriers, sporadic instances of dissection occurred in Chinese history—e.g., the famous Song-dynasty dissection of forty-six rebels in 1045 C.E. But such occasional episodes were of little consequence in medical practice. For a discussion of the lack of a Chinese anatomy, see Jia De-dao, *Concise History of China's Medicine* [95], pp. 220–222. Also see Yamada Keiji, "Anatometrics of Ancient China," *Chinese Science* 1991; 10:39–52.

4. Manfred Porkert, "Chinese Medicine: A Traditional Healing Science," in *Ways of Health*, ed. by David S. Sobel (New York: Harcourt Brace Jovanovich, 1979), p. 158. Also see Porkert, *Theoretical Foundations*, pp. 107–108. Nathan Sivin makes a similar point. "The early Chinese body was composed mainly of vaguely defined bones and flesh traversed by circulation tracts. Through these tracts vital fluids (not necessarily liquid) circulate between . . . an ensemble of systems in the center of the body that controls metabolic and other spontaneous vital processes. It would be more exact to call them ensembles of functions rather than systems. Most . . . were associated with and named after vaguely described viscera. Exactly what their physical correlates are or precisely where they are located did not mandate diligent exploration. . . . They are not so much anatomical features as offices in the central bureaucracy of the body." "State, Cosmos, and Body in the Last Three Centuries B.C.," *Harvard Journal of Asiatic Studies*, 1995; 55: 5–37, p. 12.

5. The *Nei Jing* speaks mainly of five Yin and six Yang Organs. There are several implicit references to the Pericardium as a sixth Yin Organ, but the first explicit statement is in "Difficulty 25" of the second-century *Nan Jing* or Classic of Difficulties [3], p. 66. This book is a series of eighty-one questions and answers concerning the *Nei Jing*.

6. *Su Wen* [1], sec. 3, chap. 11, p. 77.

7. This is a traditional saying that combines the meaning of several references in the *Nei Jing*, e.g., *Su Wen*, sec. 7, chap. 21, p. 139, and *Ling Shu*, sec. 4, chap. 18, p. 139.

8. *Essential Readings in Medicine* (*Yi-zong Bi-du*) by Li Zhong-zi, 1637 (Taipei: Wen-guang, 1977), p. 6. The Kidneys in the same sentence are called "the foundation of prenatal existence" (*xian-tian-zhi-ben*).

9. Beijing Institute, *Foundations* [38], p. 12.

10. *Su Wen*, sec. 7, chap. 23, p. 153.

11. This aspect of the Spleen is not directly mentioned in the *Nei Jing* but is spoken of in "Difficulty 42" of the *Nan Jing* [3]: "The Spleen binds [or wraps] the Blood" (p. 99). The word *govern* in relation to Spleen and Blood seems to have been used first by Tang Zong-hai in his medical classic *Discussion of Blood Patterns* (first published 1885) to distinguish the functions mentioned in the *Nei Jing* of the various Organs in relation to the Blood. See p. 10 of the 1977 edition [20].

12. *Su Wen*, sec. 12, chap. 44, p. 246.

13. Paraphrase of *Su Wen*, sec. 8, chap. 29, p. 180.

14. *Ling Shu*, sec. 4, chap. 17, p. 189.

15. *Su Wen*, sec. 3, chap. 10, p. 70.

16. *Ling Shu*, sec. 4, chap. 17, p. 189. The five tastes are bitter, sour, sweet, salty, and acrid.

17. *Su Wen*, sec. 3, chap. 8, p. 58. Undoubtedly, the general of the *Nei Jing* bears a resemblance to the military leader mentioned in Chapter 68 of the *Tao-te Ching*.

    A skillful leader of troops is not oppressive with his military strength. A skillful fighter does not become angry. A skillful conqueror does not compete with people. One who is skillful in using men puts himself below them.

    (Wing-tsit Chan, *A Source Book in Chinese Philosophy*, 1963, pp. 171–172.)

    François Jullien cites a classical source to point out that the traditional general "expects victory from the potential born of disposition, not from the men placed under his command." *The Propensity of Things*, 1995, p. 30. The general's strategic tool "must be as mobile as flowing water. . . What is involved is the deeper intuition that a particular disposition loses its potentiality when it becomes *inflexible* (or static). . . . It is here that strategic theory coincides with the most central idea of Chinese culture: the perpetually renewed efficacy of the course of nature, illustrated by the succession of days and nights and the cycle of the seasons. Ultimately, because the absolute causality constituted by the *Dao* never becomes immobilized in any one disposition, it remains forever inexhaustible." Ibid., pp. 33–34 [italics in the original].

18. *Ling Shu*, sec. 2, chap. 8, p. 86.

19. Various aspects of the Liver's activity are mentioned in the *Nei Jing* and other early texts. Tang Zong-hai seems to have been the first to use the expression "flowing and spreading" to summarize these functions. See his *Discussion of Blood Patterns* [20], p. 8. This expression is now standard in all modern texts.

20. Beijing Institute, *Foundations* [38], p. 13.

21. *Su Wen*, sec. 3, chap. 9, p. 68.

22. This prescription (*Xiao yan san*) was formulated by Chen Shi-Wen in his Song dynasty *Professional and Popular Prescriptions from the Taiping Era* (*Taiping Hui-min He-ji Ju-fang*) in 1151 B.C.E.

23. *Ling Shu*, sec. 2, chap. 8, p. 86.

24. Dan Bensky and Randall Barolet. *Chinese Herbal Medicine: Formulas & Strategies* (Seattle: Eastland Press, 1990), p. 271.

25. *Ling Shu*, sec. 2, chap. 8, p. 86.

26. *Su Wen*, sec. 3, chap. 10, p. 70.

27. The Chinese word *jin* is here translated as tendon. The word in its traditional clinical use does not have a precise physical correlate and can refer to any (Western-defined) tendon, ligament, or muscle that is involved in a disharmony of the Liver. The muscle of the Spleen-muscle connection can be any tendon or ligament that is involved in a Spleen disharmony. This is an example of how function and relationship are more important than precise physical substrata in Chinese medicine.

28. *Ling Shu*, sec. 4, chap. 17, p. 189.

29. Ibid. The five colors are white, yellow, red, blue-green, and black.

30. *Su Wen*, sec. 3, chap. 10, p. 73.

31. Ibid., sec. 1, chap. 1, p. 6.

32. Zhang Jie-bing, *Illustrated Wing to the Classic of Categories* [30]. This quotation is in the *Additions to Wings* (*Lei-jing Fu-yi*), sec. 3, chap. 17, p. 439. The quotation is actually about the Life Gate Fire, which Zhang Jie-bing here uses as a general expression for the Kidneys. (See note 33.) The *Nan Jing* too says, "The Kidney area is the origin of the five Yin and five Yang Organs, the root of the twelve Meridians . . . and the origin of the three Burners" ("Difficulty 8," p. 17).

33. The *Nei Jing* uses the term *ming-men* to denote the shine of eyes. Later, in "Difficulty 36" of the *Nan Jing*, the term is used to designate Kidney Yang and is identified with the right Kidney. Later medical authorities disagree as to whether the Life Gate Fire is the right Kidney only, or the Yang of both Kidneys, or just a general name for the Kidney. An interesting summary of this historical debate is included in Li Tiao-hua, *Patterns and Treatment of the Kidneys and Kidney Illnesses* [60], pp. 2–4.

34. *Su Wen*, sec. 1, chap. 1, p. 6.

35. Zhongshan Institute, *Clinical Use of Chinese Medicines* [92], p. 192. Like digitalis, aconite can be poisonous and needs to be carefully used. For a discussion on the pharmacology of aconite, see: W. Tang and G. Eisenbrand, *Chinese Drugs of Plant Origins*, pp. 19–44 and C. M. Chang and P. P. H. But, *Pharmacology and Application of Chinese Matera Medica*, pp. 668–673. (See Appendix E on adverse effects of Chinese herbs.)

36. *Su Wen*, sec. 7, chap. 23, p. 154.

37. *Su Wen*, sec. 7, chap. 23, p. 154.

38. Ibid., sec. 2, chap. 5, p. 41.

39. *Ling Shu*, sec. 4, chap. 17, p. 189.

40. *Su Wen*, sec. 3, chap. 9, p. 68.

41. *Ling Shu*, sec. 4, chap. 17, p. 189. The five tones or musical notes are called *jiao, zhi, guan, shang,* and *yu.*

42. Traditional Chinese Medical Research Institute and Guangzhou Institute, *Concise Dictionary of Traditional Chinese Medicine* [34], p. 280.

43. This phrase is standard in most recent introductory or pathology texts on traditional medicine. The earliest statement of this sort is from the *Nan Jing*: "The Kidney area is . . . the door of respiration" ("Difficulty 8," p. 17). The *Nei Jing* mentions asthma as a possible Kidney or Kidney Meridian symptom (*Su Wen*, sec. 7, chap. 22, p. 148; *Ling Shu*, sec. 3, chap. 10, p. 125). Around 280 C.E., Wang Shu-he linked asthma to a possible Kidney or Kidney Meridian disharmony in his *Classic of the Pulse* (*Mai Jing* [22]), p. 19. Chao Yuan-fang continued this tradition in his *Discussion on the Origins of Symptoms in Illness* [13] of 610 C.E., sec. 15, chap. 6, p. 89. By the time of the Ming dynasty this connection between the Kidneys and breathing was firmly and formally stated by various scholars. The quotation in the text, "The Kidneys rule the grasping of Qi," now commonly used by traditional doctors, is from *Ordering of Patterns and Deciding Treatments* (*Lei-zheng Zhi-cai*) by Lin Pei-qin. This volume first appeared in 1839 and the quotation appears in sec. 2, p. 113 (Taipei: Whirlwind Press, 1978).

44. *Ling Shu* [2], sec. 10, chap. 71, p. 475.

45. *Su Wen*, sec. 3, chap. 9, p. 67.

46. *Ling Shu*, sec. 4, chap. 17, p. 189.

47. Shanghai Institute, *Foundations* [53], p. 80.

48. *Su Wen*, sec. 20, chap. 44, p. 246, and sec. 3, chap. 10, p. 72.

49. For an interesting discussion of the comparative effects of Western and Chinese methods of treating insomnia, see Tianjin Institute, *Practical Clinical Handbook of Traditional Chinese Medicine* [56], p. 149. Also see Peng Jin, "Prof. Kong Lingxu's Experience in TCM Treatment of Insomnia," *Journal of Traditional Chinese Medicine*, 1998; 19: 175–181, Y. Lu, "Insomnia: Treatment with An Mian Tang," *Journal of Chinese Medicine*, 1999; 59: 28–33.

50. Ma Ruo-shui, *Theoretical Foundations of Traditional Chinese Medicine* [62], p. 35.

51. The Yang Organs are, in general, more susceptible to External Pernicious Influences. The Lungs are an exception. (See Appendix B.)

52. *Su Wen*, sec. 7, chap. 23, p. 155.

53. *Su Wen*, sec. 3, chap. 10, p. 72.

54. Ibid., sec. 7, chap. 21, p. 140.

55. Shanghai Institute, *Foundations* [53], p. 83.

56. For an elaborate English-language discussion of the entire question of Fluids, see Steven Clavey, *Fluid Physiology and Pathology in Traditional Chinese Medicine* (Melbourne, Australia: Churchill Livingstone, 1995).

57. *Su Wen*, sec. 3, chap. 10, p. 70.

58. Ibid.

59. The Chinese have two distinct terms for "hair": *fa*, or "head hair," and *mao*, which may be translated as "body hair" or "surface hair."

60. The effectiveness of the Chinese medical treatment may be partially related, from a Western medical perspective, to the fact that *astragulus* can excite the central nervous system (Zhongshan Institute, *Clinical Use of Chinese Medicines* [92], p. 330). Modern research has also produced evidence for the effect of *astragulus* on the common cold and the immune system, both by itself and especially in combination in the "Jade Screen," in such studies as "Effect of *Radix astragali* on the Parainfluenza I (Sendai) Virus Infection in Mice and on its Epidemiological Efficacy in the Prophylaxis of the Common Cold," JTCM, January 1980. Some of this Chinese research has been replicated in the West. For example, see D. T. Chu et al., "Immunotherapy with Chinese Medicinal Herbs I. Immune Restoration of Local Xenogeneic Graft-Versus-Host Reactions in Cancer Patients by Fractionated *Astragulus Membranaceus In Vitro*," in *Journal of Clinical and Laboratory Immunology*, 1988; 25: 119–123.

61. *Ling Shu*, sec. 4, chap. 17, p. 189.

62. Ibid., sec. 3, chap. 11, p. 78.

63. *Su Wen*, sec. 13, chap. 47, p. 262.

64. For some of the flavor of these debates, see such articles as "Tentative Discussion on the Triple Burner by Cheng Jia-zhang," SJTCM, October 1958; "Concerning the Triple Burner Dispute," JTCM, January 1959; and "Clarification of Unsolved Problems Concerning the Triple Burner," JTCM, July 1980.

65. This statement was first made in relation to the Triple Burner in "Difficulty 38" of the *Nan Jing*. Sun Si-miao, the great Tang-dynasty physician, repeated this statement and emphasized this explanation in his Thousand Ducat Prescriptions [19] (first published 652 C.E.), sec. 20, chap. 4, p. 362. All sorts of interpretations and disagreements with this idea exist in the medical literature.

66. *Su Wen*, sec. 3, chap. 8, p. 59.

67. *Ling Shu*, sec. 4, chap. 18, p. 199.

68. Ibid.

69. Ibid.

70. In the medical tradition, only secondary mention is made of the Triple Burner's digestive and Qi function. In the *Nan Jing* ("Difficulty 31"), the Triple Burner is called the "road for nutrition" and is referred to as "the beginning and end of Qi." Zhang Jie-bing, in his Ming-dynasty commentary on the *Nei Jing*, called the *Lei Jing* or Classic of Categories, says that the Triple Burner is "the commander-in-chief of all the Qi of the various Organs, the Protective Qi, Nutritive Qi, and the Meridian Qi of the Interior and Exterior, right and left, upper and lower regions" and that it "is responsible for communication among the different parts of the body"

(Zhang, Illustrated Wing [30], sec. 3, chap. 23, p. 121). Again in the *Nan Jing* ("Difficulty 66"), the Triple Burner is called the "sixth Yang Organ, responsible for supporting all the various types of Qi of the body." But the Qi and digestive functions of the Triple Burner are usually considered secondary to its Water-metabolism functions. The tradition concerning Qi is based on an unexplained, out-of-place phrase in the *Nei Jing* (*Ling Shu*, sec. 3, chap. 10, p. 131), but a comprehensive examination of the symptomology of the Triple Burner Organ (as opposed to the Meridian) in the *Nei Jing* shows it to be primarily related to Water movement (e.g., *Ling Shu*, sec. 1, chap. 2, p. 20), again confirming the central interpretation of this Organ.

71. This classic introduction was written by Lin Yi, Gao Bao-heng, and Sun Qi-guang, who were Song dynasty Imperial Medical Scholars and Librarians of the Hall of Records. This discussion appears on page 11 of Huangfu Mi's *Systematic Classic of Acupuncture* [15]. This text is the earliest acupuncture manual in existence.

4

THE MERIDIANS: THE WARP AND WOOF

and on acupuncture and herbology

The word *Meridian* as used in East Asian medicine came into the English language through a French translation of the Chinese term *jing-luo*.[1] *Jing** means "to go through" or "a thread in a fabric"; *luo* means "something that connects or attaches," or "a net." Meridians are the channels or pathways that carry Qi and Blood through the body. They are not Blood Vessels. Rather, they comprise an invisible lattice that links together all the fundamental textures and Organs. In Chinese Meridian theory, these channels are unseen but are thought to embody a kind of informational network—the Qi and Blood move along them, and a therapeutic system is conceptually organized through the details of its design. Because the Meridian system unifies all the parts of the body, it is essential for the maintenance of harmonious balance. The *Nei Jing* says: "The Meridians move the Qi and Blood, regulate Yin and Yang, moisten the tendons and bones, benefit the joints."[2]

---

*The character *jing* for Meridian is different from the term *Jing* that means Essence.

The Meridians connect the interior of the body with the exterior. (As has been said earlier, the distinction between inner and outer has more to do with significance than with place—the interior is more important than the exterior.) This is the basis of acupuncture theory, that working with points on the surface of the body will affect what goes on inside the body, because it affects the activity of the textures that are traveling through the Meridians. Every Chinese physician must have a complete grasp of the Meridian system. Most acupuncture points relate to the Meridians, and most herbs a doctor prescribes are thought to enter one or more of the Meridian pathways.

The Meridian system is made up of twelve regular Meridians that correspond to each of the five Yin and six Yang Organs, and to the Pericardium (which for the purposes of Meridian theory is an independent Organ).[3] These are sometimes called Jing Meridians. There are also eight Extra Meridians, only two of which, the Governing Vessel and the Conception Vessel,[4] are considered major Meridians. This is because they have independent points—points that are not also on any of the twelve regular Meridians. The paths of the other six Extra Meridians all intersect with these twelve Meridians and have no independent points of their own. There are also many small, finer, netlike minor Meridians, called Luo Meridians. The twelve regular Meridians along with the Governing and Conception Meridians are the fourteen major Meridians. They and the minor Meridians are the warp and woof of the body.[5]

A great number of books on Meridian theory have been published in European languages as a result of the Western interest in acupuncture. This chapter, therefore, will deal with Meridian theory only as it pertains to Chinese medical knowledge as a whole—for its use in explaining patterns of disharmony.

Meridian theory assumes that disorder within a Meridian generates derangement in the pathway and creates disharmony along that Meridian, or that such derangement is a result of a disharmony of the Meridian's connecting Organ. A disorder in the Stomach Meridian, for example, may cause upper toothache because the

Meridian passes through the upper gums, while lower toothache may be the result of a disorder of the Large Intestine Meridian. Pain in the groin may as easily result from a Liver Meridian disorder as from a disorder of the Liver itself.

Disharmonies in an Organ may manifest themselves in the corresponding Meridians. For instance, pain along the Heart Meridian may reflect Congealed Blood or Stagnant Qi in the Heart. Excess Fire in the Liver may follow the Meridian and generate redness in the eyes.

An understanding of the interconnections between fundamental textures, Organs, and Meridians informs the practices of acupuncture and herbology. These are the two main forms of treatment used in Chinese medicine, and Meridian theory allows the physician to apply them to particular patients. The goal of all treatment methods in Chinese medicine is to rebalance those aspects of the body's Yin and Yang whose harmonious proportion and movement have become disordered. Agitated activity, for instance, as in the case of inappropriate anger such as that characterized by excessive Liver activity, must be calmed. Insufficient activity, say of the Kidney Yang, must be tonified to avoid lack of sexual energy. Substances that accumulate inappropriately must be drained—as is done to correct an excess of Fluids in the abdomen. If there is not enough Qi in the Lungs, it must be replenished so that the patient does not continually catch cold. Movement must also go in the proper direction. If the Qi of the Spleen descends, causing chronic diarrhea, it must be lifted; if the Qi of the Stomach ascends, causing nausea, it must be sent down. Stagnant Qi must be moved; reckless movement of the Blood must be stabilized. Too much Cold in the Kidneys must be warmed; extra Fire in the Lungs must be cooled. Whatever is out of balance must be rebalanced. The complementary aspects of Yin and Yang must be harmonious.

The basic idea behind acupuncture (considered a Yang treatment because it moves from the exterior to the interior) is that the insertion of very fine needles into points along the Meridians can rebalance bodily disharmonies. A related technique, moxibustion, entails the application of heat from certain burning substances at the acupuncture points. The primary *moxa*, or heating substance, is mugwort—(*Artemisia vulgaris*). The action of the needles or of moxibustion affects the Qi and Blood in the Meridians, thus affecting all the fundamental textures and Organs. The needles can reduce what is excessive, increase what is deficient, warm what is cold, cool what is hot, circulate what is stagnant, move what is congealed, stabilize what is reckless, raise what is falling, and lower what is rising.

Classical theory recognizes about 365 acupuncture points on the surface Meridians of the body.[6] With the inclusion of miscellaneous points and new points used in ear acupuncture and other recent methods, the total universe has risen to at least 2,000 points for possible use.[7] In practice, however, a typical doctor's repertoire might be only 150 points.

In contemporary texts, point location is generally based on modern anatomy. For example, a manual produced by the Academy of Traditional Chinese Medicine in 1975 describes the location of a common point as "at the lateral side . . . above the transverse popliteal crease between the *musculus vastus laterali* and the *musculus biceps femoris*."[8] Classical texts, which do not reflect an interest in detailed anatomy, refer to that same point as the place where the tip of the middle finger naturally touches the thigh when the patient is standing.[9] The classical literature locates other points by means of easily defined, yet precise, bodily landmarks such as creases, bony prominences, hairlines, and places where the skin changes in color and textural quality.

Each acupuncture point has a defined therapeutic action. Each unique acupuncture point embodies a particular quality of Qi that can resonate with a disharmony and elicit a return to health. The physician chooses to work on those points that are most appropriate for treating a particular individual's pattern of disharmony. Rarely are acupuncture points used singly; a combination of points is usually chosen. A typical treatment entails the insertion of five to fifteen needles. Acupuncture needles were originally made of bronze or possibly copper, tin, gold, or silver. In earlier periods, they may have been bone, horn, or slivers of bamboo, gold, or silver. They are now made of stainless steel, are of hairlike thinness, and produce relatively little pain when inserted. The depth to which a needle penetrates depends on the particular point; needles are inserted only a millimeter or two at the finger points, but they may be placed up to three or four inches deep at the buttocks' points.

The initial modern interest in acupuncture concerned pain relief and its potential use as an analgesia and anesthetic technique. As a result, Western interest has been aimed disproportionately at applying acupuncture to pain control. A number of theories have been developed to explain the mechanisms of pain relief achieved through acupuncture.

The gate theory, for example, suggests that stimulation from the needles jams the lower nerve bundles in the central nervous system so that other pain signals—e.g., those from an incision—cannot reach the brain. This can be envisioned by imagining a telephone system in a major city: if too many individual lines are in use it is difficult for caller to get into the trunk lines and make a connection.[10]

Another theory of acupuncture anesthesia suggests that the insertion of the acupuncture needles may stimulate the release of endorphins, a class of opiates naturally produced within the brain. These substances are potent painkillers and could explain some of the pain-reducing properties of acupuncture.[11]

These preliminary findings and theories will generate further important research into the physiological mechanisms of acupuncture and its possible place in biomedicine. But these tentative theories are only of partial value because they isolate one of acupuncture's uses and ignore its many other potential clinical applications.[12] (See Appendix E for further discussion.)

While acupuncture has become well known in the West, its clinical partner, Chinese herbology, is still relatively unknown. This has led to the widespread misconception that acupuncture constitutes all of Chinese medicine. In fact, the knowledge of herbs is central to Chinese medicine. During the last two millennia, many more books have been devoted to herbology than to acupuncture. And while

Chinese physicians tend to practice both medical techniques, physicians who practice only with herbs are more numerous than those who practice only with acupuncture.[13]

The body of knowledge of Chinese herbology has been preserved in a great succession of pharmacopoeias and clinical manuals, a tradition that began during the early Han dynasty (the third century B.C.E.). The pharmacopoeias are vast catalogs of medicinal substances with therapeutic value. For example, a pharmacopoeia produced by the famous physician Li Shi-zhen, posthumously printed in 1596 C.E., included 1,892 entries. Of these, 1,173 were botanical ingredients, 444 were zoological ingredients, and 275 were derived from minerals. A recent Chinese pharmacopoeia is a massive compilation of 5,767 entries.[14] The substances commonly used in the Chinese materia medica span a great range of materials, from well-known herbs and minerals such as *ephedra* and gypsum to strange animal products such as the gallstones of a cow or dried skin secretions of a particular toad.[15]

Traditional pharmacopoeias usually define each entry in terms of how the various herbs evoke the fundamental textures and affect specific complaints. The twentieth-century pharmacopoeias also describe how the substances are understood in terms of modern pharmacology, citing active compounds, detectable biochemical effects on microorganisms, animals, and humans, and toxicity. (See Appendix E.)

After distinguishing a particular pattern of disharmony in a patient, the practitioner of traditional Chinese medicine usually chooses a prescription from a repertoire of some 1,000 common classical prescriptions that can rebalance various disharmonies. These prescriptions are learned from the great clinical manuals that exist alongside the pharmacopoeias. The formulas are coordinated matrixes that can resonate with various imbalances and elicit health. Thus, the physician is armed with knowledge that has been tested over the past centuries of Chinese medical history. Herbs are seldom used singly; they are usually combined in prescriptions containing five to fifteen substances. The dosages average three to fifteen grams per herb. Most commonly, herbs are decocted into a drink, but pills, powders, tinctures, and poultices are also widely used. Because every patient's body is unique, the physician begins with a general prescription as delineated in the classical texts, and then adjusts the mixture to the patient by adding or deleting various herbs or by manipulating the dosages of the compounds to fit the precise disharmony.

Together, acupuncture and herbology constitute the basic therapeutic modalities the Chinese physician uses to restore balance in the body. Other important Oriental techniques—massage, lifestyle advice, exercise regimes—also use the Meridians. All are thought to have therapeutic access to the body through the Meridians. The pathways of these Meridians are illustrated in Figures 3 through 16,[16] which depict both the channels within the body and the external pathways along which the acupuncture points are located. The general reader is invited to just glance at the pictures. Attention to details is unnecessary to comprehend the rest of the book.

Key to Meridian Diagrams

Solid lines are Meridians on the surface of the body.

Broken lines are Meridians inside the body.

Dots are acupuncture points on the surface of the body belonging to the Meridian.

Triangles are acupuncture points on the surface of the body belonging to other Meridians that the primary Meridian is passing through.

Numbers correspond to numbers within the caption text.

(These numbers should not be confused with those in references elsewhere in the text such as "Liver 2.")

All the Meridians, except the Governing and Conception Vessels, are assumed to have bilateral symmetry, even though only one side of the body is shown.

Representation of the internal organs is for the convenience of the modern reader. The traditional system might not be concerned with this type of anatomy.

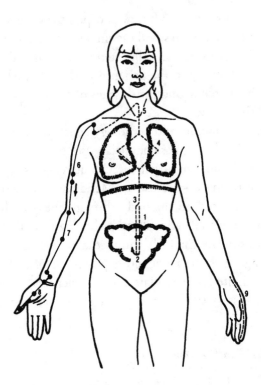

FIGURE 3 *The Lung Meridian* [*Shou-tai-yin fei-jing* 手 太 阴 肺 经]

The Lung Meridian originates in the middle portion of the body cavity (1) and runs downward, internally, to connect with the Large Intestine (2). Turning back, it passes upward through the diaphragm (3) to enter its pertaining Organ, the Lungs (4). From the internal zone between the Lungs and the throat (5), it emerges to the surface of the body under the clavicle. Descending, the Lung Meridian then runs along the medial aspect of the upper arm (6) to reach the elbow crease. From there, it runs along the anterior portion of the forearm (7), passes above the major artery of the wrist, and emerges at the radial side of the tip of the thumb (8). Another section of the Lung Meridian branches off just above the wrist and runs directly to the radial side of the tip of the index finger (9) to connect with the Large Intestine Meridian.

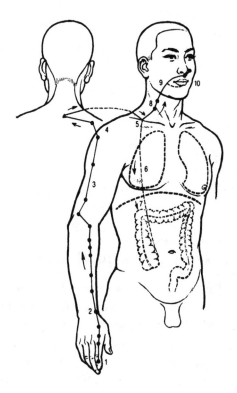

FIGURE 4 *The Large Intestine Meridian* [*Shou-yang-ming da-chang-jing* 手 阳 明 大 肠 经]

The Large Intestine Meridian begins at the tip of the index finger and runs upward along the radial side of the index finger (1) and between the thumb and index finger. It passes through the depression between the tendons of the thumb (2) and then continues upward along the lateral aspect of the forearm to the lateral side of the elbow. From there, it ascends along the anterior border of the upper arm (3) to the highest point of the shoulder (4). On top of the shoulder, the Meridian divides into two branches (5). The first of these branches enters the body and passes through the Lung (6), diaphragm, and the Large Intestine (7), its pertaining Organ. The second of these branches ascends externally along the neck (8), passes through the cheek (9), and enters, internally, the lower teeth and gum (10). On the exterior, it continues, curving around the upper lip and crossing to the opposite side of the nose.

FIGURE 5   *The Stomach Meridian*
   [*Zu-yang-ming wei-jing* 足 阳 明 胃 经]

The Stomach Meridian begins, internally, where the Large Intestine Meridian terminates, next to the nose (1). It then ascends to the bridge of the nose, meeting the Bladder Meridian at the inner corner of the eye, and emerging under the eye. Descending from there, lateral to the nose, it enters the upper gum (2) and curves around the lips before passing along the side of the lower jawbone (3) and through the angle of the jaw. It then turns upward, running in front of the ear (4) to the corner of the forehead. A branch descends from the lower jaw (5), enters the body, and descends through the diaphragm. It then enters its pertaining Organ, the Stomach, and connects with the Spleen (6). Another branch leaves the lower jaw, but remains on the surface of the body as it crosses over the neck, chest (7), and abdomen (8), and terminates in the groin. Internally, the Meridian reconstitutes itself at the lower end of the stomach and descends inside the abdomen (9) to reconnect with the external branch in the groin. From this point, the Meridian runs downward over the front of the thigh (10) to the outer side of the knee (11), and continues along the center of the front of the lower leg to reach the top of the foot. It terminates at the lateral side of the tip of the second toe. A branch deviates from the Stomach Meridian just below the knee (12) and ends at the lateral side of the middle toe. A short branch also leaves from the top of the foot (13) and terminates at the medial side of the big toe to connect with the Spleen Meridian.

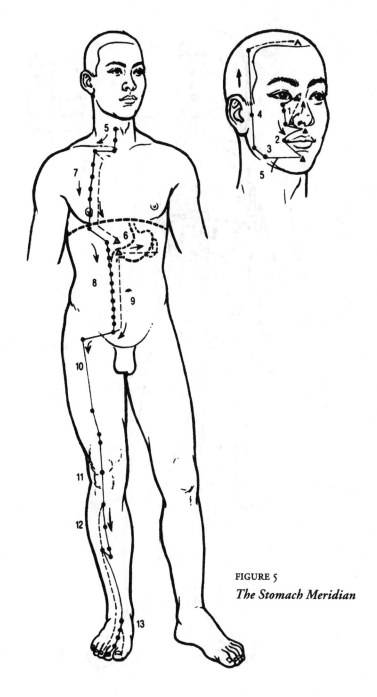

FIGURE 5

The Stomach Meridian

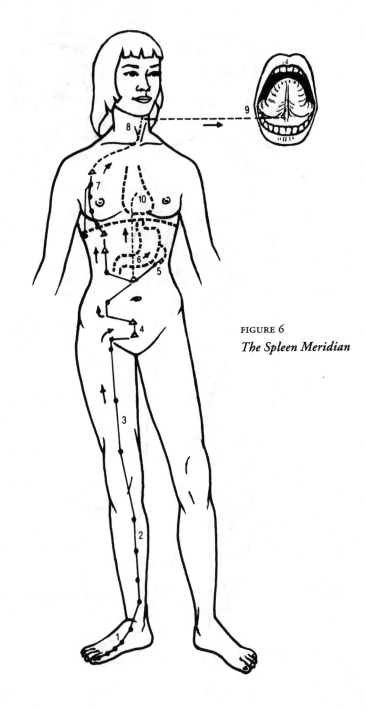

FIGURE 6

The Spleen Meridian

FIGURE 6 *The Spleen Meridian* [*Zu-tai-yin pi-jing* 足 太 阴 脾 经]

The Spleen Meridian originates at the medial side of the big toe. It then runs along the inside of the foot (1), turning in front of the inner ankle bone. From there, it ascends along the posterior surface of the lower leg (2) and the medial aspect of the knee and thigh (3) to enter the abdominal cavity (4). It runs internally to its pertaining Organ, the Spleen (5), and connects with the Stomach (6). The main Meridian continues on the surface of the abdomen, running upward to the chest (7), where it again penetrates internally to follow the throat (8) up to the root of the tongue (9), under which it spreads its Qi and Blood. An internal branch leaves the Stomach, passes upward through the diaphragm, and enters into the Heart (10), where it connects with the Heart Meridian.

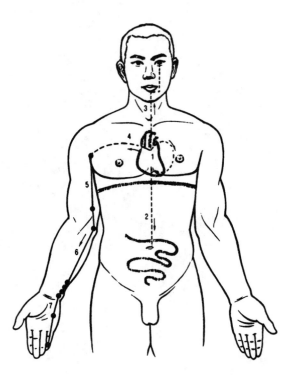

FIGURE 7 *The Heart Meridian*
[*Shou-shao-yin xin-jing* 手 少 阴 心 经]

The Heart Meridian has three branches, each of which begins in the Heart
(1). One branch runs downward through the diaphragm (2) to connect to the
Small Intestine. A second branch runs upward from the Heart along the side
of the throat (3) to meet the eye. The third branch runs across the chest from
the Heart to the Lung (4), then descends and emerges in the underarm. It
passes along the midline of the inside of the upper arm (5), runs downward
across the inner elbow, along the midline of the inside of the forearm (6),
crosses the wrist and palm (7), and terminates at the inside tip of the little
finger, where it connects with the Small Intestine Meridian.

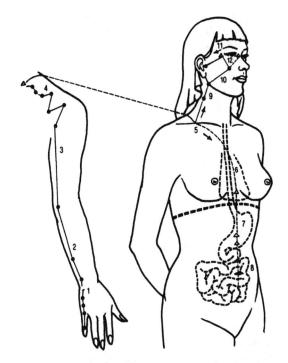

FIGURE 8 *The Small Intestine Meridian*
[*Shou-tai-yang xiao-chang-jing* 手 太 阳 小 肠]

The Small Intestine Meridian begins on the outside of the tip of the little finger, crosses the palm and wrist (1), and passes upward along the posterior aspect of the forearm (2). The Meridian continues upward along the posterior border of the lateral aspect of the upper arm (3), circles behind the shoulder (4), and runs to the center of the uppermost part of the back (where it meets the Governing Meridian). Here, the Meridian divides into two branches, one entering internally (5) to connect with the Heart (6), diaphragm, and Stomach (7), before entering its pertaining Organ, the Small Intestine (8). The second branch ascends along the side of the neck (9) to the cheek (10) and outer corner of the eye (11) before entering the ear. A short branch leaves the Meridian on the cheek (12) and runs to the inner corner of the eye, where it connects with the Bladder Meridian.

FIGURE 9 *The Bladder Meridian*
   [*Zu-tai-yang pang-guang-jing* 足 太 阳 膀 胱 经]

The Bladder Meridian starts at the inner side of the eye and ascends across the forehead (1) to the vertex of the head. From this point, a small branch splits off and enters into the brain (2), while the main Meridian continues to descend along the back of the head (3) and bifurcates at the back of the neck (4). The inner of these two branches descends a short distance to the center of the base of the neck (5), then descends parallel to the spine (6). A branch splits off, entering the body in the lumbar region and connecting to the Kidney (7) and its pertaining Organ, the Bladder (8). The outer branch traverses the back of the shoulder (9), descends adjacent to the inner branch and the spinal cord, and crosses the buttocks (10). The two branches continue downward, descend the posterior aspect of the thigh (11), and join behind the knee. The single Meridian now continues down the back of the lower leg (12), circles behind the outer ankle, runs along the outside of the foot (13), and terminates on the lateral side of the tip of the small toe, where it connects with the Kidney Meridian.

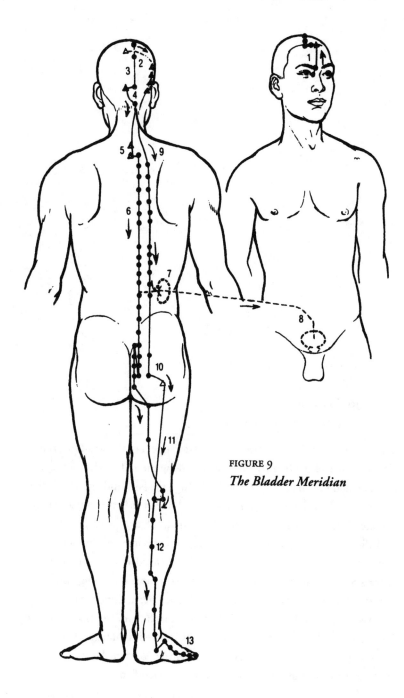

FIGURE 9
The Bladder Meridian

FIGURE IO *The Kidney Meridian*
  [*Zu-shao-yin shen-jing* 足少阴肾经]

The Kidney Meridian starts from the inferior aspect of the small toe, runs across the sole of the foot (1), and emerges along the arch of the foot (2) to circle behind the inner ankle and pass through the heel. It then ascends the medial side of the lower leg (3) to the medial side of the knee crease, climbs upward along the innermost aspect of the thigh (4), and penetrates the body near the base of the spine (5). This branch connects internally with the Kidney (6), its pertaining Organ, and with the Bladder (7), before returning to the surface of the abdomen above the pubic bone and running upward over the abdomen and chest (8). Another branch begins inside at the Kidney (6), passes upward through the Liver (9) and diaphragm, and enters the Lung (11). This branch continues along the throat (10) and terminates at the root of the tongue. A smaller branch leaves the Lung (11), joins the Heart, and flows into the chest to connect with the Pericardium Meridian.

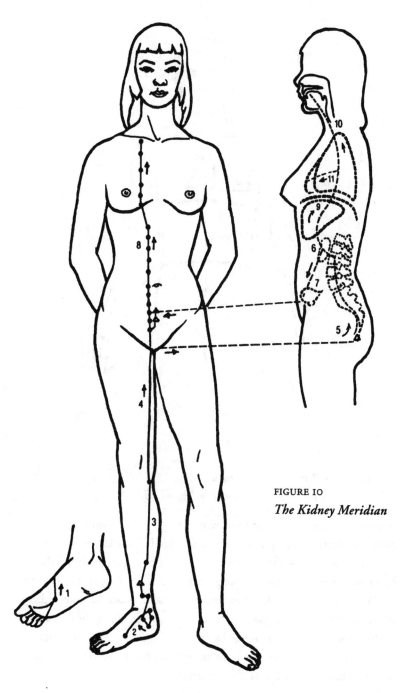

FIGURE 10
The Kidney Meridian

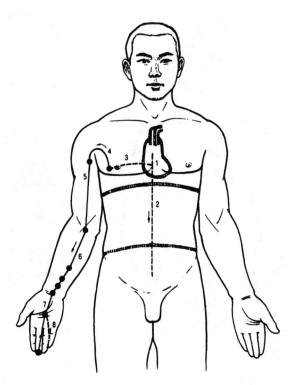

FIGURE II *The Pericardium Meridian*
[*Shou-jue-yin xin-bao-jing* 手厥阴心包经]

Beginning in the chest and in its pertaining Organ, the Pericardium (1), this Meridian descends through the diaphragm (2) to link the Upper, Middle, and Lower portions of the Triple Burner. A second internal branch of the Meridian crosses the chest (3), emerging to the surface at the area of the ribs. The Meridian then ascends around the armpit (4) and continues down the medial aspect of the upper arm (5) to the elbow crease. It runs further down the forearm (6) to the palm of the hand (7), ending at the tip of the middle finger. A short branch splits off from the palm (8) to connect with the Triple Burner Meridian at the end of the ring finger.

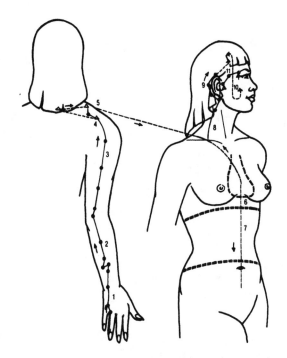

FIGURE 12 *The Triple Burner Meridian*
[*Shou-shao-yang san-jiao-jing*
手 少 阳 三 焦 经]

Beginning at the outside tip of the ring finger, the Triple Burner Meridian proceeds over the back of the hand (1) and wrist to the forearm (2). It runs upward, passing around the outer elbow, along the lateral aspect of the upper arm (3), to reach the posterior shoulder region (4). From here, the Meridian travels over the shoulder (5) and enters into the chest underneath the breastbone. An internal branch passes from this point through the Pericardium, penetrates the diaphragm (6), and then proceeds downward (7) to unite the Upper, Middle, and Lower Burners. Another, exterior branch ascends toward the shoulder and runs internally up the neck (8). It reaches the posterior border of the ear (9) and then interiorly circles the face (10). A short branch originates behind the ear, penetrates the ear, and emerges in front of the ear (11) to reach the outer end of the eyebrow and connect to the Gall Bladder Meridian.

FIGURE 13   *The Gall Bladder Meridian*
[*Zu-shao-yang dan-jing* 足少阳胆经]

The Gall Bladder Meridian begins at the outer corner of the eye (1), where two branches arise. One branch, remaining on the surface, weaves back and forth on the lateral aspect of the head before curving behind the ear (2) to reach the top of the shoulder. It then continues downward, passing in front of the underarm (3) and along the lateral aspect of the rib cage (4) to reach the hip region. The second branch internally traverses the cheek (5) and proceeds internally through the neck (6) and chest (7) to reach the Liver and its pertaining Organ, the Gall Bladder (8). Continuing downward, this branch emerges on the side of the lower abdomen, where it connects with the other branch in the hip area (9). The Meridian then descends along the lateral aspect of the thigh (10) and knee to the side of the lower leg (11) and further downward in front of the outer ankle. It crosses the top of the foot (12) and terminates at the lateral side of the tip of the fourth toe. A branch leaves the Meridian just below the ankle to cross over the foot (13) to the big toe, where it connects with the Liver Meridian.

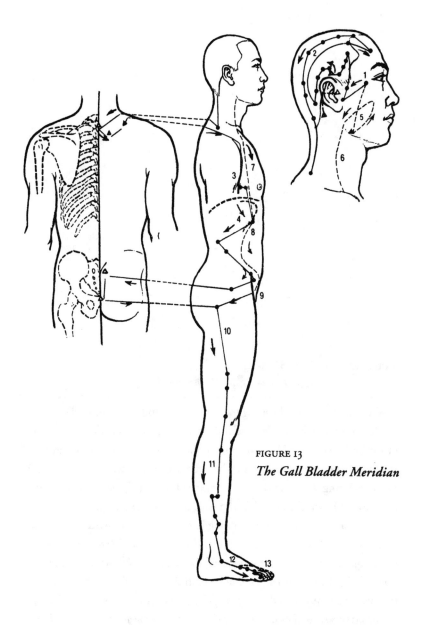

FIGURE 13

The Gall Bladder Meridian

FIGURE 14 *The Liver Meridian*
   [*Zu-jue-yin gan-jing* 足厥阴肝经]

Beginning on the top of the big toe, the Liver Meridian traverses the top of
the foot (1), ascending in front of the inner ankle and along the medial aspect
of the lower leg (2) and knee. It runs continuously along the medial aspect of
the thigh (3) to the pubic region, where it encircles the external genitalia (4)
before entering the lower abdomen. It ascends internally (5), connects with its
pertaining Organ, the Liver (6), and with the Gall Bladder, and scatters
underneath the ribs (7) before pouring into the Lungs (8), where it connects
with the Lung Meridian (Fig. 3). The entire cycle of the Meridian system
begins anew here. Reconstituting itself, the Meridian follows the trachea
upward to the throat (9) and connects with the eyes (10). Two branches leave
the eye area: One descends across the cheek to encircle the inner surface of
the lips (11); a second branch ascends across the forehead (12) to reach the
vertex of the head.

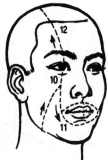

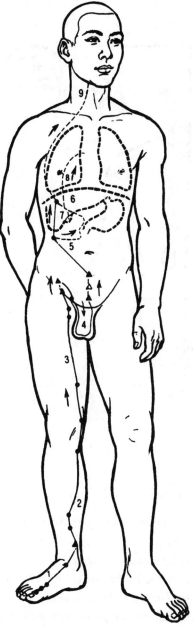

FIGURE 14

The Liver Meridian

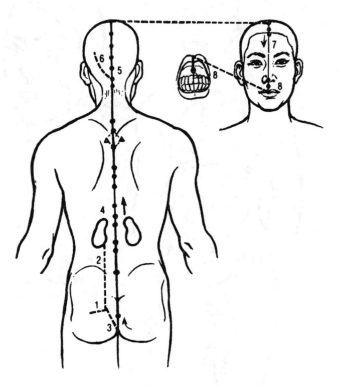

FIGURE 15 *The Governing Vessel* [*Du-mai* 督 脉]

The Governing Vessel begins in the pelvic cavity (1). An internal branch ascends from here to the Kidney (2). Another internal branch descends to emerge at the perineum (3) and pass through the tip of the coccyx. Ascending along the middle of the spinal column (4), it reaches the head (5) to penetrate into the brain (6). The main branch continues over the top of the head, and descends across the forehead (7) and nose to end inside the upper gum (8).

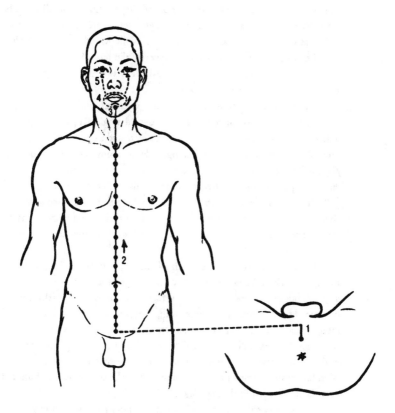

FIGURE 16 *The Conception Vessel* [*Ren-mai*]

The Conception Vessel begins in the pelvic cavity, emerges at the perineum between the anus and external genitalia (1), and runs forward across the pubic region. It ascends along the midline of
the abdomen (2), chest, and throat to the lower jaw (3), where it penetrates internally to encircle the lips (4) and send a branch to
the eyes (5).

NOTES

1. "Channel" is in fact a better translation of *jing-luo* than "Meridian." The word *channel* is closer to the Chinese, suggesting a three-dimensional conduit that contains some kind of substance, while Meridian implies only a two-dimensional grid. In this book, however, the term *Meridian* has been used in order to avoid the confusion of using a new term.

2. *Ling Shu* [2], sec. 7, chap. 49, p. 340.

3. Until recently the most common speculation was that Meridians were a hypothetical construct that linked earlier discovered single acupuncture points. These points had supposedly been empirically tested from as early as the late Stone Age. Recent archeological findings in Hunan province of intact pre–*Nei Jing* medical manuscripts put Chinese medical history in general, and Meridian development in particular, in a different light. (These books are known collectively as the Han Ma-wang Burial Mound Silk Books. A collection of the most intact texts has been published and is titled after the largest manuscript, *Prescriptions for Fifty-Two Illnesses* (*Wu-shi-er Bing-fang*) [Beijing: Wenwu Press, 1979].)

   In the two texts concerned with Meridians, only eleven Meridians are mentioned. These Meridians are not connected internally or to each other in a system but seem suspended on the surface of the body. Their pathways and directions are different from those in the *Nei Jing*, and they are not named after or related in any way to internal Organs. In one of the texts some of the Meridians (the text calls them "mai" or vessels) have such symptomatic names as the "tooth vessel," "ear vessel," and "shoulder vessel." In general, this early Meridian system seems primitive compared to the one of several hundred years later recorded in the *Nei Jing*.

   The relationship between Meridian and points is given an interesting twist by these early texts. No points are mentioned, just entire Meridians, portraying zones of influence, needing stimulation by moxibustion. This evidence suggests Meridians existed before points. For an English discussion and translation, see Donald Harper, *Early Chinese Medical Literature: The Mawangudui Medical Manuscripts.* (London: Kegan Paul, 1998.)

   These new glimpses into the past are reminiscent of Sigerist's speculation on medicine's development in an even earlier period of human history:

   An individual hurts his leg and spontaneously without thinking he rubs it. . . . Another individual suffers from lumbago, crawls to the fire and once he feels the heat the pain becomes more tolerable. . . . We can well imagine that early man suffering an acute pain in the stomach felt impelled to act, pressed his epigastrium with both hands, applied heat or cold, drank water or some decoction until he felt relieved. Pain, in other words, released a series of instinctive reactions, some of which were more effective than others. With developing civilization men learned to differentiate between treatments, became aware of them, remembered them and passed them on. [Henry E. Sigerist, A History of Medicine, *vol. 1, pp. 115–117.]*

For another perspective on the origins of acupuncture, see D. C. Epler, "Bloodletting in Early Chinese Medicine and its Relation to the Origin of Acupuncture," in *Bulletin of the History of Medicine,* 1980; 54: 337–367.

The controversy concerning the origins of acupuncture is likely to continue. In fact, the original speculation that acupuncture points preceded the development of Meridian theory has received a boost with the recent recovery of several prehistoric mummies with well-preserved tattoos. These tattoos have numerous demarcation points on the body that do not seem to have decorative importance and seem to clearly overlap well-know acupuncture points. A series of clever histological investigations of the tattoos and radiological studies of the mummies themselves indicate that the so-called "Icemen" were familiar with a simple form of symptomatic acupuncture. This recent evidence raises the possibility that acupuncture may have originated in the Eurasian continent at least two thousand years earlier than previously thought. See: L. Dorter, M. Moser, F. Bahr, K. Spindler, E. Egarter-Vigl, S. Guillén, G. Dohr, and T. Kenner, "A Medical Report from the Stone Age?" *Lancet* 1999; 354: 1023–1025.

4. The Chinese character (*ren*) for this Meridian means "responsibility," probably implying responsibility for the Yin Meridians. The word also has the connotation of conception (pregnancy), which is where the common English translation comes from.

5. The convention of speaking of fourteen Meridians begins with Hua Shou's Elaboration of the Fourteen Meridians [14], first published 1341 C.E. In this treatise, for the first time, the Governing Vessel and Conception Vessel were separated from the eight Extra Meridians and included with the regular twelve Meridians.

6. The *Nei Jing* abstractly and theoretically states that there are 365 points (*Su Wen,* sec. 15, chap. 58, p. 291), but only mentions 160 points by name in all of its discussion. The number of regular acupuncture points was clarified and increased throughout Chinese history. The table in note 9 summarizes this historical progression (based on a comparable chart in Shanghai Institute, Study of Acupuncture Points [86], p. 4). Also, it should be noted that massage, cupping, and scarification (*gua sha*) of Meridian points are also critical acupuncture techniques. See A. Nielsen, *Gua Sha: A Traditional Technique for Modern Practice,* Edinburgh: Churchill Livingstone, 1995; Ilkay Z. Chirali, *Traditional Chinese Medicine: Cupping Therapy,* Edinburgh: Churchill Livingstone, 1999. Cupping and scarification

were once historically important in Western medicine. For remarks on medical amnesia and cupping see: Ted J. Kaptchuk, "Consequences of Cupping," [Letter] *New England Journal of Medicine*, 1997; 336: 1009.

Qigong, is another imortant healing modality in modern China. Under the rubric of this label exists a multiplicity of techniques which represent a fusion of health-longevity practices and an amalgam of various Chinese religious ideas. Fundamentally, *qigong* has to do with cultivating a "mindful body" or an "embodied mind" to influence the movement, quality and/or quantity of Qi within a person. Using breathing, intention, visualization based on traditional Chinese physiology, meditation, and exercise, it is thought that Qi can be precisely manipulated. Some practitioners claim to "emit" it to others.

Qigong, which can function as a kind of "secular religion," has come to occupy a critical place in a modern China, especially after Deng Xiaoping's rise to power in the 1980s. (Sometimes *qigong* is referred to as the "fifth modernization.") Depending on which version of *qigong* is selected, health or religion can be emphasized by different degrees. In many ways, *qigong* is a continuity of earlier Chinese historical forms of Taoist "inner alchemy." In some forms, it also creatively borrows Western ideas in order to garb itself as a scientifically validated medical system or an acceptable "scientific religion." For example, most *qigong* adepts claim that the existence of Qi has been scientifically and experimentally proven and that it resembles magnetism, electricity, or some kind of subatomic particle. It is also possible that *qigong* has been influenced by such Western movements as mesmerism and magnetic healing via routes that allowed neurasthenia to become an important discursive feature of Chinese health awareness. For an overview of *qigong* with a medical emphasis see: K. M. Sancier, "Medical Applications of *Qigong*," *Alternative Therapies*, 1996; 2: 40–46 and Ching-Tse Lee and Ting Lei, "*Qigong*" In: W. B. Jonas and J. S. Lewin (eds.) *Essentials of Complementary and Alternative Medicine*. Philadelphia: Lippincott Williams and Wilkins, 1999. For examples of scientific studies of *Qigong* see: Shenghan Xu, "Psychophysiological Reactions Associated with *Qigong* Therapy," *Chinese Medical Journal*, 1994; 107: 230–233 and Kwok Cho Tang, "*Qigong* Therapy—Its Effectiveness and Regulation" *American Journal of Chinese Medicine*, 1994; 23: 245–242; Zhang Mingsu and Sun Xinggyuan. *Chinese Qigong Therapy*, Jinan: Shandong Science and Technology Press, 1988. For an historical-sociological perspective on *qigong* see: Kunio Mirua, "The Revival of Qi: *Qigong* in Contemporary China," in: Livia Kohn (ed.) *Taoist Mediation and Longevity Techniques*. For an anthropological account see E. Hsu, *The Transmission of*

Chinese Medicine, 1999. For a discussion of religious-medical healing in Japan that roughly parallels the *qigong* phenomena in China see: Winston Davis, *Dojo: Magic and Exorcism in Modern Japan*. Stanford: Stanford University Press, 1980. For examples of Western movements synthesizing an amalgam of religion, science, and health care see: Robert C. Fuller, *Mesmerism and the American Cure of Souls*, Philadelphia: University of Pennsylvania Press, 1982. For a discussion of how spiritual materialism can be a critical force in modern Western health movements see: Ted J. Kaptchuk and David M. Eisenberg, "The Persuasive Appeal of Alternative Medicine," *Annals of Internal Medicine* 1998; 129: 1061–1065.

"Bonesetting" and spinal manipulation have also had a long tradition as part of East Asian therapeutics, see: Y. K. Li, S. Z. Zhong, "Spinal Manipulation in China," *Journal of Manipulative and Physiological Therapeutics*, 1998; 21: 399–401.

7. For a fairly comprehensive presentation of the outside-Meridian points, see Hao Jin-kai, Illustrative Charts of Extra Meridians Acupuncture Points [76]. For a discussion of modernization in acupuncture and the development of new points, see Elizabeth Hsu, "Innovations in Acumoxa: Acupuncture Analgesia, Scalp and Ear Acupuncture in the People's Republic of China," in *Social Science and Medicine* 1996; 42: 421–430.

8. Academy of Traditional Chinese Medicine, *An Outline of Chinese Acupuncture* (Beijing: Foreign Languages Press, 1975), p. 181. This text also locates the point in the traditional way.

9. The earliest stated location of this point (Gall Bladder 31, *Feng-shi*, Wind Market) is in Wang Shu-chuan, Classic of Nourishing Life with Acupuncture and Moxibustion [21] (first appeared 1220 c.e.), p. 73. The oldest location of a point would usually be presented in Huang-fu Mi, Systematic Classic of Acupuncture [15], which first appeared in c. 282 c.e. This text gives the earliest systematic presentation of acupuncture that includes point location, but it does not include Gall Bladder 31.

Historic Progression of Meridian Points

SOURCES	POINTS: Single	Bilateral	Total
Nei Jing	25	135	160
Systematic Classic of Acupuncture (c. 282 c.e.)	49	300	349

continued

Historic Progression of Meridian Points (continued)

| | **POINTS:** | | |
SOURCES	Single	Bilateral	Total
Illustrated Classic of Acupuncture Points as Found on on the Bronze Model (1026 c.e.) and Elaboration of the Fourteen Meridians (1341 c.e.)	51	303	354
Classic of Nourishing Life with Acupuncture (1220 c.e.) and Great Compendium of Acupuncture (1601 c.e.)	51	308	359
Golden Mirror of Medicine (1742 c.e.)	52	308	361

10. The gate theory was postulated by Ronald Melzack and Patrick Wall ("Pain Mechanisms: A New Theory," *Science*, 1965; 150: 971–979). Though still controversial, it is a plausible mechanism to integrate disparate information about pain perception. As a comprehensive theory it explains that the pain sensation is not the product of a single nerve system, but that each specialized portion of the entire nervous system contributes to the pain experience. One of the central assertions of the gate control theory is that there exists a spinal gating mechanism in the dorsal horns, the substantia gelatinosa, that regulates the amount of information conveyed from the peripheral nerve fibers to spinal cord transmission cells. These cells in turn activate central nervous system structures such as the thalamus, responsible for expressions of pain. The gating mechanism is thought to transmit more sensory pain information as the proportion of small diameter (A-delta or C) fibers firing exceeds the amount of large diameter (A-beta) fiber activity. Melzack considers acupuncture a form of hyperstimulation analgesia, where the acupuncture pain relief is thought to be due to this phenomenon of inhibition of pain by stimulation of large fiber activity. (See R. Melzack and S. G. Dennis, "Neurophysiological Foundations of Pain" in *The Psychology of Pain*, edited by R. A. Sternback (New York: Raven Press, 1978.) For a more recent discussion see H. J. McQuay and R. A. Moore. *Evidence Based Resource for Pain Relief*, Oxford: Oxford University Press, 1998. For a social-historical discussion of the gate theory see Isabelle Baszanger, *Inventing Pain Medicine: From the Laboratory to the Clinic*, New Brunswick, NJ: Rutgers University Press, 1998.

11. The first evidence that neurochemicals were released by acupuncture came in 1974 from a controlled experiment in which pairs of rats were connected serially through their circulatory systems. An acupuncture needle applied to the point Large Intes-

tine 4 (*He-gu*) in one rat raised the pain threshold in *both* rats. Also, the effect of acupuncture in one rabbit could be transferred to another rabbit by cerebrospinal fluid. In 1976, it was reported that substances that were blocked by morphine antagonists were released with acupuncture. A group of substances, identified chemically as peptides and called endorphins, was then localized in the pituitary gland. The *New England Journal of Medicine* (Feb. 3, 1977) reported that the most potent of the endorphins "is 5,000 to 10,000 times more potent than morphine." Moreover, it said that endorphins lead to the release of ADH (antidiuretic hormone) from the posterior pituitary and facilitates the release of FSH (follicle stimulating hormone) and ACTH (adrenocorticotropic hormone) from the posterior pituitary. This group of chemicals appeared to function through the limbic-hypothalamus-pituitary axis. See: G.T. Lee, "A Study of Electrical Stimulation of Acupuncture Locus Tsusanli (St-36) on Mesenteric Microcirculation," *American Journal of Chinese Medicine*, 1974; 2: 53–66; J. S. Han, "Physiology of Acupuncture: Review of Thirty Years of Research," *Journal of Alternative and Complementary Medicine*, 1997; 3: Supp 1: S101–S108; A. Goldstein, "Opioid Peptides Endorphins in Pituitary and Brain," *Science* 1976; 193: 1081–1086; S. H. Snyder, "Opiate Receptors in the Brain," *New England Journal of Medicine*, 1977; 296: 266–271.

Dr. Bruce Pomeranz and a group at the University of Toronto verified and expanded on these findings by studying the responses of animals to painful stimuli after acupuncture. They found that after an induction period of twenty minutes, recordings from the pain-responsive nerve cells in the spinal cord are reduced; that there is an increase in the pain threshold, equated with analgesia, which can be blocked by naloxone (a morphine antagonist), thus implying the presence of endorphins; and that, depending on the frequency of stimulation, at least two different hormonally induced systems may be involved. This relation between acupuncture analgesia and the endorphin system has caused a great deal of excitement in the field of scientific investigation of acupuncture. Dr. Pomeranz has further supported the theory of endorphin relatedness by experimenting with strains of mice deficient in opiate receptors. Unlike their normal counterparts, these mice do not develop analgesia with acupuncture. Additional evidence was produced by using dextronaloxone, the stereoisomer of the active compound levonaloxone, which does not fit into the receptor site and does not block the analgesic effect of acupuncture. See: B. Pomeranz et al., "Acupuncture Reduces Electrophysiological and Behavioral Responses to Noxious Stimuli: Pituitary is Implicated," *Experimental Neurology*, 1977; 54: 172–178; R. S. Cheng and B. Pomeranz, "Electroacupuncture Analgesia Could Be Mediated by at Least Two Pain-Relieving Mechanisms; Endorphin and Non-Endorphin Systems," *Life Sciences*, 1979; 25: 1957–1962; B. Pomeranz and D. Chiu, "Naloxone Blockade of Acupuncture Analgesia: Endorphin Implicated," *Life Sciences*, 1976; 19: 1757–1762; J. M. Peets and

B. Pomeranz, "cxbk Mice Deficient in Opiate Receptors Show Poor Electroacupuncture Analgesia," *Nature*, 1978; 273: 675–676; R. S. Cheng and B. H. Pomeranz, "Electroacupuncture Analgesia Is Mediated by Stereospecific Opiate Receptors and Is Reversed by Antagonists of Type I Receptors," *Life Sciences*, 1980; 26: 631–638.

Human clinical studies of experimentally induced pain and acupuncture analgesia have confirmed that there is an increase in the pain threshold as well as a decrease in the desire to report a stimulus as painful. Evidence also seems to indicate that acupuncture analgesis is blocked by the addition of the opioid antagonist naloxone. Also monoamines (serotonin, dopamine, and noradrenaline) have been implicated in acupuncture analgesia. Serotonin, for example, appears to be important at both the spinal cord and brain levels since acupuncture analgesia is sharply reduced if biosynthesis is blocked, the receptor is blocked, or the neurons destroyed. On the other hand, dopamine and noradrenaline appear to antagonize acupuncture analgesia in the brain and potentiate it in the spinal cord. J. S. Han has also reported cross-tolerance between electroacupuncture and morphine, anatogonism of acupuncture analgesia with brain microinjection of naloxone, attenuation of acupuncture analgesia with brain microinjection of endorphin antibodies, and selective release of enkephalins and dynorphins into cerebrospinal fluid (CSF) following electroacupuncture. D. J. Mayer, D. D. Price, A. Rafii, "Antagonism of Acupuncture Analgesia in Man by the Narcotic Antagonist Naloxone," *Brain Research*, 1977; 121: 368–372; C. R. Chapman, M.E. Wilson and J. D. Gehrig, "Comparative Effects of Acupuncture and Transcutaneous Stimulation on the Perception of Painful Dental Stimuli," *Pain*, 1976; 2: 265–283; 9: 183–197; X. H. Chen and J. S. Han, "All Three Types of Opioid Receptors in the Spinal Cord Are Important for 2/15 Hz Electroacupuncture Analgesia," *European Journal of Pharmacology*, 1992; 211: 203–210; J. S. Han, "Acupuncture Activates Endogenous Systems of Analgesia," In: *NIH Consenses Development Conference on Acupuncture*, Bethesda, MD: NIH, 1997; J. S. Han, *The Neurochemical Basis of Pain Relief by Acupuncture: A Collection of Papers, 1973–1987, Beijing Medical University*. Beijing: Chinese Medical Scientific Publishers, 1987.

More recent evidence supports the notion that one of the mechanisms of acupuncture may be a form of neuroelectric stimulation for the gene expression of neuropeptides. Gao reported changes in μ opioid receptor expression of oncogenes and opioid peptide genes in response to electroacupuncture. (M. Gao et al., "Changes in μ Opioid Receptor Binding Sites in Rat Brain Following Electroacupuncture," *Acupuncture & Electro-Therapeutics*; 1997 22: 161–166.) in H. F. Guo et al., "Brain Substrates Activated by Electroacupuncture (EA) of Different Frequencies (II): Role of Fos/Jun Proteins in EA-Induced Transcription of Preproenkephalin and Preprodynorphin Genes," *Molecular Brain Research*; 1996 43: 167–173.

Recently, the availability of functional Magnetic Resonance Imaging (fMRI) has begun to demonstrate that acupuncture has regionally specific, quantifiable effects on relevant structures of the human brain. Cho and colleagues stimulated an acupuncture point located in the lateral aspect of the foot (Bladder 67) related to vision and showed that it activated an accipital lobes region observed with fMRI that was the same area activated by stimulation of the eye by directly using light. Stimulation of non-acupuncture points 2 to 5 cm away from the vision-related points on the foot failed to activate the occipital lobes. (Z. H. Cho et al., "New Findings of the Correlation Between Acupoints and Corresponding Brain Cortices Using Functional MRI," *Proceedings of the National Academy of Sciences,* 1998; 95: 2670–2673.

For detailed summaries of modern research into the potential scientific mechanisms of acupuncture, see Bruce Pomeranz and Gabriel Stux (eds.), *Scientific Bases of Acupuncture,* (Berlin: Springer-Verlag, 1989); Alan Bensoussan, *The Vital Meridian: A Modern Eploration of Acupuncture* (London: Churchill Livingstone, 1991); Bruce Pomeranz, "Scientific Research Into Acupuncture for Relief of Pain," *Journal of Alternative and Complementary Medicine,* 1996; 2: 53; O. B. Wilson, "Biophysical Modeling of the Physiology of Acupuncture," *Journal of Alternative and Complementary Medicine,* 1997; 3 Supp 1: 25–39; L. F. He, "Involvement of Endogenous Opioid Peptides in Acupuncture Analgesia," *Pain* 1987; 31: 99–121; G. A. Ulett, J. S. Han and S. P. Han, "Traditional and Evidence-Based Acupuncture: History, Mechanisms and Present Status," *Southern Medical Journal* 1998; 91: 115–120.

12. The mechanism by which acupuncture may function is an ongoing recearch agenda. The available modern research from China on the effects and applications of acupuncture from a basic science approach are not well presented and are poorly designed by Western standards (with the important exceptions noted in the previous note). A summary of this Chinese research appears in Shanghai Institute, *Acupuncture* [85], pp. 399–408. The English translation of this text by O'Connor and Bensky (Chicago: Eastland Press, 1981) is excellent. This section is chapter 10. It catalogs studies on animals and humans performed in modern China. The results are wide-ranging, with all the physiological systems undergoing change. A very small sample of the results is as follows:
a. Needling acupuncture point Stomach 36 (*Zu-san-li*) strengthens intestinal peristalsis (muscle contractions in animals, barium transit time in humans). Other points relax the intestines. Using a more refined methodology, some of these findings have been replicated in Western laboratories. See H. O. Jin et al., "Inhibition of Acid Secretion by Electrical Acupuncture Is Medicated via Beta-Endorphin and Somatostatin," *American Journal of Physiology,* 1996; 271: G524–G530. For evidence based on human studies in the West, see Y. Li et al., "The Effect of Acupuncture on Gastrointestinal Function and Disorders," *American Journal of Gas-*

troenterology 1992; 87: 1372–1381; and for animal studies see S. G. Dill, "Acupuncture for Gastrointestinal Disorders," *Problems in Veterinary Medicine*, 1992; 4: 144–154.

b. Needling Large Intestine 4 (*He-gu*) and Triple Burner 5 (*Wai-guan*) causes vasodilation and lowers blood pressure. Needling Pericardium 6 (*Nei-guan*) causes vasoconstriction, helpful in hypotensive states.

c. The heart rate is able to be regulated; a fast beat can be slowed, a slow one can be increased. The general tendency is to reduce heart rate and strengthen cardiac muscle contraction.

d. Beedling Stomach 36 (*Zu-san-li*) and Large Intestine 4 (*He-gu*) increases the level of 17-hydroxycorticosteroids in the blood, sometimes by a factor of two or three. These levels are maintained for a considerable time.

e. The Shenyang Scientific Medical Research Institute, using direct measurement methods, found that the ACTH content of the blood of white rats rose markedly after they received electro-acupuncture.

f. Levels of oxytocin, vasopressin, norepinephrine, follicle stimulating hormone, and prolactin are affected when different points are needled.

g. The immune system is stimulated. Patients with bacillary dysentery show an increase in phagocytosis three hours after acupuncture treatment, which peaks twelve hours after treatment. The effect was greatest with electric acupuncture (a modern technique of hooking the needle to a low-voltage electric current), less sustained with regular acupuncture, and even less with moxibustion alone.

In rabbits, leukocyte counts increase with acupuncture treatment, peaking in three hours.

h. After needling numerous points, acetylcholine concentration in the brain is increased in animals (compared with controls). This indicates an inhibitory state, as in analgesia and anesthesia.

The summary of acupuncture research in China is *Developments in Acupuncture Research* (*Zhen-jiu Yan-jiu Jin-Zhan*), ed. by Traditional Chinese Medicine Research Institute (Beijing: People's Press, 1981). For a summary of the status of acupuncture science research on animals in the West see S. Andersson and T. Lundeberg, "Acupuncture from Empiricism to Science: Functional Background to Acupuncture Effects in Pain and Disease," *Medical Hypotheses* 1995; 45: 271–281.

13. Herbology clearly becomes the dominant tendency of Chinese literate medicine from the Tang Dynasty (618–907 C.E.) onward. The early period seems more concerned with acupuncture. For example, the *Nei Jing* mentions only two herbal prescriptions. Increasingly acupuncturists in the West are using herbs. For example, a report from the United Kingdom shows that 45.5 percent of acupuncturists used herbs. Y. Jin, M. I. Berry and K. Chan, "Chinese Herbal Medicine in the United Kingdom," *Pharmaceutical Journal*, 1995; 255: R37.

14. Jiangsu New Medical Institute, *Encyclopedia of the Traditional Chinese Pharma-copoeia* [32].

15. The toad is *Bufu bufu gargarizens* which has actions that resemble digitalis. For extensive scientific discussions on the pharmacology of this Chinese substance and most other herbs see: H. M. Chang and P. P. H. But, *Pharmacology and Application of Chinese Materia Medica*, vols. 1–2. Some important Western drugs have even been developed from Chinese herbalism. Ephedrine is the most well known and entered the modern Western pharmacopoeia via early-twentieth-century research on the Chinese herb *ephedra* (C. P. Li, *Chinese Herbal Medicine* [Washington, D.C.: John E. Fogarty International Center, U.S. Dept. of HEW, NIH, 1974], p. 5).

16. Figures 3–6 are based on diagrams appearing in Academy of Traditional Chinese Medicine, *An Outline of Chinese Acupuncture* (Beijing: Foreign Languages Press, 1975). The earliest description of Meridian pathways, but without all the points, is the *Ling Shu*, sec. 3, chap. 10.

ORIGINS OF DISHARMONY: STORMY WEATHER

or when a cause is not a cause

In my early student days in China, I worried that the Chinese perception of disease—the ideas as well as the vocabulary—was not only unusual and mysterious, but also just plain silly. It seemed too simple or quaint to talk, as the Chinese do, of Dampness, Wind, or Heat as generative factors in illness. Then one night, while I was having dinner with the Chinese family I lived with, a woman at the table excused herself because of a "head Wind." That incident made me realize how culturally relative my medical perceptions were. To my Chinese friends, the idea of head Wind was not at all outlandish—it was as grounded in reality as the Western concept of the flu. Chinese ideas represent a different way of detecting and organizing information about health and disease.

Chinese medicine and Chinese philosophy, as we have seen, do not concern themselves very much with cause and effect, or with trying to discover *this* cause that begets, in linear progression, *that* effect. Their concern is with relationships, with the pattern of events. Thus, their idea of the way illness begins is very different from the Western view.

In fact, the Chinese do not have a highly developed theory for the origins of disease. They conceive of certain factors that affect a person, factors that could be described in the Western vocabulary as causes. It is therefore tempting to the Western mind to describe them as such, but to the Chinese these generative influences are not exactly causes. Take Dampness, for example. In China, as in the West, ordinary people might say that someone became ill because he or she went out in the rain or because she lives in a damp basement. But to the Chinese, dampness precipitates only a pattern of Dampness; there is no distinction between the illness itself and the factor that "caused" it. The question of cause becomes incidental. In this sense, the word *cause* is almost a synonym for *effect*. In Chinese pattern-thinking (further explained in Chapter 7), what might at first seem to be a cause becomes part of the pattern, indistinguishable and inseparable from the effect. Pattern-thinking subsumes the cause, defining it in terms of the effect and making it part of the total pattern. What we in the West call a cause has little importance in Chinese thought. For Qi and its resonance operational system, the cause, the process, and the outcome merge. The lines of causality are bent into circles.

Nevertheless, the general population in China, and its medical practitioners, when asked "Why is there disharmony?" speak of at least three categories of precipitating factors in illness. These are environment, emotional responsiveness, way of life, and heredity.

The general population, including doctors, will sometimes think of these factors as causes. People assume that Dampness, for instance, can "cause" illness in some people at certain times. Besides the physician, friends, relatives, and neighbors might advise a person to wear a raincoat or to move out of a damp basement.

In the narrower, more precise and refined realm of medicine, pattern-thinking about illness is more complex and nuanced than it is in the general society. To the physician, the view of Dampness, for example, as a cause of disease is less important than two other ways of thinking about it. The physician would first take note of the wet basement as a simple fact, a piece of information, a sign to be considered along with other signs. He may tell the patient to move (i.e., he may treat the Dampness as a cause), but his main concern would be to place this sign into the patient's total configuration of signs— including color of face, pulse, tongue, emotional ambiance, and so forth. The physician would see Dampness as one element of a pattern of disharmony and would not necessarily single it out as a cause needing treatment. The Dampness is just part of the picture. Other people living in the wet basement may not get sick. So something else is going on to make the patient sensitive. The physician's gaze inevitably goes to the complete arrangement of signs. If the patient can't move out of the basement, the doctor would try to reharmonize him or her so as to eliminate the sensitivity to Dampness. And even if the patient could change homes, he or she would still need reharmonizing to deal with the pattern carried within that is susceptible to Dampness. Chinese medicine refuses to see Dampness as an isolatable entity.

The amount of attention given to such relationships leads to the second and more important way a Chinese physician understands Dampness—as both an individual and a universal pattern. Dampness is a pattern of qualities and events that becomes an emblematic representation, a "diagnostic" image of internal disharmony or an internal meteorological report. Dampness means the human landscape is "boggy." The person is a microcosm manifesting the same configuration of signs as does the macrocosm. Dampness in the environment is wet, heavy, sodden, and lingering; Dampness in the body makes a person heavy, bloated, and slow. If one's internal pattern is very "swampy," one can manifest such bodily signs without ever having been exposed to a drop of external moisture. It is important to note that the Dampness outside the body may precipitate a condition of Dampness within the body, but exposure in a causal sense is unnecessary. One is more likely to have a Damp illness in London, but it is still possible in Arizona. Dampness is recognized by what is going on inside, not by knowledge of external exposure. The condition is not *caused* by Dampness; the condition *is* Dampness. The cause is the effect; the line is a circle. The physician sees the bodily pattern as a miniature form of the more general natural image, and because the patterns of the body and of nature are similar, they share an identity of resonating equivalence.

In answer to the question "Why do people get sick?" the Chinese can answer that precipitating factors in one of the three categories—environment, emotion, and way of life—generate illness. But although one or another of these factors may be present at the beginning of an illness, that factor is never seen as separate from the illness. It is part of the web, one of the signs and symptoms the Chinese physician weaves into a diagnosis.

⊣ THE SIX PERNICIOUS INFLUENCES [*liu-yin*]

The six Pernicious Influences are the meteorological factors that play a part in disease. They include six climatic phenomena—Wind, Cold, Fire or Heat, Dampness, Dryness, and Summer Heat[1]—and are also called the six Evils (*liu-xie*).[2] An "internally generated" Pernicious Influence tends to be an assessment of a protracted disharmony and a description of a chronic condition; an "externally generated" Influence tends to be a statement of exposure and imply a sudden onset of illness. As infectious and contagious diseases become a less prominent aspect of health care for significant parts of the world, Internal Pernicious Influences has become the dominant discussion in East Asian medicine.

An Internal Pernicious Influence is a description of a long-term illness or constitutional pattern of disharmony.[3] The Internal Pernicious Influence, which has the name of an atmospheric condition that is considered to be out of control, is a metaphoric representation of "bad weather" that persists in the human terrain. The disharmonious climate has the sense that the Yin-Yang balance has been disrupted and distorted. The label means that the everyday life of a human being and the particular kind of weather manifest similar signs and symptoms, share a resonance of Qi.

When the body is weakened by an imbalance of Yin and Yang, a climatic phenomenon can be said to "invade" the body and become a Pernicious Influence. This is an important Chinese explanation for diseases with sudden onset (e.g. a cold or flu) or dramatic changes in what is typical behavior for a person. It is also a statement that the microcosm is affected "directly" by the macrocosm. When there is such an incursion, the Chinese believe that the body undergoes a conflict between the Pernicious Influence and the Normal Qi. The first encounter of the invading Influence is with the body's Protective Qi. If the Protective Qi is strong, the Influence is expelled and the individual recovers. But if the Qi is weak, or the Pernicious Influence is very strong, the illness develops and goes deeper, becoming more involved with the internal Organs.

Illnesses generated by any of the Pernicious Influences that have invaded the body usually come on suddenly, with no warning. They are characterized by aversion toward the particular Influence (e.g., fear of cold, dislike of wind), fever, chills, body aches, and general malaise. These symptoms are understood to be the result of Normal Qi and Protective Qi attempting to expel the Influence. When a Pernicious Influence invades the body, from the outside, it is called an External Pernicious Influence. All the Pernicious Influences, however, are really models or images for human processes that mimic climatic conditions, and share similar resonance. In the following description of each Influence, both the internal and external aspects are discussed.

Dampness [*shi* 湿]

Dampness is wet, heavy, and slow; it is Yin. Human activity should ceaselessly transform from one state to another; when it gets "bogged down" Chinese medicine sees Dampness. Dampness accumulates, has poor and unclear boundaries, and tends to be "sticky." Dampness is heavy, turbid, and lingering; it has a kind of "soft" overstability. Dampness tends to move downward, and so the *Nei Jing* states that "the lower body is the first area affected by Dampness."[4] When a person experiences Dampness, the head may feel dull—"as if in a sack," the Chinese say. The limbs may feel heavy and sore, and the person will express a dislike for damp environments. Excretions and secretions associated with Dampness are copious and often turbid, cloudy, or sticky, like "sand" in the eyes, cloudy urine, heavy diarrhea, heavy vaginal discharge, or fluid-filled or oozing skin eruptions. Dampness can easily obstruct the movement of Qi, producing fullness of the chest or abdomen and dribbling or incomplete urination or defecation. Dampness can penetrate the Meridians, affecting the limbs and causing heaviness, stiffness, or soreness of the joints.

Dampness resonates with and most easily affects the Spleen. The Spleen rules "the raising of the pure," and transforms the valuable components of food and drink into Qi and Blood. This transmutation depends on a "vaporization" process that requires a dry environment. A traditional Chinese saying sums this up as "The Spleen likes Dryness."[5] The Spleen is therefore especially sensitive to Dampness. Dampness can readily "distress" the Spleen and interfere with its "raising" of pure foods and fluids. This can be seen in signs such as loss of appetite, indigestion, nausea, diarrhea, and abdominal edema. At the same time, however, other Spleen disharmonies, because they prevent the raising or transforming of Fluids, can allow extra moisture to linger in the body, leading to a condition of Dampness elsewhere in the body.

Dampness may affect the Spleen's Consciousness of Potentials (Yi) and creates a morass of a different set of "boggy" problems. In this situation, a person might ruminate easily, constantly worry, be unable to make a decision, help others in a kind of "clinging" way, easily succumb to the "holding on" component of jealousy, be over-sympathetic, be trustworthy and nurturing to others to the point of self-destructiveness, notice that experiences that once were exciting become burdensome, be unable to "let go" or prioritize excessive responsibilities, obsess over ideas, be compulsive, or experience mental unclearness or "flabbiness."

External and Internal Dampness are distinguishable primarily by their speed of onset. External Dampness will be acute and accompanied by other External signs, but will easily turn into Internal Dampness. And Internal Dampness will make a person more susceptible to External Dampness. Either type of Dampness lingers and stagnates, and even External Dampness can last a relatively long time.

CLINICAL SKETCH *Two patients have painful, vesicular lesions on their bodies. The first patient has the eruptions on his face, the second patient has them on her lower trunk. A biomedical doctor diagnoses both conditions as herpes zoster and prescribes analgesics for the pain, as there is no especially effective biomedical treatment for the virus causing the disease. The patients go to a Chinese doctor, who will probably recognize overlapping (they both have red, painful, and swollen eruptions, which is Heat) but distinct patterns of disharmony (they are located in different places). The patient with face blisters will be seen to have more of a Wind component while the patient whose eruptions are on the lower trunk will be considered to have a Dampness component because of its being in the lower part of the body. The treatments will differ accordingly. This illustration is based on the incident mentioned in the Introduction to the first edition. If these Chinese treatments prove to be effective in randomized controlled clinical trials, it may be because some of the herbs used to treat this condition have demonstrated the ability to inhibit virus in vitro.[6] Also it seems that selecting an herbal treatment solely on the basis of biomedical knowledge would probably have been less effective than combining the herbs according to traditional methods.[7]*

Mucus (*tan*) is a form of Internal Dampness. It is a "concentrated" chronic Dampness and is seen in conjunction with a great many disharmonies.

The term *Mucus* includes the Western meaning of a secretion of the mucous membranes visible, for instance, in the form of phlegm. But it also has other characteristics and connotations that make it an entirely different concept from that of Western physiology. Mucus generally arises with disharmonies of the Spleen or Kidneys that affect the movement of Water in the body. Such a condition allows

Dampness to linger, and the Dampness may condense, creating Mucus. Mucus is thick and heavy, heavier than Dampness. It can more easily cause obstructions and can generate lumps, nodules, or tumors.

When Mucus disturbs the Consciousness of Potentials (Yi), the signs will resemble a more exaggerated and focused Dampness. Symptoms can include mental confusion, extreme obsessive ideation, repetitive and fixed ruminations, and even loss of contact with reality and delusions. (Some of this symptomology overlaps with a joint Spleen/Heart pattern; see Chapter 8). Mucus affecting the Heart Spirit alone will lead to inappropriate or bizarre behavior, stupor, or comalike states. When Mucus collects in the Lungs, there may be coughing with heavy expectoration or deeply entrenched grief. Mucus in the Meridians may result in numbness, paralysis, or the development of nodules and soft mobile tumors. Mucus in the throat can cause the sensation of a lump in the throat. An examination of the tongue and pulse will tell a physician whether or not Mucus is present in a disharmony. A thick, "greasy" coating on the tongue or a slippery pulse are the two most important signs. (See Chapter 6) Whenever there is Mucus, it implies Dampness.

Wind [feng 风]

Wind is quick, light, and dry; it is Yang. Human activity should have times of stillness and stability; when there is disturbance with excess movement, Chinese medicine often sees Wind. Wind is the Qi of distorted locomotion. Wind in human activity resembles Wind in nature. It produces change and urgency in what would otherwise be smooth and even, and it causes things to appear and disappear rapidly. Wind affects the body just as it moves the branches and leaves of a tree; things are pushed or become helter-skelter.

Wind (especially Internal Wind) resonates with and most easily affects the Liver. A healthy Liver creates the ambience of smooth and relaxed movement. A distortion in the Liver creates irregular, disjointed, turbulent, and chaotic movement for the Liver itself and

nurturing. Often Cold and Dampness appear simultaneously or mutually generate one another.

Internal Cold is related to insufficient Yang and is associated with the Kidneys, since the Kidneys have the Life Gate Fire and are the source of the person's Yang. Internal Cold often is evident when the Kidneys' functions become weak and the person feels cold. In this case, Cold signs include frail legs and back, frequent urination and edema (Fire unable to control Water), needing extra blankets at night, failure to develop or thrive, or lack of sexual desire. If Cold affects the Will, a person can be deeply passive and fearful, susceptible to a collusion of the Will (having another Will take over his own), or feel excessively guilty (taking responsibility for actions that he or she did not intend or had no responsibility for causing). Cold also resonates with the Spleen (the Spleen needs the Kidneys' Fire to function); when this happens, Cold and Dampness usually coexist because the Spleen is sensitive to Dampness.

External Cold disharmonies, like all External Pernicious Influences, come upon the person suddenly. They are usually accompanied by the fear of cold, as well as chills, mild fever, headache, and body aches. Usually the chills are more pronounced than the fever, and the fever is interpreted as the body's effort to expel the External Influence. This type of External Cold usually belongs to the Lungs.

CLINICAL SKETCH *A male patient complains of difficulty in urinating and of dribbling urine, problems that gradually become more frequent over several years. A Western physician diagnoses a prostate condition (benign prostatic hypertrophy). The patient visits a Chinese physician, who notices that his face is pale and he is wearing a lot of sweaters. The patient tells the physician that he has always disliked cold and that he sleeps curled up. These and other signs, such as a deep, slow pulse and a pale, moist tongue, point to a pattern of Internal Cold. Treatment might include moxibustion, stimulation by burning mugwort, at such points as Governor Vessel 4 (Ming-men, Life Door) and Kidney 2 (Ran-gu, Blazing Valley) in order to strengthen the Kidney Qi. The physician might also prescribe decoctions containing praying mantis cocoons, as they enter the Kidney Meridian and strengthen or tonify the Life Gate Fire.*[14]

Heat [*re* 热] *or Fire* [*huo* 火]

The terms *Heat* and *Fire* can be used interchangeably, although Heat usually connotes an External Pernicious Influence and Fire an Internal Pernicious Influence. Fire, however, is also a normal characteristic of the body. It is the body's Yang aspect, as opposed to the Yin, one of the two bodily principles that must be kept in balance. The Fire that is the normal Yang of the body should not be confused with Fire Pernicious Influence. The difference is a matter of proportion or location in the human landscape.

Heat or Fire, because of its characteristic of being hot and active, is a Yang phenomenon. Its signs within the body resemble its manifestations in nature. When Heat Pernicious Influence is present, the whole body or portions of it feel hot or appear hot. The person affected by it dislikes heat and has a preference for cold. He or she will display such signs as high fever, a red face, red eyes, and dark, reddish urine. Heat can also collect in small areas of the body's surface, creating Fire Poison (what in the West would be called inflammation). Its symptoms are carbuncles, boils, reddish ulcers, or other skin lesions that are red, swollen, raised, and painful. Secretions and excretions related to Heat or Fire Pernicious Influence tend to be sticky and thick and to feel hot: cough with thick yellow mucus or stools with mucus and blood accompanied by burning sensation in the anus. Heat or Fire Pernicious Influences can also dry out bodily matter and deplete the Fluids. Thus, a dry tongue, unusual thirst, dry stools, or scanty urination are other possible signs of the presence of this Influence.

Heat Pernicious Influence, being a Yang phenomenon, induces movement, as does Wind. Wind is more mobile, however, and its movement is trembling or spasmodic, sudden or abrupt. Heat, on the other hand, is said to induce "reckless movement," especially of Blood and Heart Spirit. In the Blood, such movement often leads to hemorrhaging and red skin eruptions. In the Heart Spirit, "reckless movement" may be recognized by confused speech or delirium, for instance, in a patient with a high fever. External Heat or Fire disharmonies are marked by high fever, headache (since Heat rises), swollen and sore throat, dry mouth, great thirst, desire for cold, occasional bloody sputum, skin eruptions, irritability, or delirium. There is usually a higher fever with Heat than with Cold and only slight or no chills, more headaches, and fewer body aches. This is because Heat tends to rise and it obstructs the Meridians less than Cold does. As with the other External Pernicious Influences, the onset of illness is usually sudden.

Internal Heat or Fire develops from disharmonies of the Yin and Yang of the various Organs and takes multiple forms. It will be discussed in Chapter 7.

CLINICAL SKETCH *A patient suddenly gets a high fever and a severe sore throat. She has a red face, a dry, hacking cough, and no fear of cold. A Western physician takes a throat culture and discovers the presence of Group A Betahemolytia strep-tococcus. Antibiotic drugs are prescribed, with good results. If the same patient had gone to a Chinese physician, he very likely would have diagnosed a Heat Pernicious Influence. Herbs like* Coptis *and* Scutellena, *which disperse and cool Fire, would have been prescribed. The results probably would have been adequate though not as dependable as the antibiotic treatment. Modern research shows, incidentally, that both* Coptis *and* Scutellena *inhibit the growth of streptococcus bacteria. Acupuncture treatment, such as needling Large Intestine 4 (He-gu, Adjoining Valleys), to cool Fire, would in this case have offered some symptomatic relief and heightened the body's resistance, but would have been less effective than herbs.*[15]

Dryness [*zao* 燥] *and Summer Heat* [*shu* 暑]

Dryness and Summer Heat are two distinct Pernicious Influences, but they are much less important than Wind, Cold, Heat, and Dampness. This is because they are less frequently used as a description of the inner environment and other influences can represent them. In clinical practice they are even more overlooked than they are in the traditional theory.

Dryness Pernicious Influence is a Yang phenomenon. It is also closely related to Heat. Dryness and Heat are on a continuum, with the Dry end emphasizing dehydration and the Heat end emphasizing redness and hotness. Thus, Dryness is accompanied by dry nostrils, lips, and tongue, cracked skin, and dry stools.

External Dryness often interferes with the circulating and descending functions of the Lungs, manifesting perhaps a dry cough with little phlegm, thirst, bleeding nose, or chest pain, as well as the signs of suddenness, fever, body aches, and other symptoms characteristic of the External Pernicious Influences. The common disharmonies that involve Internal Dryness will be discussed in Chapter 8.

Summer Heat is purely an External Pernicious Influence that always results from exposure to extreme heat. Its symptoms include sudden high fever and heavy sweating. Summer Heat easily injures the Qi, causing exhaustion, and depletes the Fluids. It often occurs together with Dampness.

· The six Pernicious Influences, Internal or External, can never be seen in isolation from the body. They can only be recognized by the signs and symptoms that accompany them. And those signs and symptoms are part of a human pattern that is greater than any one Pernicious Influence. The Dampness or the Wind-Cold that begins a disharmony is part of the disharmony itself, and the disharmony contributes to the condition of Dampness or Wind-Cold. The linear idea of cause and effect becomes a circle in Chinese medicine, because Chinese pattern-thinking subsumes all the pieces into a more important whole.

Dampness or Wind-Cold or other climatic phenomena are finally descriptions of human landscapes, metaphors that relate what's going on in the body to its complement in the universe. As causes, they are secondary to the overall pattern. In fact, in some cases, exposure to Dampness may generate a Cold condition, or exposure to Cold may generate a Wind-Heat condition. And if someone has been exposed to Dampness but manifests a Heat pattern, then Heat is what counts. Treatment will be for Heat, not for Dampness. In biomedicine, it is often impossible to treat a condition without knowing the cause; in Chinese medicine, the treatment is always for the condition itself, regardless of the "cause." The Pernicious Influence, as a cause, is unimportant.

An individual may have tendencies toward a certain state—one person is usually Cold or Damp, while another is Hot or Dry. Each of these people will receive a Pernicious Influence in his or her own way, so that it will become part of that person's unique pattern. The Pernicious Influence does not have any characteristics that belong to it alone and that are not defined by its manifestations in a particular person.

The Pernicious Influence can only influence—it cannot determine. And with all the elements that are considered in Chinese medicine, it is just one piece, another sign to be woven into the pattern.

—| THE SEVEN EMOTIONS [*qi-qing* 七 情]

Ordinary Chinese speak of emotions as "causes" of disease. But emotions are "causes" in the same way as the Pernicious Influences. Excessive anger, worry, or stress can cause illness in the same way that living in a damp basement can be hazardous. In this sense, emotions have a proximal causal relation to disharmony. But more important, emotions share the circular logic of Chinese medicine: the cause is also the outcome. Emotions could be considered prominent "atmospheric" phenomena of the human landscapes. Emotions are a generating influence, but ultimately they are another sign to be understood as part of the human landscape.

The Chinese recognize that emotional responsiveness is a critical component to healthy human life.[16] But the passions also easily lose their proportion and become a "cause" and an important sign of a pattern of disharmony. An emotion in excess, an inappropriate reaction, a self-destructive passion, an emotional response out of proportion to a situation, or a single automatic habitual response to many different life events all can be signs that the human being has lost his or her capacity for harmonious reactivity.

The *Nei Jing* cites seven basic emotions that particularly affect a person and that are still considered most important: elation, anger, sadness, grief, worry, fear, and fright. The differences between sadness and grief, fear and fright, appear to be of degree; sometimes these pairs are combined as one emotion. Of course, emotional qualities are not in themselves pathological, and all of them appear in healthy individuals. It is only when an emotion is either excessive or insufficient over a long period of time, or when it arises very suddenly with great force, that it can generate imbalance and illness. And the reverse is also true: somatic states can generate unbalanced emotional states.

Emotional excess or insufficiency acts on the Qi and on the other fundamental textures. The *Nei Jing* states that "excess elation is associated with slow and scattered Qi; excess anger induces the Qi to ascend; excess sadness and grief weakens the Qi; excess worry generates 'knottedness' or 'stuckness'; fear results in descending Qi; and fright induces chaotic Qi."[17]

The seven emotions are also thought to correlate with the five Yin Organs: worry with the Spleen, anger with the Liver, fear and fright with the Kidneys, elation with the Heart, and sadness and grief with the Lungs. Disharmonies in one of these Organs tend to produce an imbalance in the corresponding emotion and vice versa. Excessive worry, for example, may result in stagnation of the Qi or Dampness, thereby disturbing the Spleen's function of transforming food and leading to such abdominal symptoms as stomach distention or poor digestion. When excessive anger affects the Liver, there may be signs such as dizziness, chest congestion, or a bitter taste in the mouth. Excessive sadness or grief may weaken the Lung Qi, while great fear can make Kidney Qi descend, even to the point of causing a person to lose control of urination. Excessive elation can scatter the Heart Qi and cause confused behavior.

The five basic emotions share a connection with the five Spirits and the five virtues. The passions are a kind of "deformed" virtue sharing identical resonances but existing in a chaotic or unstructured form. The five Spirits should be able to harness the five emotions and allow their energy to become virtues. Worry and excessive pondering is distressing, but it can be the basis for envisioning new possibilities in the world. Worry is transformed by the Consciousness of Potentials (Yi) into creativity and faithful support. Anger is a sensitivity to others but can also be an especially potent foundation for human kindness. The Non-Corporeal Soul (Hun) transforms assertiveness and awareness of others into benevolence. Fear detects the unknown, but it has the same energetic quality that is sensitive to and can embrace Wisdom and the trust of faith. The Will transmutes angst into wisdom. The awareness of loss and the experience of grief is not far removed from a cherished and awesome recognition of completion. The Corporeal Soul (Po) turns sadness into preciousness and beauty. The potential disruption of elation can easily become the warmth of human contact. The Heart Spirit finds the genuine connection in elation. This transformation of emotional Qi into a virtue with a similar quality of Qi at a more coherent level of organization often requires an inner effort of self-reflection. It may benefit from the assistance of herbs and acupuncture.

In the over 2,000 years of Chinese medical writings on the emotions, as with every topic, there has been a diversity of opinions and serious debate. One of the most interesting discussions, both theoretically and therapeutically, can be found in the writings of the greatest physician of the Tang dynasty, Sun Si-miao (590–682 C.E.). Some of his notions have an astonishingly modern ring, and it is worth transmitting the bottom line of his insight: people suffer illness "because they do not have love in their life and are not cherished."[18] His ideas on love were not systematized into the seven emotions theory but have found a place in therapeutics and the discussion of the patient-physician relationship. (See Chapter 9.)

CLINICAL SKETCH *This case is drawn from the author's personal practice files. A young 33-year-old woman returned to my office after having been successfully treated ten years previously for primary amenorrhea. She was recently diagnosed with inoperable uterine cancer. After extensive chemotherapy and radiation, the cancer had spread to the lungs. She had pain in the chest and a dry, weak cough.*

She was tired. She was doing a myriad of other "unconventional" interventions. She wavered between being hopeful that alternative therapies would save her life and facing her death. She felt deep sadness and anger. Fear was much less prominent. Some of these feelings were directed at the cancer; much was directed at her partner and her father. We discussed her healing strategy and how I might fit in. Regrettably, I told her that I had no solutions for the physical disease of cancer but was willing to try and help her as much as I could. I gave her herbs and acupuncture for the chest pain and cough. I gave her tonic herbs for her Deficient Qi. Luckily, both problems responded quickly. I also included Lung herbs (e.g., Ophiopagon japonicus) and acupuncture points (e.g., Lung 3, Tian Fu, Celestial Mansion) for the grief and Liver herbs (e.g, Paeonia lactifora) and acupuncture points (e.g., Gall Bladder 44, Qiao-yin, Portal Yin) for anger. She thought these treatments helped as well; she felt a renewed sense of awe toward life and felt more kind toward others. Her physical condition continued to deteriorate, but she maintained her determination. She invited me to her wedding, which turned out to be both very beautiful and tragically sad. Her father was there and on his own initiative told me that his daughter had forgiven him for his years of earlier neglect. He cried quite a bit. Her family invited me to the funeral several weeks later. I felt fortunate to have been able to spend time with her at the end of her life. I hope my treatments helped.

⊣ WAY OF LIFE [*bu-nei-wai-yin* 不 内 外 因]

This category of precipitating factors is traditionally called "not External, not Internal." In other words, it includes those factors that are neither Pernicious Influences (External) nor emotions (Internal). To the West, these are usually considerations of lifestyle, and so they have been categorized as such. This category also includes inherited constitution and disposition.

A discussion of lifestyle and medicine poses a special problem. Lifestyle is not the province of medicine alone, but is also the concern of the culture as a whole and all its members. What is considered harmonious, valuable, and correct in medicine may be an unexamined cultural belief that has been incorporated into the medical system. Sometimes it is simple to distinguish a deeply held cultural prejudice and a principle that is more exclusively a medical issue. For example, the great physicians of the Far East usually believed rice to be the "central" grain for human life. Obviously, this recommendation would be seen as too parochial for Westerners. Or a more extreme example would be the notion accepted by the authors of the *Nei Jing* that honoring an emperor is a positive value with health benefits. Clearly, this is a societal norm that has adopted a medical guise. Lifestyle, much more than any other medical consideration, can easily carry the imprint of such unexamined cultural biases. This caveat notwithstanding, lifestyle must necessarily be a major clinical consideration for the East Asian physician, whether practicing in the East or West. How a person lives is a critical piece of the landscape. But the physician's perception, judgment, or recommendation must be carefully considered and must be in the context of a patient's own unique culture, history, and individual options. In "cross-cultural" medicine, the practitioner must avoid his or her cultural preconceptions. This is especially true because physicians have enormous and disproportional power and must avoid imposing their own personal judgments.

Lifestyle, like Dampness or anger, must be seen in a two-pronged manner. On the one hand, the discussion may be about "cause," but, on the other hand, the discussion is very much a description of behavior, a sign of activity, that needs to be integrated into a perception of a pattern.

Diet

Diet is considered an important influence on health and illness in Chinese medicine, and many books are devoted to dietary considerations. Because the Stomach receives food and the Spleen is responsible for transforming it into Qi and Blood, these two Organs are most affected by diet.

Irregularity in quantity or quality of food, or in time of eating, can disrupt bodily harmony. Insufficient food or lack of proper food can mean that insufficient raw material reaches the Spleen. There will then be Deficient Qi and Blood, in the whole body or in certain Organs. Excess food that obstructs the Stomach's "ripening" and the Spleen's "transforming" is called "Stagnant Food" and may lead to such symptoms as distension, sour belching, or diarrhea.

A predilection for certain types of food can also generate disharmony. The Chinese say that too much raw food can strain the Yang aspect of the Spleen and generate Internal Cold Dampness resulting in such signs as abdominal pain, diarrhea, or weakness. Fatty and greasy foods, alcohol, or sweets can produce Dampness and Heat. Improperly cleaned food may injure digestion. Different tastes resonate with different organs.

The Chinese people know many types of food, combinations of foods, and methods of preparation that are sometimes prescribed in medical literature and practice. This book is not primarily concerned with therapeutics, so Chinese dietary suggestions are not discussed. Diet, more than most other therapies, is strongly tied to a society's particular customs and habits. The physician needs to be culturally sensitive, as most Chinese dietary concepts are not easily transferable to Western culture. No Chinese book could tell Westerners what to eat for breakfast—Westerners would probably not be able to find the ingredients or prepare them, nor would many of them want to eat the result. And the Chinese could never give a reasoned opinion, based on empirical experience, on precisely when to eat or not to eat lasagna.

Sexual Activity

Sexuality and sexual activity are powerful factors in health and illness. Sexuality is deeply personal, steeped in pervasive cultural norms and often influenced by power and class position. Social constraints and moral judgments can be hidden as medical or "natural" facts. Separating what is medical from what is a more "arbitrary" imposition of society can be difficult if not impossible.[19]

Like any society, China's relationship to sexuality has been complex. Attitudes toward various forms of sexual behavior—such as same-sex relationships (ancient China's elite, like classical Greece, was often homosexually centered), sexual versus reproductive relationships, autoeroticism, masturbation, transsexualism, fetishism—and the essential question of how to balance duty and pleasure varied tremendously and differentially influenced medical texts.[20] The discussion of what is "proper" sexuality often merges with what is "healthy" sexuality; medical knowledge often masks social constraints and culturally contrived norms. The bottom line, however, is that the East Asian physician recognized sexuality as a basic and fundamental force in the human landscape.

Chinese medicine considered that, to the extent that sexuality has an intimate relationship to reproduction, its roots lie in the Kidney's Essence (Jing). Sexual dysfunction can be a sign of Kidney disharmony as well as lead to Kidney disharmony. The dynamic of sexuality and reproduction depends on healthy Essence and the balance of the Kidney's Fire and Water. Disharmonious sexuality—diminished or exaggerated libido, painful or uncomfortable sexual intercourse, inability to have sexual relations, premature ejaculation, inability to reach sexual climax—can lead to disharmony or be a symptom of Kidney Essence disharmony.

But sexuality (and especially in its relationship to sensuality) is modulated by all the Organs. For example, the Spleen allows sexuality to be nurturing, the Liver allows it to be assertive, and the Heart allows it to be affectionate and warm. Spleen disharmony can be associated with inappropriate obligation and loyalty; Liver sexuality can be overly or insufficiently aggressive, and Heart sexuality can be recognized by an overindulgence in seduction or constantly feeling disconnected.

Physical Activity

The category of physical activity includes general life activity. All life activity, to the Chinese, should point toward the goal of living in harmonious balance with the seasons and one's own constitution and stage of life. Yang times—morning, spring, youth—should be active

periods in a person's life; Yin times—evening, winter, old age—
should be quiescent periods. The *Nei Jing*, for instance, mentions
that in the winter one should "go to sleep early but arise late" and
remain dormant "like someone with private intentions or as if one's
intentions were already fulfilled."[21]

Physical activity is important to harmonize the flow of Qi and
Blood and to develop strength in the body. Excessive labor, however,
can strain the Spleen's ability to produce Qi and Blood, leading to
deficiencies of these fundamental textures. The body must rest, but
excessive ease or slothfulness can weaken the vitality of Qi and
Blood. Excessive use of a particular part of the body—a barber's
hand, for instance, or a singer's voice—can lead to strain and disharmony. In some cases, the physician will suggest a change of lifestyle,
but often this is impossible. In the case of a singer, for instance, the
physician would prescribe treatments so that continual use of the
voice would not throw the body out of balance; the physician would
create a balance within the given constraints of a person's unique
options.

An inappropriate lifestyle can be both a generative factor of
disharmony and a manifestation of disharmony itself. Inappropriate
lifestyle accompanies disharmony; there is no beginning or end. A
person who is always "running around" may drain the Qi of the various Organs, or conversely may be manifesting hyperactivity of those
Organs. Someone who is always "sitting around" can cause the Qi
and Blood to stagnate or may be manifesting depressed activity of
the Organs.

Chinese medical practitioners are always concerned with the
maintenance of health. The *Nei Jing* poetically says: "To administer
medicine after an illness begins is . . . like digging a well after becoming thirsty or casting weapons after a battle has been engaged."[22]
Patients are often taught correct diet, proper attitudes, and healthful lifestyles. The central concern is always balance, rhythm, and
harmony. Food, for instance, should be prepared and eaten in balance. Leafy green vegetables, a Yin substance, should be cooked

with ginger, which is Yang. T'ai Chi exercises encourage rhythmic and controlled movement. Adolescents are expected to have different emotional attitudes than the elderly. Frail people should do less demanding work than people with robust constitutions.

Recommendations of this type are not made only by doctors. The determination of what is or is not a healthful lifestyle is made by the society at large and becomes part of a cultural model of "how to live." The theory and practice of health are thus also the concern of philosophers, educators, cooks, homemakers, parents, grandparents, neighbors, and friends. Obviously, physicians must always be careful not to abuse their position of power and "cultural" authority with their patients.

Miscellaneous Factors

The Chinese also recognize several other precipitating factors in illness (which, strangely, belong in the "not External, not Internal" category). These include burns, bites, parasites, and trauma—sudden, easily identifiable conditions and proximal causes of disease. Although these factors can be readily thought of as causes, the Chinese physician must nevertheless consider how they interact with other bodily signs and symptoms, and must discern a pattern to reharmonize. Even a snakebite or a burn cannot be isolated from the rest of a person's being. The miscellaneous factors are extensively dealt with in the therapeutic literature but are not essential to the understanding of the Chinese medical view.

All of the precipitating factors discussed in this chapter would be called causes in the West. But it must be stressed again that in Chinese medicine, a distinct and separable cause is unimportant; the relationships within a pattern are crucial. Any one factor is, finally, another piece of the whole. And the complete patient is treated, never for the cause, but for his or her unique configuration of signs and symptoms. The idea of causality in Chinese medicine is ultimately a means for identifying and qualifying the important relationships between environment, emotional character, personal lifestyle, and health and illness.

NOTES

1. Different historical periods have emphasized different Pernicious Influences in the theory and clinical practice. The *Nei Jing*, for example, deals extensively with Wind but briefly with Fire. Cold, in this earlier period, is usually considered the source of febrile illnesses. Later periods will emphasize Heat. For a discussion, see Jia De-dao's *Concise History of China's Medicine* [95], 1979, pp. 66–69, 194. For a discussion of how the concept of Wind changes from pre–*Nei Jing* times until the Han period, see Paul Unschuld, *Medicine in China*, 1985, pp. 67–72; and Shigehisa Kuriyama, "The Imagination of Winds and the Chinese Conception of the Body," in *Body, Subject and Power in China*, Zito and Barlow (eds.), 1994.

2. Besides the Pernicious Influences, there is the concept of Pestilences—*li-qi* or *yi-qi*. Pestilence is considered an additional External Pernicious Influence. It is first mentioned in the *Su Wen* (sec. 21, chap. 71), but the idea was not fully developed until Wu You-xing wrote his Discussion of Warm Epidemics [25] in 1642 C.E. In that book, he discussed "warm epidemics" or "pestilence" as separate from climatic conditions but able to affect even the healthiest body with great virulence. However, appropriate treatment methods are still based on determining which of the six Pernicious Influences the Pestilence resembles.

3. The understanding of External and Internal aspects of a Pernicious Influence varies with historical period. An example of the discussion concerning this problem in relation to Wind and apoplexy appears in Shanghai Institute, *Lecture Notes on Traditional Chinese Internal Medicine* [54], p. 162.

4. *Su Wen*, sec. 8, chap. 29, p. 180.

5. Beijing Institute, *Foundations* [38], p. 57.

6. An excellent discussion of herpes zoster appears in Guanganmen Hospital, "Collected Clinical Experiences of Zhu Ren-kang," *Dermatology* [73], pp. 70–76. Only one of the prescriptions recommended for herpes zoster does not include some herbs listed in Chen Xin-qian, *Pharmacology: New Edition* [71], pp. 121–131 as inhibiting the growth of virus. The main herbs are *Baphicacanthes cusia*, *Taraxacum mongolicum*, and *Portulaca oleracea*. All these herbs are considered useful in cooling Heat. For an English discussion of herpes zoster, see De-hui Shen, Nissi

Wang, and Hsiu-fen Wei, *Manual of Dermatology in Chinese Medicine*, Seattle: Eastland Press, 1996.

7. The hospital that edited Dr. Zhu's cases (see note 6) reported that in the 144 cases of herpes zoster treated by traditional methods between January 1974 and June 1975, a noticeable and significant reduction of length of illness and severity of pain was observed as compared with cases treated with Western methods or those receiving no treatment ("Collected Clinical Experiences of Zhu Ren-kang," *Dermatology* [73], p. 76).

8. *Su Wen* [1], sec. 12, chap. 42, p. 236.

9. Ibid., sec. 12, chap. 42, p. 238.

10. Ibid., sec. 8, chap. 29, p. 180.

11. Reports such as "Analysis of Effectiveness of Traditional Chinese Herbal Medicines in 150 Cases of Influenza and Preliminary Analysis of 1006 Cases Using Acupuncture for Treatment of Influenza," in *Journal of Traditional Chinese Medicine* (JTCM), February 1960, indicate that traditional methods of treatment can sometimes be effective. For a discussion of acute respiratory infections and Chinese herbs see C. Liu and R. M. Douglas, "Chinese Herbal Medicines in the Treatment of Acute Respiratory Infections: A Review of Randomized and Controlled Clinical Trials," *Medical Journal of Australia*, 1998; 169: 579–582.

12. *Su Wen*, sec. 11, chap. 39, p. 218.

13. Ibid., sec. 22, chap. 74, p. 539.

14. For an interesting clinical report on how Chinese medicine views and treats swollen prostate, see "Preliminary Experience in Combining Traditional Chinese and Western Medicine to Treat Swollen Prostate in Sixty-Five Cases," JTCM, February 1980, pp. 34–35. In this patient group four main types of patterns were discovered: a Damp-Heat pattern; a Deficient Yin pattern; a Deficient Yang pattern (as in the example given); and a Deficient Spleen Qi pattern. Using only Chinese herbal medicines, results based on subjective reports showed that forty patients recovered normal urination, eleven improved, and nine had no change. (The biomedical treatment involved use of a catheter when necessary.) For further examples of the Chinese treatment of BPH see: J. M. Jia, "Observation on Effect of Xiaolong Tongbi Capsule in Treatment of Benign Prostatic Hypertrophy and Study on Its Mechanism," JTCM, 1998; 39: 664–667 and S. Ge and F. Meng, "Acupuncture in the Treatment of Chronic Prostatitis: A Report of 350 Cases," *International Journal of Clinical Acupuncture*, 1991; 2: 19–23.

15. For a discussion of the antibiotic effects of the two herbs mentioned, see Shanghai First Medical Hospital, *Clinical Handbook of Antimicrobial Medicines* [82], pp. 77–78. The possible mechanism of acupuncture's role in infectious illnesses is not so well described in the literature as the probable herbal mechanisms. However, some research has been reported, as in "Role of Humoral Immunity in Acute

Bacillary Dysentery Treated with Acupuncture," JTCM, April 1980. This study reports that acupuncture on humans produced marked increases in the level of immunoglobulin, total complements, specific antibodies, fecal SIgA, and the bactericidal properties of plasma. The same article reports that according to analysis of serum lysozyme and the phagocytosis of reticuloendothelial cells of the liver in rabbits, acupuncture appears to stimulate and strengthen humoral immunity.

16. Any discussion of emotions in East Asia must consider the complex cross-cultural questions embedded in the continuum and interaction of the psyche and soma. As we have noted before, East Asian medicine has always recognized the psychosomatic assumption that psychological and physiological processes are interactive and have a shared clinical significance. For example, on a very simple level, Oriental medicine can see anxiety and heart palpitations, fear and sweating, revulsion and nausea, anger and changes in metabolism, despair and sighing as being emotional and physical concomitants of a single yin-yang manifestation. Nevertheless, Eastern and Western people may tend to experience different ends of this continuum in their actual lives. What may be a single "energetic" phenomenon in Oriental medical theory may appear to be a different experience for people in different cultures. Any discussion of emotions must ultimately take this question into account. For an insightful phenomenological discussion concerning the unique and distinct manner psychological and somatic symptoms are linked and buried in the Chinese medical semantic network, see Thomas Ots, "The Angry Liver, the Anxious Heart and the Melancholy Spleen: The Phenomenology of Perceptions in Chinese Culture," *Culture, Medicine and Psychiatry* 1990; 14: 21–58.

Probably the most important discussion in the cross-cultural psychiatry literature in relationship to emotions in East Asia is the question of somatization (communicating or experiencing psychological discomfort through a somatic medium). It is often the case that illness complexes that are recognized in the West as primarily affective emotional disorders are often experienced as being somatic in the East. This inquiry has mostly been in terms of contemporary Asian people and the applicability of Western-defined psychological symptomology or disease categories. Most cross-cultural studies seem to corroborate Tseng's early conclusion that "Chinese patients tend to somatize their emotional conflicts." (W. S. Tseng, "The Nature of Somatic Complaints Among Psychiatric Patients: The Chinese Case," *Comprehensive Psychiatry*, 1975; 15.) Kleinman has confirmed these notions: "minor psychiatric problems—depression, anxiety reaction, hysteria, psychophysical reactions, etc.—are most commonly labeled as medical (physical) illnesses. That is, the secondary physical complaints accompanying the psychological disorders are labeled as medical problems, while the psychological issues are systematically left unlabeled." (Arthur Kleinman, "Depression, Somatisation and the New Cross-Cultural Psychiatry," *Social Science and Medicine*, 1977; 11: 3–10, p. 6.) In contemporary China it has often been noted that "the Chinese medical care system does not recognize and deal with psychosocial issues in illness, nor does it give much attention to any mental disorder other than schizophrenia." (David Mechanic and Arthur Kleinman, "Ambulatory Medical Care in the People's Republic of China: An Exploratory Study," *American Journal of Public Health*, 1980, 70: 62–68, p. 65.) And as Lau states: "depressive illness often passes unrecognized in domiciliary practice, because of its tendency to hide behind a facade of somatic symptoms that command the patient's as well as the doctor's attention." (B. Lau et al., "How Depressive Illness Presents in Hong Kong," *Practitioner*, 1983: 227: 112–115, p. 112.) With the exception of studies like the Ots study mentioned above, very little work has been done to systematically investigate this issue in the context of East Asian medicine or East Asian medical history. For a student of Chinese medicine, this cross-cultural issue is apparent when he makes his first visit to China for further study. First-hand clinical experience frequently prompts Western observers to remark, "It seems as if all the patients have read the textbooks." Patients in China often report "neat" problems with details concerning particulars of perspiration, gradations of thirst, various tastes in the mouth and other description that are routine components of health care discourse in China. (See Chapter 6.) People have learned to monitor themselves on this level and this is what doctors elicit. Little psychological or existential detail is involved. Practitioners in the Orient "choose to focus on somatic complaints as a point of departure for therapeutic intervention. Dealing directly with psychological and social factors would destroy rapport and minimize cooperation." (Margaret Lock, "The Organization and Practice of East Asian Medicine in Japan: Continuity and Change," *Social Science and Medicine* 1980; 14B: 345–253, p. 251.) Practitioners in the West seem to have learned to make cross-cultural adjustments. See, for example, Linda Barnes, "The Psychologizing of Chinese Healing Practices in the United States," *Culture, Medicine and Psychiatry*, 1998; 22: 413–443.

17. *Su Wen*, sec. 11, chap. 39, p. 221.

18. Sun Si-miao, *Supplemental Wings to the Thousand Ducat Prescriptions (Qian-jin Yi-fang)*. Beijing: People's Press, 1982 (682 C.E.), vol. 15, p. 166. Love is not usually thought of as a positive feeling, cognitive state, or passion in Chinese thought with the exception of the Mohist idea of "universal love" (*bo ai*). The Confucian ideal of human kindness (*ren*) is much more critical in medical thinking. See Yu-lan Fung's *A History of Chinese Philosophy* for a discussion of the Mohist idea of love.

19. Malinowski long ago noted that "not even the simplest need, nor yet the physiological functions most independent of environmental influences can be regarded as completely unaffected by culture. . . . There is no human activity which we could regard as purely physiological that is "natural." Bronislaw Malinowski, *A Scientific Theory of Culture and Other Essays*, Chapel Hill: University of North Carolina Press, 1944, p. 69. The interpenetration of "natural being" with culture

is developed by such inquiries as Helmuth Plessner, *Laughing and Crying: A Study of the Limits of Human Behavior*, Evanston: Northwestern University Press, 1970; F. J. J. Buytendijk, *Prolegomena to an Anthropological Physiology*, Pittsburgh: Duquesne University Press, 1974.

20. For a discussion of the position of homosexuality in Chinese history, see Bret Hinsch, *Passions of the Cut Sleeve: The Homosexual Tradition in China*, Berkeley: University of California Press, 1990. For English discussions on the diversity of sexual attitudes and practices in historical China, see R. H. van Gulik, *Sexual Life in Ancient China*, Leiden: E. J. Brill, 1974; Fang Fu Ruan, *Sex in China: Studies in Sexology in Chinese Culture*, New York: Plenum Press, 1991; N. H. van Staten, *Concepts of Health, Disease and Vitality in Traditional Chinese Society: A Psychological Interpretation*, Wiesbaden, Germany: Steiner, 1983; and T'ien Ju-K'ang, *Male Anxiety and Female Chastity: A Comparative Study of Chinese Ethical Values in Ming-Ch'ing Times*, Leiden: E. J. Brill, 1988; Douglas Wile, *Art of the Bedchamber*, Albany: State University of New York Press, 1992. For an English-language discussion of contemporary Chinese sexuality besides the Fang Fu Ruan book cited above, see William R. Jankowiak, *Sex, Death, and Hierarchy in a Chinese City: An Anthropological Account*, New York: Columbia University Press, 1993.

21. *Su Wen*, sec. 1, chap. 2, p. 11.

22. Ibid., p. 14.

6

THE FOUR EXAMINATIONS: SIGNS AND SYMPTOMS

and Aristotle and Lao Tzu revisited

The first five chapters discussed the vocabulary and ideas behind the Chinese weaving of patterns. Now the theories of fundamental textures, Organs, Meridians, and Pernicious Influences must become concrete. How do these ideas work when they are applied to a specific patient? How do they enable a physician to perceive a pattern of disharmony? What does the doctor look for, and how are the more important clues distinguished from the less important? How does the doctor begin to deal with all the signs and symptoms a patient presents?

In this chapter, we will follow the procedure a novice physician uses with a patient. We will see the way Chinese physicians examine patients—what they look for, how they judge the significance of what they see, how they interpret the signs and symptoms. These pieces—the stones, mountains, mist, and pebbles of the landscape—can include a wide range of data—physical frame, style of movement, pain, moods, pulse, and many other signs. When these bits and pieces of information are put together, they create the image of a disharmony. In Chapter 9, we will examine an alternative method that is related to how a seasoned and veteran physician might work.

But the very process of examining the pieces of a pattern poses a problem: What do we make of a piece in a system that says that only the whole can determine the meaning of the piece? Before we go on to the examinations, therefore, we should look again at the philosophy that informs Chinese medicine so that our customary Western viewpoint will not interfere with our understanding.

As has been said, Chinese philosophy and medicine are based on Taoist consciousness[1] and on Yin-Yang theory, which imply a world view very different from that of the West. The Chinese could never produce an Aristotelian, and would be hard pressed to accept Aristotle's famous law of contradiction: "There is a principle in things, about which we cannot be deceived but must always, on the contrary, recognize the truth—viz., that the same thing cannot at one and the same time be and not be, or admit any other similar pair of opposites."[2] This principle, that *A* cannot be *not A*, became the cornerstone of all Western logic. Yet little trace of it can be found in either Taoist thought or Chinese medical writings.

A very different spirit informs the Chinese view of knowledge and being. Lao Tzu, the earliest Taoist sage, formulated this understanding of the nature of reality:

> *To be bent is to become straight.*
> *To be empty is to be full.*
> *To be worn out is to be renewed.*
> *To have little is to possess.*[3]

Chuang Tzu, the Taoist philosopher, says:

> *When there is life there is death, and when there is death there is life. When there is possibility, there is impossibility, and when there is impossibility, there is possibility. Because of the right, there is wrong, and because of the wrong, there is right. . . . The "this" is*

also the "that." The "that" is also the "this."... Is there really a
distinction between "that" and "this"?... When "this" and "that"
have no opposites, there is the very axis of Tao.[4]

Change and transformation are the only constants for the Chinese; things (*A* and *not A*, "this" and "that") can simultaneously be and not be. Yin and Yang produce each other, imply each other, and finally *are* each other.

There was at least one pre-Socratic Western philosopher, Heraclitus, who seems to have developed a view of the universe comparable to that of the Taoists. The fragments of his writings that have come down to us set forth his ideas:

The attunement of the world is of opposite tensions,
    as is that of the harp and bow.[5]
The road up and the road down is one and the same.
    The beginning and end are common.[6]
That which is at variance with
    itself agrees with itself.[7]
Cold things become warm, warmth cools,
    moisture dries, the parched get wet.
    It scatters and gathers, it comes and goes.[8]

This Heraclitean notion of primitive flux is very close to that of the Tao. But Heraclitus represents only one skein of Western thought. The dominant ideas were those of Aristotle and his followers, for whom the primary consideration was how things emerge from such flux and achieve distinct existence. The flux had to be differentiated, carved into distinct categories, before there could be reality as Aristotle conceived it. The Aristotelian emphasis on form derives from this concern.

The Chinese, however, never thought of the Tao, or flux, as a vicious undertow from which things must fight free and distinguish themselves. To them, the flux is a vast harmony that embraces all things. They do not ask of an entity how well it measures up to the pure form prescribed for it, but rather what is its relationship to other entities. It is not important or even necessary that every entity attain pure form, but it is important that every entity have a place in the overarching pattern of existence.

In the nineteenth century, Hegel finally confronted and denied Aristotle's law of contradiction and developed the theory that has come to be known as Hegelian dialectics. For Hegel, the intricacies of relationship override the Aristotelian concern that *A* not be confused with *not A*. *A* can, in fact, be other than *A*, depending on its place in an overall schema. These ideas are so similar to those of Chinese philosophy that Hegelian and Chinese thought have often been compared.[9]

But Chinese and Taoist philosophy are not exactly the same as Hegelian dialectics. The Chinese, for example, never elaborated their intuition of the dialectical process into a philosophy of reason as Hegel did. They went no further than to make simple refinements in Yin-Yang theory. They never tried to tame the elusive and changeable qualities of the Tao. The word *Tao*, although sometimes translated as "the Way," cannot really be translated into satisfactory English, and even its meaning in Chinese frustrates the attempt to pin it down. "The Tao that can be told of is not the Tao. The Name that can be named is not the constant name."[10] And so the Chinese have developed ways of alluding to the Tao—in aphorisms, parables, and tales that are more like poetry than like the systematic presentations of Western thought.

But the Tao is not poetry either; to see it as such is also to lose it. The Tao, as the ultimate reality, can be apprehended—in medicine, for instance—but that apprehension has to take place within the context of flux, interconnectedness, and dynamism. The Tao comes to stand for something that does not deny reason, but always manages to remain just outside its grasp. (See Chapter 9.)

The Chinese emphasis on interconnectedness and change takes on a very specific character in the context of medicine. When the young Chinese physician examines a patient, he or she plans to look at many, many signs and symptoms and to make of them a "diagnosis," to see in them a pattern. Each sign means nothing by itself and acquires meaning only in its relationship to the patient's other signs. What it means in one context is not necessarily what it means in another context.

When statements are made in this chapter, therefore, they are always modified by the word *usually*. This is because no statement is going to be specifically true and applicable in every case. In a landscape painting, a mountain *usually* denotes Yang because it is big and hard; but in a picture that focuses on an ocean, mountains may appear in the distance, thus denoting Yin because they are relatively small and passive. The meaning of the mountains is determined by context.

The same is true of the body. A "rapid" pulse, for example, is considered a sign of Heat. The correspondence between rapid pulse and Heat is about as rigid a correspondence as can be found in Chinese medicine. Yet there are cases in which even a rapid pulse can have a different or opposite meaning. A patient may be lying listlessly in bed, covered by many blankets. He is short of breath, his face is pale, and his body is puffy. He has no appetite, his stools are watery, and he has a pale, moist, swollen tongue. These symptoms make up a pattern of Deficiency/Cold disharmony, a Yin disharmony—even though his pulse is 120 beats per minute. In this case, the abnormally fast pulse, usually a sign of extreme Heat, or Yang, signifies extreme weakness, or Yin. *A* is usually *A* but sometimes it is *not A*.

In Chinese medicine, as in Chinese philosophy, one cannot understand the whole until one knows the parts and cannot understand the parts without knowing the whole. Learning a detail, *A*, for instance, is not worth much until the full circle of Chinese medicine has been traveled, at which time *A* will show itself to be rich and useful. The part can only be known when the whole is apparent. This dialectic, this circularity, is a kind of catch-22, but it is also a central aspect of the medicine's artistry. The Chinese interplay of whole and parts does not lend itself to booklike elucidation; the sequential, linear book form can only attempt to approach the intricacies of the Chinese system. But the nature of the difficulty, at least, can be made explicit.

The Chinese resistance to revealing fixed or essential forms has another implication that is worth noting. The word *diagnosis* is sometimes used in this book as a convenience for the reader. As we have said before, for Chinese medicine, *pattern* is a better translation because it has an important implication. For the Chinese, a pattern or a diagnosis is mainly an emblematic category that allows for an exchange of words. It is not meant as a label for people. It has no existence as an abstract "truth" that exists independent of the patient. As the anthropologist Judith Farquhar has noted in other domains of Chinese medicine, such statements "function as allegorical resources for clinical thinking."[11] The pattern description has meaning in practice, not as a fixed ontological entity. As the medical scholar Arthur Kleinman has described, they are "a serious attempt to codify complex, subtle, interactive views of experience into therapeutic formulations that claim contextual rather than categorical application."[12] They are tentative, meant to be tested in practice. The Chinese physician realizes that they are a limited attempt to capture what is necessarily intangible.

Before reading the rest of the chapter, the reader, especially the casual one, should be alert to another potential problem. The rest of this chapter assigns a common interpretation to representative pieces of the human terrain. For some general readers, these descriptions may be tedious. It is worth knowing that it is not necessary to retain or memorize any of the details. One can just skim the information in this chapter and still easily follow the rest of the book's attempt to explain pattern perception.

⊣ THE FOUR EXAMINATIONS [*si-jian* 四 诊]

The neophyte Chinese physician encounters a patient in four stages. (Chapter 9 discusses experienced physicians.) The four stages are called the Four Examinations,[13] because each one focuses on a different way of recognizing signs in a patient. The Four Examinations are Looking, Listening and Smelling (these two words are the same word in Chinese), Asking, and Touching. The physician completes each of the Examinations, gathering signs to weave into the final "diagnosis."

The signs themselves may fall neatly into place, pointing unanimously to a particular disharmony. Or they may seem to contradict each other, requiring the physician to interpret closely and carefully before making a determination. Some signs—like those of the pulse or tongue—are more important than others and are given greater weight. They bring the bodily landscape into focus. Some signs— like headache or blood in the urine—are looked on more as complaints beneath which a disharmony is lurking and are given little diagnostic weight. These complaints demand interpretation and clarification from accompanying signs and symptoms. A complaint is the problem that brings a person to a physician; the patient will usually mention his or her complaint. A sign, however, is something that the doctor looks for but that the patient would not necessarily know or talk about. There are a countless number of possible signs, symptoms, and complaints; this discussion is limited to those signs that are most characteristic of Chinese diagnosis and that make the most important contribution to pattern discernment.[14] The chapter also tends to emphasize somatic signs because these are considered easier for a beginner to learn. Other perceptions and signs that have to do with overall impression or "gestalt" are accurately accessible to only experienced physicians (see Chapter 9.)

An individual sign or symptom may point to a particular Organ or to a quality of disharmony. This chapter describes signs that point to the most commonly found qualities of patterns, the basic shades. The major qualities, of course, are Yin and Yang. Disharmonies always involve imbalances of Yin and Yang. For additional refinement, the Yin-Yang archetypes are often broken down into subcategories: Deficiency and Excess, and Cold and Hot. When the reference is to proportion of textures, Deficiency is the Yin aspect and Excess the Yang; with reference to temperament and level of activity, Cold is Yin and Hot is Yang. The terms *Cold* and *Hot*, of course, designate normal aspects of the body, as well as environmental factors (Pernicious Influences) and qualities of disharmony. Their meanings in any given situation can be distinguished only by the context in which the words are used, but in this chapter they will be considered as qualities of disharmony.*

Looking [*wang-zhen* 望诊]

The first stage of the Four Examinations is Looking. In the Looking Examination, the physician attends to at least four characteristics that are visible to the eye. The first is general appearance, including the patient's physical shape, the patient's manner, the way he or she behaves during the clinical encounter, and the quality of the patient-physician interaction. The second is facial color. The third characteristic is the tongue, including the material of the tongue itself, the coating of the tongue, and its shape and movement. The fourth is the bodily secretions and excretions. These characteristics are presented in the order of observation by the physician. In order of their importance to the novice doctor, however—that is, how much weight they are given when the doctor begins to discern patterns—they are: tongue, facial color, secretions and excretions, and appearance. (Chapter 9 will upset any such ordering.)

Appearance   The patient's physical shape is an indication of his or her health. A person whose appearance is strong and robust is likely

---

*The reason for this apparent lack of precision in terminology lies in the nature of the Chinese language. In this ideographic language, there are relatively few words, and each character has a wide semantic range. A word can be a noun, adjective, or verb depending on its context. There are no verb tenses or moods. The shade or actual meaning of a word is determined by context. Thus a word such as *Heat* can be used to mean the body's normal Heat, or can be a Pernicious Influence, or a quality of disharmony, or the name of a pattern of disharmony. Although there is ambiguity in the Chinese language, however, there is also the possibility of expressing subtle and elusive shades and fusions of meaning.

to have strong Organs. When disharmonies occur in such a person, they are likely to be those of Excess. A weak-looking, frail individual is more likely to have weak Organs and therefore to have disharmonies of Deficiency.

Someone who is overweight is often prone to Deficient Qi, all the more so if he or she tends to be pale and swollen. Heaviness can also be a sign of tendency toward Excess Mucus or Dampness. A thin person, especially one with a sallow complexion, narrow chest, and dry skin—a dried prune appearance—is often prone to Deficient Yin or Blood. Great wasting of flesh in the course of a long illness suggests that the Essence is exhausted.

For acute illnesses, signs of shape are generally the least reliable aspects of a patient's appearance. For chronic illnesses, they show long-term predispositions to certain kinds of disharmony.

The *Nei Jing* states, "Yang is movement, Yin is quiescence."[15] This is the key to examining a patient's manner and emotions. A person who is agitated, outward, talkative, aggressive, and irritable is usually manifesting a Yang tendency. A passive, inward, quiet manner is usually Yin. Heavy, forceful, ponderous movement is typically part of a disharmony of Excess; frail and weak movement usually indicates a Deficiency. Quick movement is usually part of a Heat pattern; slow, deliberate movement is generally part of a Cold pattern. If the patient, when in bed, stretches his feet, removes the covers, or moves away from heat, he may well be suffering from a Heat disharmony. If, on the other hand, the patient curls up in bed, likes to be covered, or wants to be near heat, the doctor would suspect a Cold condition. The assessment of the patient-physician interaction is critical for Chinese medicine, but its "method" is often transmitted to the aspiring physician only during clinical training. It is considered difficult to write about and capture. But some examples are helpful. (More details will be discussed in Chapter 9.) From a modern Western perspective, this examination of the clinical encounter is often dismissed as "subjective," but from the Chinese viewpoint, it may be the only aspect of the human landscape that the practitioner actually witnesses. Every nuance of the interaction, any subtle shift in appearance can contribute to the physician's overall interpretation. For example, if the patient tries to take care of the physician, the physician suspects Dampness. If the patient cannot explain the symptoms clearly, Mucus is probably present. If the physician feels unreasonably pressured by the patient, a Liver excess is likely. If the patient presents complaints with deep angst that seems disproportionately fearful, a Kidney disharmony may be lurking. If the patient seems extremely shy or vulnerable, easily blushes, or touches the wrist of the physician in an effort to make human contact, the Heart Organ is likely to have a disharmony. This type of awareness can be endlessly refined. For example, the physician can pay attention to how the patient reacts to various emotional attitudes he or she intentionally "gives" in the encounter; a patient who becomes especially attentive or reactive to slight shifts in emphasis during the encounter may reveal much of the underlying pattern. A patient's sensitivity to the physician's expression of worry or sympathy may mean Spleen, a reaction to assertiveness implies the Liver, heightened responsiveness to fear may reveal the Kidneys, inappropriate shifts in discussion relate to the Heart, and a deep and easy recognition of sadness may indicate a Lung disharmony.

Facial Color   The color of the face, its expressiveness, and its moistness are closely related to the body's Qi and Blood. The *Nei Jing* states that "all the Qi and Blood of the Meridians pour upward into the face."[16] Normal and healthy facial color obviously depends on a person's racial and ethnic origin, climatic conditions, and occupation. In general, however, a healthy face is shiny and moist. If an individual is ill, but the face appears healthy, it suggests that the Qi and Blood are not weakened and that the illness is not serious. A withered face implies weakness of the vital textures and a less favorable prognosis. Abnormal facial colors have definite clinical significance. White is associated with disharmonies of Deficiency or of Cold. A bright white face with a puffy, bloated appearance is a sign of Deficient Qi or Deficient Yang. If the white face is lusterless and withered, it signifies Deficient Blood. Sometimes the face is white when there is pain. Red appears with Heat and Fire. When the entire face is red, it is a sign of Excess Heat. The words *Heat* and *Fire* refer to the same phenomenon, but the word *Heat* is usually used to talk about external Heat, while *Fire* is used to talk about internally generated Heat. Yellow indicates Dampness or Deficiency. A yellow face is especially related to Internal Dampness produced by a weak Spleen not "raising the pure fluids." When the entire body, including the eyes, is yellow, the symptom is always seen as indicating a Damp condition. If the yellowness tends toward bright orange, the Dampness is also Hot and is called Yang jaundice; if the yellow is pale, it is a sign of Cold Dampness and is called Yin jaundice. A pale yellow face without brightness may be a sign of Deficient Blood.

Qing is an important color in Chinese culture and medicine. The Chinese describe it as "the color of a dragon's scales." It is translated as "blue-green," although connoting many shades between blue and green. Blue-green indicates stagnation or obstruction of Blood and Qi (Congealed Blood and Stagnant Qi). It is usually associated with patterns of Excess. Because the Liver rules flowing and spreading, and because Wind is associated with Liver disharmonies, Qing also appears when there is Liver disharmony or Wind. In the case of extreme obstruction, Qing may acquire a purplish tinge.

Darkness or Black is associated with Deficient Kidneys and Congealed Blood. This color often arises after a prolonged chronic illness. The blackness may be especially evident under the eyes.

Tongue Observing the tongue is one of two pillars of the Four Examinations;[17] the other is feeling the pulse. One elderly Chinese physician, a teacher of the author, described the tongue as a piece of litmus paper that reveals the basic qualities of a disharmony. Many signs may be interpreted only when the entire configuration can be seen, but the tongue interpretation is always essential. It is often the clearest indication of the nature of a disharmony and its pattern, reliable even when other signs are vague and contradictory.

When talking about the tongue, Chinese physicians make a distinction between the tongue material and the coating of the tongue.

The Chinese word for the tongue coating can best be translated as "moss" or "fur." The tongue material and tongue moss are treated as two separate elements of tongue examination.

The tongue material can be various shades of red and can have varying degrees of moisture.

A normal tongue is pale red and somewhat moist. The characteristic healthy color is the result of abundant Blood carried to the tongue by smoothly moving Qi. If the tongue maintains its normal color during an illness, it is a sign that the Qi and Blood have not been injured. A pale tongue is less red than a normal tongue, and indicates Deficient Blood or Deficient Qi. A dry, pale tongue is more likely to be Deficient Blood; if it is wet, it is more likely to be Deficient Qi.

A red tongue is redder than a normal tongue, and points to a Heat condition in the body.

A scarlet tongue is deeper red than a red tongue, and points to an extreme Heat condition. In a disharmony characterized by External Heat, it indicates that Heat has entered the deepest levels of the body.

A purple tongue usually indicates that the Qi and Blood are not moving harmoniously and that there is a pattern of Stagnant Qi or Congealed Blood. A pale purple tongue means the obstruction is related to Cold; reddish-purple is a sign of Heat-related injury to the Blood or Fluids. In general, if the lack of flow is due to Cold, the tongue will appear moist. If it is due to Heat, the tongue will appear dry. A purple tongue may also be associated with the Liver's failure to flow or spread properly.

A tongue with a dark tinge signifies some form of stagnation.

The coating, fur, or moss on the surface of the tongue is the result of Spleen activity. During its vaporization of pure essences, the Spleen also causes small amounts of impure substances to ascend, like smoke. These substances come out in the tongue. Some medical literature, in fact, refers to tongue moss as "smoke." The moss is thus intimately related to digestion and can reflect the state of the digestive system. Other activities of the body also leave impressions on the moss—evidence of bodily states—that are visible to the physician.

The tongue moss covers the whole surface or patches of the surface of the tongue. It can vary in thickness, color, texture, and general appearance. In a healthy individual the density of moss is relatively uniform, although it may be slightly thicker in the center of the tongue. The moss is thin, whitish, and moist, and the tongue material can be seen through it.

A thin moss can be normal, but during an illness it may be a sign of Deficiency. A very thick moss is nearly always a sign of Excess.

Moss that is puddled with moisture is a sign of Excess Fluids, usually due to Deficient Yang (or Fire, the body's internal Heat), but is also a possible sign of other patterns, such as Dampness.

Moss that is very dry or sandpaperlike is a sign of Excess Yang or Fire, or of Deficient Fluids.

A moss that appears firmly implanted on the tongue body, like grass sprouting from the ground, signifies strong Spleen and Stomach Qi. Moss that appears to be floating on the surface of the tongue is a sign of weak Spleen and Stomach Qi.

A greasy moss appears to be a thick, oily film covering the tongue or a portion of it. It can resemble a layer of white petroleum jelly or butter, and is a sign of Mucus or Dampness in the body. A pasty moss, which is greasy but somewhat thicker (the Chinese say it looks like the lumpy result of mixing oil and flour), signifies extreme Mucus or Dampness.

When the moss seems to have been removed so that the tongue or a portion of it appears shiny, it is called "peeled tongue"—described by Chinese texts as resembling the flesh of an uncooked chicken after the skin has been removed. A peeled tongue may be a sign of Deficient Yin or Fluids, or of Spleen Qi too weak to raise smoke.

White moss, though also the color of normal moss, can appear in illness. It may signify Cold, especially if there is excessive moisture in the tongue material. But if the white moss resembles cottage cheese (or, as the Chinese say, unshaped tofu), it signifies Heat in the Stomach.

A yellow moss points to Heat: the deeper the yellow, the greater the Heat.

A black or gray moss is a sign of either extreme Heat or Cold—extreme Heat if the tongue material is red, extreme Cold if it is pale.

The shape and movement of the tongue are also considered. A normal tongue is neither too big nor too small for the mouth, looking neither swollen nor shriveled. It should move with flexibility but not uncontrollably, and it should not slant in any particular direction. The normal tongue should be a smooth piece of flesh without cracks, and although it may have raised papillae, it should have no red pimples or eruptions.

The swollen tongue is puffy with scalloped edges, as though it had been imprinted by the teeth. The usual origin of a swollen tongue is Deficient Qi or Excess Fluids. In rare instances, however, it may be part of a pattern of Excess Heat, in which case the tongue body will also be very red.

A thin tongue is slender, smaller than a normal tongue, and is usually a sign of Deficient Blood or Fluids.

A stiff tongue lacks flexibility, resembling, as the Chinese say, "a piece of wood." This type of tongue usually implies a Wind Pernicious Influence or Mucus obstructing the Heart Qi.

A trembling tongue seems to wiggle uncontrollably. When this type of tongue is pale, it is a sign that Qi is insufficient to regulate proper movement. If the tongue is red, the diagnosis is usually Internal Wind moving the tongue.

A tongue that lolls like a panting dog's is most often a sign of Heat.

A contracted tongue that cannot be stretched out is usually seen in serious situations. When the accompanying tongue color is pale or purple, Cold is probably contracting the body. If a contracted tongue is swollen, it usually signifies Mucus or Dampness. If the tongue material of a contracted tongue is red, it is a sign that Heat has injured the Fluids.

Cracks on the tongue are common and are considered normal if they have been present since birth. If, however, they develop during an illness, they are a sign of chronic and severe illness. The exact interpretation depends on the tongue color. Cracks in a red tongue are usually a sign of Heat injuring the Fluids or of Deficient Yin; cracks in a pale tongue signify Deficient Blood and Qi.

Red eruptions, pimples, or thornlike protrusions on the tongue, redder than the occasional raised papillae of the normal tongue, are usually signs of Heat or of Congealed Blood.

These signs often occur on only certain portions of the tongue. For example, the center of the tongue alone may be thickly coated, or only the sides of the tongue might be red, or a crack might appear just at the tip. For such cases particular areas of the tongue are said to correspond to particular Organs. Figure 17 illustrates these correspondences, which are helpful but are *never* considered absolute.

FIGURE 17 *Areas of the Tongue and Corresponding Organs*

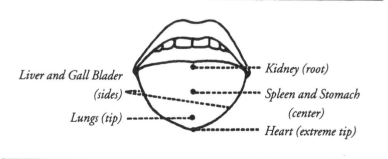

Liver and Gall Blader (sides) — Kidney (root)
Spleen and Stomach (center)
Lungs (tip) — Heart (extreme tip)

Secretions and Excretions The principal secretions and excretions are phlegm, vomit, urine, and stool. Because phlegm and vomit may be seen by the physician, they are considered part of the Looking

Examination. Urine and stool are usually discussed with the patient and are therefore covered in the Asking Examination.

Clear, thin phlegm exuding from the nose and throat is usually part of a Cold pattern. If the phlegm is yellow and sticky, it is a sign of Heat. Sticky yellow looks concentrated or "cooked." A large amount of phlegm easily coughed usually indicates Dampness. Bloody phlegm is commonly a sign of Heat injuring the Lungs.

Thin, watery, clear vomit usually signifies a Cold pattern and Deficient Stomach Qi, as does the vomiting of undigested food without a sour taste in the mouth. Sour-tasting vomit usually indicates Stomach Heat. Yellow, bitter-tasting vomit is a sign of Liver Heat or Gall Bladder Heat.

Listening and Smelling [wen-zhen 闻 诊]

This Examination deals with a number of common signs, all about equally important in the weaving of a diagnosis.

Voice and respiration are the first. Coarse, strong respiration may signify Excess. Weak respiration or shortness of breath, accompanied by weak, low voice and little speech, suggests Deficiency. A sudden loss of voice suggests an External Pernicious Influence, while chronic loss of voice is usually a sign of Deficiency. Wheezing most often suggests Mucus.

A heavy cough or a sudden and violent one is a sign of Excess. A dry, hacking cough suggests Heat or Dryness. A weak cough is usually part of a Deficiency pattern.

Chinese medicine distinguishes between two main kinds of bodily odors that are present during illness. These smells are difficult to describe, and so the Chinese physician relies heavily on experience when interpreting them. One odor is characterized as foul, rotten, and nauseating, like the odor of rancid meat or rotten eggs. Such an odor signifies Heat. The second odor is less nauseating but more pungent or fishy, and may seem to hurt the nose. It is like the smell of fumes from bleach, and indicates Cold and Deficiency.

Asking [*wen-zhen* 问 诊]

In the third of the Four Examinations, the physician asks questions, as would a Western doctor, to discover important but not readily apparent information. Of course, many, many questions may be asked, but only those that are most common and that are essential for beginners to learn pattern perception are discussed here. These cover the following topics: sensations of cold or hot; perspiration; headaches and dizziness; quality and location of pain; urination and stool; thirst; appetite and tastes; sleep; gynecological concerns; and personal background (including medical and psychosocial history). Questions about hot and cold, pain, and medical history are generally the most important. The other signs discovered by Asking may contribute necessary shadings to a pattern, but these signs are rarely decisive.

The order of the questions presented here follows a traditional gradation that is used to help beginning students learn how to think in terms of patterns.[18] They range from the simplest to more complex. The purpose is to provide building blocks for the development of pattern recognition. An experienced physician ignores this order or the entire idea of a fixed set of questions and instead facilitates a natural give-and-take. For an "old-timer," the clinical "story" comes out in a soul-to-soul encounter (see Chapter 9).

Sensations of Cold and Hot   In general, Cold corresponds to Yin and Hot to Yang, for internally generated disorders. Subjective sensations of Heat, feeling warm to the touch, or a dislike of hot weather or hot places can be a sign of Heat. Cold is signified by the opposite—constant chills or a preference for warm places, for instance.

Acute fevers of external origin fall into the special category of febrile illnesses. Until very recently, such illnesses were always considered life-threatening and were in fact a major cause of death. Fevers are therefore a central focus of most Chinese medical texts, as they are in the writings of Hippocrates and in other early medical traditions. (Febrile illnesses are the subject of Appendix A.)

When a patient has a sudden fever together with chills, it indicates that the body's Qi is attempting to expel an External Pernicious Influence; it is not necessarily a sign of Cold. If the fever persists but the chills disappear, the illness is said to have gone deeper and the fever is a sign of Heat. A low-grade fever especially noticeable in the afternoon or heat felt only in the palms of the hands, soles of the feet, and the sternum (known collectively to the Chinese as the "five hearts") indicates insufficient Yin.

If the patient has no fever yet fears Cold, he or she is usually suffering from Deficient Yang or Deficient Qi, especially if the condition is chronic. Interestingly, whether or not blankets make the patient any warmer is a helpful diagnostic distinction. If blankets increase the patient's warmth, the disharmony is probably in Internal Deficiency of Yang. If not, the disorder may be an invasion of an External Cold Pernicious Influence.

Perspiration Perspiration occurs when the pores are open but not when the pores are closed. Both these conditions are affected by various disharmonies. If a patient perspires in the daytime even though he or she engages in little or no physical activity (spontaneous sweating), it indicates that Protective Qi is not properly regulating the pores and that there may be a pattern of Deficient Yang or Deficient Qi. Excessive perspiration during sleep (night sweating), however, signifies Deficient Yin.

If no perspiration occurs during an illness with fever and other signs of an External Pernicious Influence, the Pernicious Influence is probably Cold that has obstructed the pores. If there is perspiration during such an illness, it suggests External Heat opening the pores, or perhaps a Deficiency of Qi hampering the proper regulation of the pores. The choice between these two possibilities would be based on other signs. If the fever breaks after perspiration, the Pernicious Influence has been expelled.

Headaches and Dizziness Headaches may accompany any of the patterns of disharmony, but some broad distinctions between types of headaches can be helpful. Sudden headaches often appear with External Pernicious Influences, which disturb the Yang or Qi of the head. Chronic headaches more often accompany Internal disharmonies. Severe headaches may be a sign of Excess, while slight, annoying headaches are usually signs of Deficiency. The Organ most associated with headaches is the Liver, because Liver Qi often rises when the Liver is in disharmony. A physician may consider the exact location of a headache significant, since it corresponds to the Meridian that passes through that part of the head and thus to the rest of the system connected by that Meridian.

Dizziness, like headaches, can be part of any pattern of disharmony. Although it is most frequently seen in patterns of Deficient Yin or Blood, it always depends on the rest of the configuration for interpretations.

Pain After Cold and Hot, this is the next most important subject of the Asking Examination. In fact, pain is often the patient's chief complaint, the thing that brought him or her to the physician. Pain manifesting in a particular part of the body indicates a disharmony in that area. Pain in the chest, for instance, indicates disharmony in the Heart or Lungs; pain of the flank and rib cage indicates Liver and Gall Bladder disharmony; pain in the epigastrum (solar plexus) indicates Stomach and Spleen disharmony; abdominal pain above the navel indicates disharmony of the Spleen and Intestines; abdominal pain around and below the navel indicates disharmonies of the Intestines, Bladder, Uterus, or Kidney; groin, genital-area, and hypogastrium (lower abdomen) pain indicates Liver Meridian disharmony; and lower back pain signals Kidney disharmony.

The Chinese physician is also concerned with a patient's description of the exact quality of his or her pain. Table 2 summarizes the significance and type of disharmony associated with some common qualities of pain.

TABLE 2 *Signification of Qualities of Pain*

QUALITY OF PAIN	SIGNIFICATION
Diminished by heat	Cold
Diminished by cold	Heat
Relieved by touch or pressure	Deficiency
Aggravated by touch or pressure	Excess
Diminishes after eating	Deficiency
Increases after eating	Excess
Increases in humid weather	Dampness
Accompanied by bloating or sense of fullness	Stagnant Qi
Sharp and stabbing, usually fixed in location	Congealed Blood
Sensation of heaviness	Dampness
Moves from place to place	Wind or Stagnant Qi
Slight and accompanied by fatigue	Deficient Qi or Dampness

The time between the start of the pain and when the patient finally makes the effort to see the physician can be important. If the duration is short, the pain is likely to be "shallow" and more easily treated. If the interlude is longer, the pain may have become an integral part of the patient's negotiations in the world. The deeper pain entwines in his or her life and often requires treatment directed at the Inner Organs, emotions, and Spirit.

Urine and Stool Chinese physicians do not generally take urine or stool samples for examination; they get the information they need from the Asking Examination.

A patient whose urine is clear usually has a Cold pattern, while dark yellow or reddish urine indicates Heat. Copious urine and frequent nighttime urination suggest that the Kidneys are not properly vaporizing Water and point to Deficient Kidney Qi. Scanty urination is usually a sign of some type of Excess, such as Dampness or Heat obstructing the Bladder Qi, although it can be a sign of

Deficient Fluids. Frequent, scanty, dark, and painful urinations indicate Dampness and Heat in the Bladder. Inability to complete urination, dribbling, or a lack of force in urination often signifies Deficient Qi, Cold, or Dampness.

Infrequent, dry, or hard stools can be part of a configuration of Heat Excess, but, depending on the accompanying signs, may also signify Deficient Fluids or Deficient Qi. Frequent watery or unformed stools usually signify Deficient Yang, Deficient Qi, or Dampness. Urgent diarrhea, especially when yellowish and accompanied by a burning sensation in the anus, is a sign of Heat or Liver excess. Stools that are first dry and then wet suggest Deficiency. Undigested food in stools often signifies Deficient Yang of the Spleen.

Thirst, Appetite, and Tastes   Chinese physicians commonly ask patients whether they are thirsty. This is because thirst is often a sign of Heat, while lack of thirst often signifies Cold. Thirst without desire to drink is a sign of Deficient Yin or of Dampness.

Appetite disorders (e.g., eating too much or too little) usually signify a Stomach or Spleen disharmony due to Deficient Qi or Dampness.

Unusual tastes in the mouth may also indicate disharmony. A bitter taste suggests Heat, most commonly as a condition of the Liver or Gall Bladder. A sweet pasty taste suggests Damp Heat in the Spleen. Foul tastes often mean Liver or Stomach Heat, while salty taste sensations may indicate Kidney disharmony. Inability to distinguish tastes is usually part of a pattern of Deficient Spleen Qi.

Sleep   In keeping with their emphasis on balance, the Chinese believe that people should have just enough sleep. Too little or too much indicates imbalance and disharmony.

Insomnia is described in Chinese texts as "Yang unable to enter Yin"—the active unable to become passive. This usually means that Blood or Yin or both are Deficient and incapable of nourishing the Spirit stored in the Heart. There is therefore a relative excess of Yang, which is not balanced and is unable to quiet down. Excess Yang or Fire in any other Organ can also cause insomnia. The constant desire to sleep, or excessive sleep, is often a sign of Deficient Yang, Deficient Qi, or Dampness.

Gynecological Concerns   Chinese physicians routinely ask female patients about gynecological matters.[19] If a woman's menstrual periods arrive earlier than usual, it may signify that Heat is causing reckless movement of Blood or that Deficient Qi cannot govern Blood. The accompanying signs would make a distinction easy to arrive at. A red tongue would mean Heat; a pale tongue would mean Deficient Qi. Late menstrual periods suggest Deficient Blood or Cold causing Stagnation. Irregular menstruation is often a sign that Liver Qi is not moving harmoniously.

Excessive menstrual flow may signify Heat in the Blood or Deficient Qi. Insufficient flow or lack of menses (except during pregnancy) may mean Deficient Blood, Cold obstructing the Blood, or Congealed Blood. Pale and thin menstrual blood points to a Deficient condition. Very dark blood suggests Heat, and blood that is purplish, especially if clotted, may indicate Congealed Blood.

Copious, clear or white, and thin discharges (leukorrhea) usually signify Deficiency and Dampness. Discharges that are thick and yellow, or accompanied by itching or soreness of the vagina, are often signs of Heat and Dampness.

Personal Background   The Chinese physician wants to have a complete medical history of each patient. This is because patterns may reappear time after time, pointing to various irregularities or body activities, and because previous disharmonies may be affecting the patient's health. The patient's history is an additional sign in the diagnosis. The physician's general rule is that acute illnesses are associated with patterns of Excess, and chronic illnesses with patterns of Deficiency. Older people tend to have Deficiency patterns, whereas younger people are inclined toward Excesses. A family medical history can also be very helpful in terms of hereditary diseases.

At this point in history, all East Asian physicians would necessarily also take an inventory of the patient's biomedical status, both in terms of diseases and treatments. Oriental medicine can no longer function in an isolated context. Part of the process of moving West has meant a clear recognition of the values of the West. Medically and morally, an Oriental physician needs to know when conventional medical approaches might be more desirable. Knowing when more information is needed and when not to treat a patient or when to treat a patient in conjunction with other practitioners has become a necessary skill for any Oriental physician who practices in the contemporary health world. In some situations, the Oriental practitioner finds great value in a biomedical diagnosis. The refinements of sensory discrimination and early disease detection available through sophisticated Western technology can add significantly to the understanding of the patient's condition. Sometimes an x-ray, MRI, or laboratory report is more sensitive and accurate than the best Oriental physician. Another important reason for taking a biomedical history is that medications and other treatments can alter the appearance of important signs such as tongue and pulse. Furthermore, potential herb-drug interactions require vigilance. For the traditional practitioner, this new domain of inquiry has become another critical piece of the patient's landscape. While biomedicine can creatively add to information that is important to discern a pattern, this knowledge does not transform the Chinese medical work of detecting a unique set of Yin-Yang relationships. (See Appendix E.)

In a chronic situation or for a condition that will require a lengthy course of treatment, the physician needs to be deeply acquainted with the patient. Inquiry concerning life behaviors such as the balance of activity, rest, diet, and food habits is important. Even more critical, the physician needs to know what animates a person, "what makes him or her tick," what are the sources of strength and weakness, and what gives his or her life purpose and meaning. This deeper layer of a person, usually involving the Spirit, can sometimes reveal the clearest delineation of a pattern. The physician may need to know about significant relationships, sources of pleasure and self-worth, major disappointments, major successes, important learning experiences, and how a person managed earlier illness. Major illness is an uninvited opportunity for self-revelation and growth, and the physician must be alert to this possibility in the current situation. The physician cannot be afraid to ask "heavy" questions—"are you thinking or dealing with the possibility of death? disability? being a burden? losses? unfinished work or relationships?" The responses (whether in words, emotions, or muscular postures) can reveal the character of the human landscape, the deepest layers of Yin and Yang. (See Chapter 9.)

During the personal background part of the interview, the physician also needs to discuss the patient's preferences, expectations, and beliefs. Not only do they help reveal the energetic configuration of people, they all can be a major determinant of the physician's explanation, therapeutic strategy, and the final outcome of the patient-physician exchange.

Touching [qie-zhen 切诊]

The last of the Four Examinations, in modern East Asia, is conventionally considered the most important. (See Chapter 9 for an alternative approach.) Part of it involves touching different parts of the body and various acupuncture points. This is another way to get at information sometimes discovered by asking such questions as: Is the skin cold, hot, moist, or dry? Is pain diminished or aggravated by pressure? But the heart of the Touching Examination is the feeling of the pulse, a procedure far more complex than what we know in the modern West.

Taking the pulse is such an important feature of China's medicine that Chinese patients often speak of going to the doctor as "going to have my pulse felt." Indeed, pulse taking approaches the subtlety and complexity that bespeaks an art. It requires thorough training, great experience, and the gift of sensitivity. When the physician takes a pulse, he or she is alert to a tremendous array of

FIGURE 18 *Pulse Taking, Chinese Style*

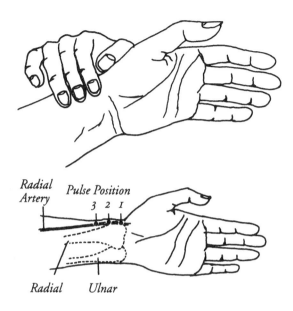

sensations that must be expertly understood and arranged as a unity—the "feel" of an individual pulse.

Although a pulse can be felt at various points on the body, Chinese medicine emphasizes taking it at the radial artery near the wrist.[20] Ideally, both patient and physician are relaxed. The *Nei Jing* suggests that early morning, when the body is calmest, is the best time to feel a pulse. The physician places his or her middle finger parallel to the lower knob on the posterior side of the radius (radial eminence). The index finger will then naturally fall next to the wrist, and the ring finger will fall next to the index finger. (See Figure 18.) The pulse can thus be felt in three positions on each wrist: The index finger touches the body at the first position, the middle finger touches at the second position, and the ring finger at the third position.

Chinese pulse theory gives meaning to the pulse as it is felt in each position on the wrist, but we will assume for now that the three fingers all feel the same thing and that the pulse is the same on each wrist. The pulse is palpated at three levels of pressure: superficial, middle, and deep. At the first or superficial level, the skin is lightly touched; at the second or middle level, a moderate amount of pressure is applied; at the third or deep level, the physician presses quite hard.

A normal or harmoniously balanced pulse is felt mainly at the middle level. Normal speed is between four and five beats per complete respiration (one inhalation and one exhalation), amounting to about seventy to seventy-five beats per minute. The quality of a normal pulse is elastic and "lively," neither hard and unyielding nor flaccid and indistinct. The normal pulse may vary, however. An athlete's normal pulse may be slow; a woman's pulse is usually softer and slightly faster than a man's; children's pulses are faster than adults'; a heavy person's pulse tends to be slow and deep, while a thin person's is more superficial.

Disharmonies in the human landscape leave a clear imprint on the pulse. Classical Chinese texts reflect a centuries-old effort to classify the basic pulses with their associated disharmonies. The codifications and discussions variously cite twenty-four, twenty-seven, twenty-eight, or thirty pulse types.[21] In the following discussion, twenty-eight classical pulses are presented in the traditional order, described, and illustrated.[22] These types are really general categories that rarely correspond exactly to a given individual's pulse, which is most often a combination of types.

Types of Pulse   The first eighteen types of pulse, described below, are the most important and indicate the primary disharmonies. The distinctions between pulses that are most commonly made by physicians are depth (the level at which the pulse is perceptible), speed, width, strength, overall shape and quality, rhythm, and length.

Depth A *floating* pulse (*fu mai*) is "higher" than normal; that is, although distinct at a light or superficial level of pressure, it is less perceptible when palpated at the middle and deep levels. This pulse signifies an External Pernicious Influence, suggesting that the disharmony is in the superficial parts of the body where Protective Qi is combating the External Influence. A floating pulse is classified as Yang because its exteriorness corresponds to a primary Yang characteristic. A floating pulse frequently occurs without any other signs suggesting External Influences. In this case, if it is also without strength, the floating pulse signifies Deficient Yin. This is because the pulse is active or "dancing," a sign of relative Excess Yang and therefore of Deficient Yin. If the pulse is floating but has strength, and again no External Influences are present, it may be a sign of Interior Wind.

A *sinking* or *deep* pulse (*chen mai*) is distinct only at the third level, when heavy pressure is applied. It indicates that the disharmony is Internal, or that there is obstruction. It is accordingly classified as Yin.

FIGURE 19 *Floating Pulse/Sinking Pulse*

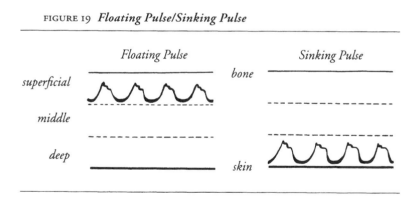

Speed A *slow* pulse (*chi mai*) is one that has fewer than four beats per respiration. It is a sign of Cold retarding movement or of insufficient Qi to cause movement. It is described as Yin.

A *rapid* pulse (*shu mai*) is one that has more than five beats per respiration. It indicates that Heat is accelerating the movement of Blood. It is accordingly a Yang pulse.

FIGURE 20 *Slow Pulse/Rapid Pulse*

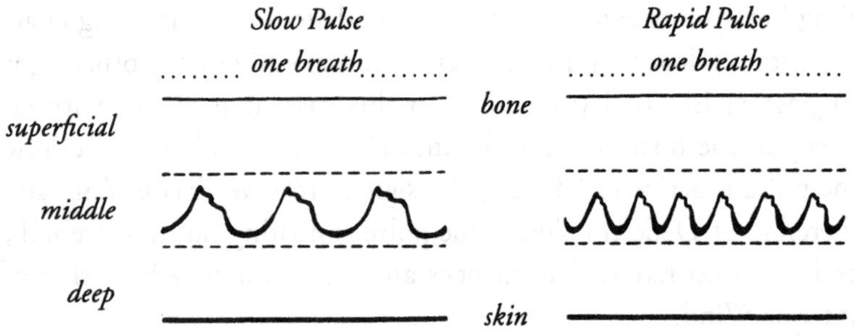

Width A *thin* pulse (*xi mai*) feels like a fine thread but is very distinct and clear. It is a sign that the Blood is Deficient and unable to fill the pulse properly. Often the Qi is also Deficient. This pulse is described as Yin.

A *big* pulse (*da mai*) is broad in diameter and very distinct, and suggests Excess. It is commonly felt when Heat is present in the Stomach or Intestines, or both. It is a Yang pulse.

FIGURE 21 *Thin Pulse/Big Pulse*

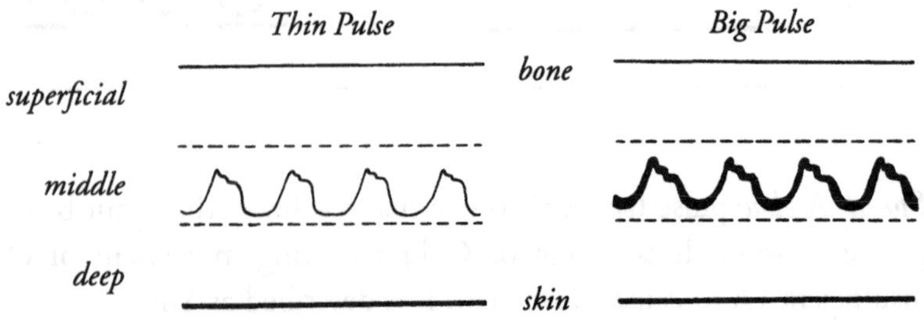

Strength An *empty* pulse (*xu mai*) is big but without strength. It feels weak and soft like a balloon partially filled with water. It is usually felt at the superficial level and is often slower than normal. An empty pulse signifies Deficient Qi and Blood, and is considered a Yin phenomenon.

A *full* pulse (*shi mai*) is big and also strong, pounding hard against the fingers at all three depths. It is a sign of Excess and is classified as Yang.

FIGURE 22 *Empty Pulse/Full Pulse*

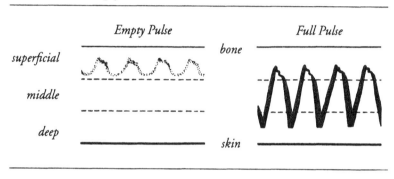

Shape A *slippery* pulse (*hua mai*) is extremely fluid. It feels smooth, like a ball bearing covered with viscous fluid. Classical texts compare it to "feeling pearls in a porcelain basin." A contemporary Chinese physician says it "slithers like a snake." It is a sign of Excess, usually of Dampness or Mucus. This pulse often occurs in women during pregnancy, when extra Blood is needed to nourish the fetus. (Touching pregnant women's pulses is one way to get the feel of this pulse. A slippery pulse is considered "Yang within Yin." (This type of classification will be discussed in Chapter 7.)

A *choppy* pulse (*se mai*) is the opposite of a slippery pulse. It is uneven and rough, and sometimes irregular in strength and fullness. Chinese texts liken it to "a knife scraping bamboo or a sick silkworm eating a mulberry leaf." When this pulse is also described as

FIGURE 23   *Slippery Pulse/Choppy Pulse/Wiry Pulse/Tight Pulse*

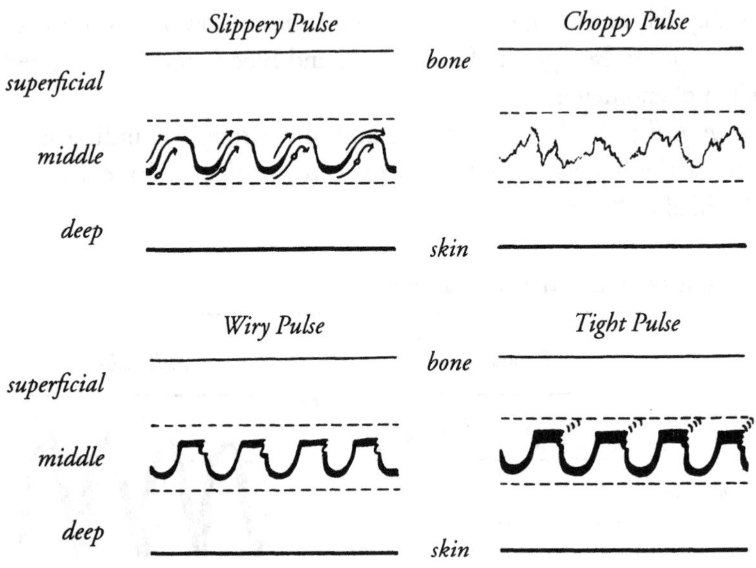

being thin, it is a sign of Deficient Blood or Deficient Jing. It can also be a sign of Congealed Blood. Sometimes a choppy pulse is irregular in rhythm. In this case it is called "the three and five not adjusted"—meaning that there are sometimes three beats per breath and sometimes five beats per breath. This is usually a Yin pulse.

A *wiry* pulse (*xuan mai*) has a taut feeling, like a guitar or violin string. It is strong, rebounds against pressure at all levels, and hits the fingers evenly. But it has no fluidity or wavelike qualities. It signifies stagnation in the body, usually related to a disharmony that impairs the flowing and spreading functions of the Liver and Gall Bladder. It is a Yang pulse.

A *tight* pulse (*jin mai*) is strong and seems to bounce from side to side like a taut rope. It is fuller and more elastic than the wiry pulse. Vibrating and urgent, it seems faster than it actually is. This pulse is associated with Excess, Cold, and Stagnation. It is considered Yang within Yin.

Length A *short* pulse (*duan mai*) does not fill the spaces under the three fingers and is usually felt in only one position. It is often a sign of Deficient Qi and is classified as Yin.

A *long* pulse (*chang mai*) is the opposite of a short pulse. It is perceptible beyond the first and third positions; that is, it continues to be felt closer to the hand or up toward the elbow. If it is of normal speed and strength, it is not considered a sign of disharmony. But if it is also tight and wiry, it points to Excess and is considered a Yang pulse.

FIGURE 24 *Short Pulse/Long Pulse*

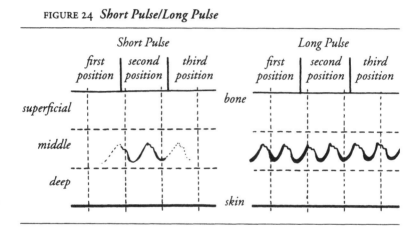

Rhythm A *knotted* pulse (*jie mai*) is a slow, irregular pulse that skips beats irregularly. It is a sign of Cold obstructing the Qi and Blood, though it may also indicate Deficient Qi, Blood, or Jing. This pulse is often a sign of the Heart not ruling the Blood properly, and the more interruptions in rhythm, the more severe is the condition. A knotted pulse is classified as Yin.

A *hurried* pulse (*cu mai*) is a rapid pulse that skips beats irregularly. It is usually a sign of Heat agitating the Qi and Blood, and is considered a Yang Pulse.

An *intermittent* pulse (*dai mai*) usually skips more beats than the previous two pulses, but does so in a regular pattern. It is often associated with the Heart, signifying a serious disharmony, or it can signal an exhausted state of all the Organs. It is a Yin pulse.

The knotted, hurried, and intermittent pulses are sometimes congenital, in which case they are not necessarily considered signs of disharmony.

FIGURE 25 *Knotted Pulse/Hurried Pulse/Intermittent Pulse*

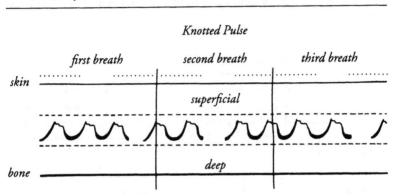

continued

FIGURE 25 *Knotted Pulse/Hurried Pulse/Intermittent Pulse (continued)*

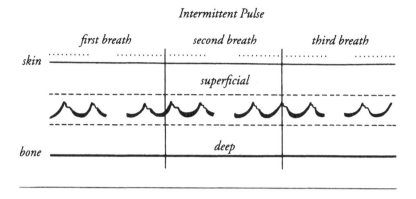

Intermittent Pulse

Moderate Pulse A *moderate* pulse (*huan mai*) is the healthy, perfectly balanced pulse—normal in depth, speed, strength, and width. It is quite rare, and pulse discussions list it as secondary. For a Chinese physician to issue a clean bill of health, a patient does not have to have this pulse. In fact, healthy people seldom do have it. Everyone's "normality" or "balance" has a certain constitutional and age-linked disposition toward Yin or Yang disharmonies, and each person's "normal" pulse will reveal this propensity. For perceiving disharmonies, the significance of a moderate pulse lies in the way it combines with other signs. If signs of Dampness are present, for instance, this pulse, which is sometimes considered slightly slippery, may reinforce a diagnosis of Dampness.

FIGURE 26 *Moderate Pulse*

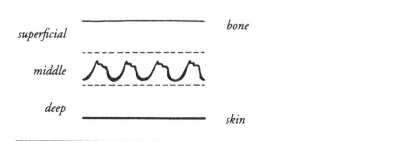

Other Pulses The other ten classical pulse types are combinations and refinements of the previous eighteen and are generally considered less important. They are, however, readily discernible by the experienced physician and are useful in determining precise shades of significance in a diagnosis.

A *flooding* pulse (*hong mai*, Figure 27) surges with the strength of a big pulse to hit the fingers at all three depths, but it leaves the fingers with less strength, like a receding wave. It signifies that Heat has injured the Fluids and Yin of the body. It is considered Yin within Yang.

FIGURE 27 *Flooding Pulse*

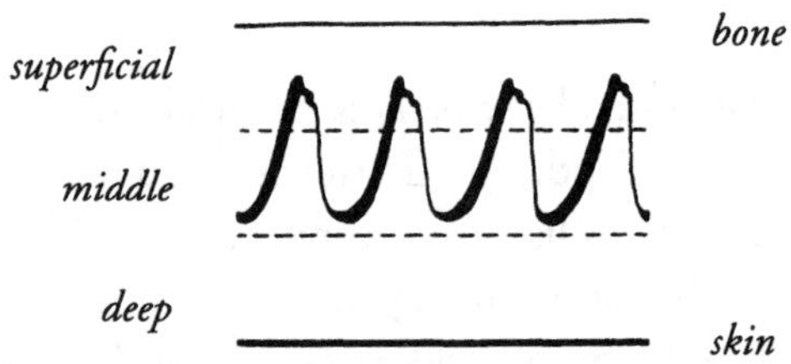

A *minute* pulse (*wei mai*, Figure 28) is extremely fine and soft, but lacks the clarity of the thin pulse. It is barely perceptible and seems about to disappear. This pulse signifies extreme Deficiency and is classified as Yin.

FIGURE 28 *Minute Pulse*

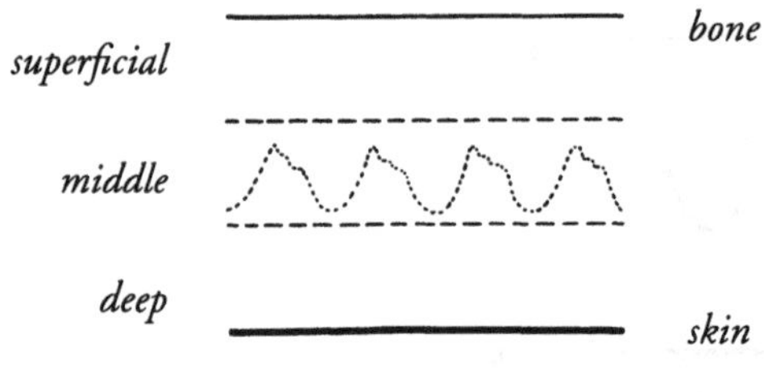

A *frail* pulse (*ruo mai*, Figure 29) is soft, weak, and somewhat thin. It is usually felt at the deep level. It is like an inverted empty pulse, but signifies a more extreme Deficient Qi condition because the Qi cannot even raise the pulse. A frail pulse is a Yin pulse.

FIGURE 29 **Frail Pulse**

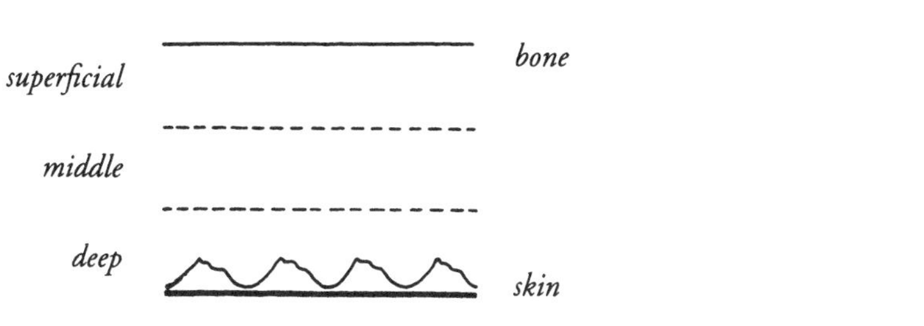

superficial		bone
middle		
deep		skin

A *soggy* pulse (*ru mai*, Figure 30) is a combination of the thin, empty, and floating pulses. It is extremely soft, is less clear than a thin pulse, and is perceptible only in the superficial position. The slightest pressure makes it disappear. A soggy pulse feels like a bubble floating on water. It is a sign of Deficient Blood or Jing and sometimes of Dampness. It is a Yin pulse.

FIGURE 30 **Soggy Pulse**

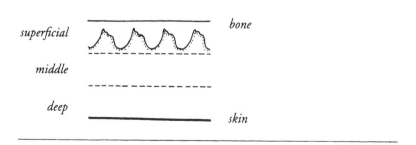

A *leather* pulse *(ge mai,* Figure 31) is a combination of the wiry and floating pulses, with aspects of the empty pulse. It feels like the tight skin on the top of a drum. It is a sign of Deficient Blood or Jing, and is classified as a Yin pulse.

FIGURE 31 *Leather Pulse*

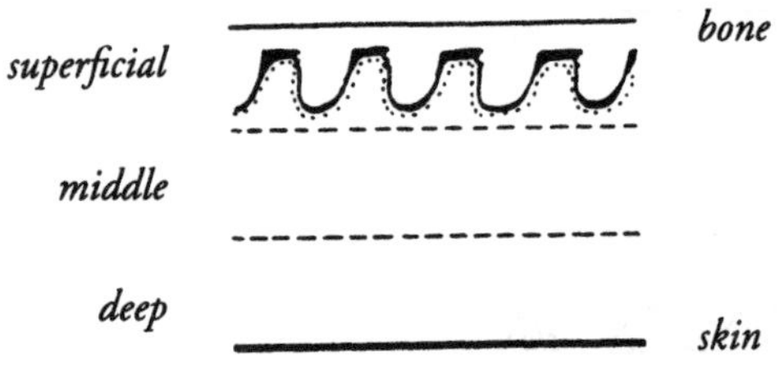

A *hidden* pulse *(fu mai,* Figure 32) is an extreme form of the sinking pulse. Intense pressure must be applied to feel it. If a hidden pulse is strong, it is usually a sign of Cold obstructing the Meridians. If it is weak, it signifies Deficient Yang that cannot raise the pulse. Hidden pulses are described as Yin.

FIGURE 32 *Hidden Pulse*

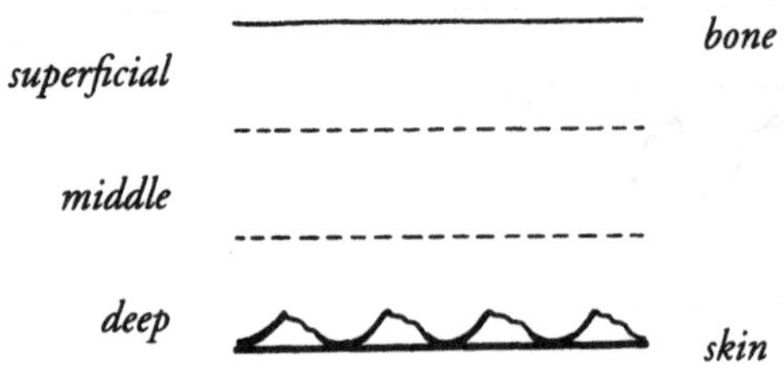

A *confined* pulse (*lao mai*, Figure 33), also known as a *prison* pulse, is the opposite of the leather pulse and is a form of the hidden pulse. It is very deep and wiry, and usually long and strong. A confined pulse is a sign of obstruction due to Cold, and is considered Yang within Yin.

FIGURE 33 *Confined Pulse*

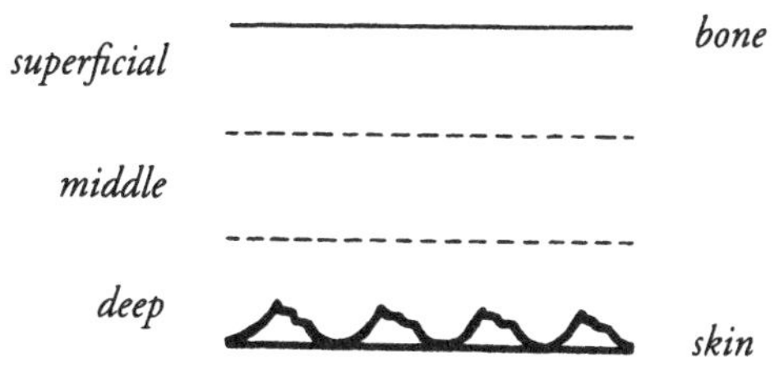

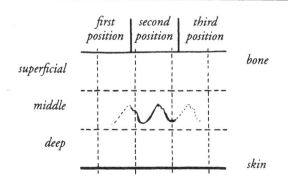

A *spinning bean* or *moving* pulse (*dong mai*, Figure 34) is a combination of the short, tight, slippery, and rapid pulses. It is felt in only one position and is said to be "incomplete, without a head and tail, like a bean." It signifies an extreme condition and is rarely seen. It usually occurs in cases of heart palpitations, intense fright, fever, or pain. It is a Yang pulse.

FIGURE 34 *Spinning Bean Pulse*

A *hollow* pulse (*kong mai*, Figure 35) feels like the stem of a green onion—solid on the outside but completely empty within. It is often a floating pulse as well. A hollow pulse implies Deficient Blood and is often seen after great loss of Blood. It is considered Yin.

FIGURE 35   *Hollow Pulse*

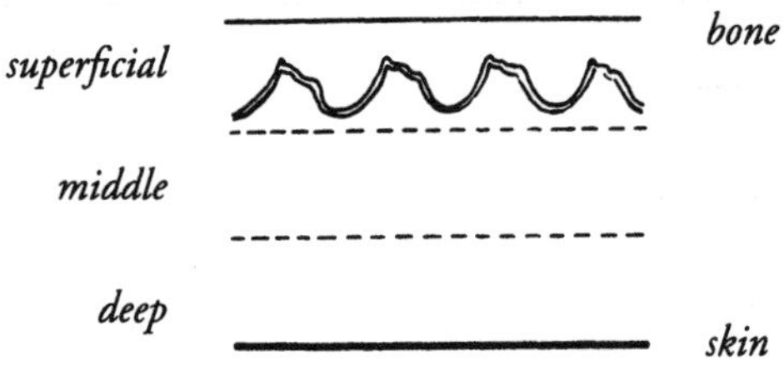

A *scattered* pulse (*san mai*, Figure 36) is similar to an empty pulse because it is floating, big, and weak. It is larger and much less distinct than the empty pulse, however, and tends to be felt primarily as it recedes. It is a sign of serious disharmony—Kidney Yang exhausted and "floating away." A scattered pulse is classified as Yin.

FIGURE 36   *Scattered Pulse*

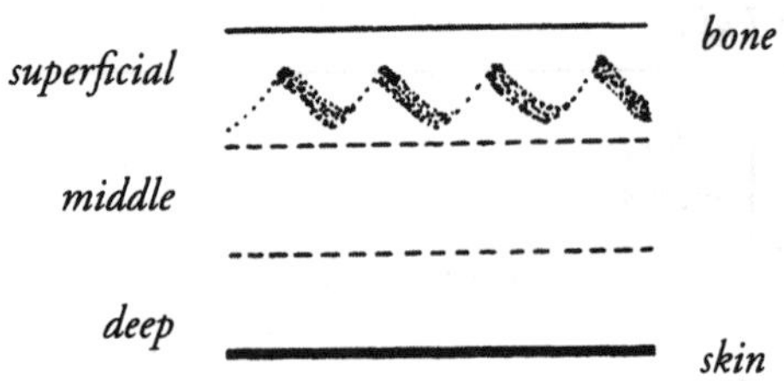

For purposes of this general description of the pulses, we have assumed that all three fingers are feeling the same pulse. In practice, however, each finger feels something slightly different. The two wrists will also give different readings. The three pulse positions on the two wrists are thought to correspond to certain Organs, indicating disharmonies in those Organs. Although there has been disagreement in China about the exact correspondences, Table 3 illustrates the system most commonly used in China today. (See Appendix C for a historical overview of opinions on the pulse position correspondences.) The correspondences are generally said to be the same at all three pressure levels, although in a more complex view, the superficial level correlates with the Yang Organs, while the deep level correlates with their coupled Yin Organs. (See Table 1 in Chapter 3.)

TABLE 3 *Pulse Position Correspondences*

POSITION	LEFT WRIST	RIGHT WRIST
First position	Heart	Lungs
Second position	Liver	Spleen
Third position	Kidney Yin	Kidney Yang (Life Gate Fire)

The twenty-eight basic pulses can be felt at three levels, in three positions, and on two wrists. Already the feeling of a pulse is quite complicated. But when we realize that the twenty-eight pulses are more often found in combination than in their pure form, and that the characteristics of even one pulse type may vary from position to position or from wrist to wrist, it is clear that the system is extremely complex, capable of infinite refinement. Pulse diagnosis is a very sophisticated art. It demands subtlety on the part of the physician to discern the relative importance of each variable and to make an intelligent and precise diagnosis—to weave a useful pattern.

This chapter has described some of the more common signs and symptoms that a physician uses to perceive a pattern. It must be repeated that we have described only the pieces of the patterns—and that for Chinese, thought and medicine pieces have no meaning outside of the whole. Any of the signs mentioned here can have a different signification, depending on the rest of the configuration. For example, the sign of thirst or a dry tongue points to Heat or Deficient Yin. This sign has this signification because it usually appears in a configuration with other Heat signs. But if the person with a dry mouth feels cold, is pale, tired, weak, emotionally flat and low-keyed, has a pale tongue and a slow, weak pulse, the dryness changes its meaning. It becomes a sign of extreme Deficiency with an inability to raise Water. The context defines the piece. Seeing the part simultaneously with the whole is one aspect of the artistry of Chinese medicine. There are no straight lines—no "this" means "that"—just cloudlike patterns that continuously change their shape.

NOTES

1. "Chinese medicine . . . has been fostered and brought to maturity by what for want of a better term we may call 'Taoist consciousness.'" Manfred Porkert, "Chinese Medicine: A Traditional Healing Science," in *Ways of Health*, ed. by David S. Sobel (New York: Harcourt Brace Jovanovich, 1979), p. 150. The importance of Confucian ideas and other traditions should not be forgotten. See Paul Unschuld, *Medicine in China*, 1985.

2. Aristotle, "Metaphysics," in *The Basic Works of Aristotle*, ed. by Richard McKeon, book 11, chap. 5, p. 856.

3. Chap. 23 of the *Tao-te Ching*, in Chan, *Chinese Philosophy*, p. 151.

4. Chuang Tzu in Chan, *Chinese Philosophy*, p. 183.

5. Jones, *Hippocrates and Heraclitus with an English Translation*, vol. 4, p. 489.

6. Ibid., p. 493.

7. Ibid., p. 485.

8. Ibid., p. 483.

9. See, for example, Needham, *Science and Civilization*, vol. 2, pp. 201, 291, 303, 466, 478; Chan, *Chinese Philosophy*, pp. 173, 183; Fung Yu-lan, *A History of Chinese Philosophy*, vol. 1, p. 185, and vol. 2, p. 212.

10. Chap. 1 of the *Tao-te Ching*, in Chan, *Chinese Philosophy*, p. 139.

11. Judith Farquhar, *Knowing Practice: The Clinical Encounter of Chinese Medicine*, p. 28.

12. Arthur Kleinman, *Writing at the Margin*, p. 29. François Jullien's assessment of categories in Chinese thought generally is also pertinent: "It is a temporary means for the mind to represent reality, one that simplifies as it illuminates." *The Propensity of Things*, p. 11.

13. The earliest reference to a method of Four Examinations is in the biography of the legendary physician Bian Que that appears in the Historical Records (*Shi Ji*) written in the early Han dynasty. This biography, part fact and part fiction, takes place during the Warring States period of the fifth century B.C.E. and contains valuable information about Chinese medicine that may even predate the *Nei Jing*. The earliest reference to a clear procedure of Four Examinations is in "Difficulty 61" of the *Nan Jing* [3].

14. One of the most complete compilations of signs and symptoms is the volume, more than a thousand pages long, called the Dictionary of Sources of Disease [35] by Wu Ke-qian. Other such compilations can be found in the Bibliography.

15. *Su Wen* [1], sec. 2, chap. 7, p. 53.

16. *Ling Shu* [2], sec. 1, chap. 4, p. 39. The Chinese character *se* is here being translated as facial color. For an important discussion on the meaning of this word in Chinese medicine see Shigehisa Kuriyama, *The Espressiveness of the Body,* 1999, pp. 173–192. Kuriyama prefers "facial expression" as a translation and also points to the notion that "se" in the earliest Chinese dictionary means "the spirit (Qi) [that appears] in the forehead." For Kuriyama, "se" is related to "raised eyebrows, a glimmer in the eyes, pursed lips, the lack of flush of color." All these doubtless form part of what we take in. But mostly, we don't attend to them separately and consciously, any more than we read a book letter by letter. Rather, what we see, or think we see—it is often difficult to be sure—are hesitation or impatience, despair or longing, shiftiness or candor. That is, we gaze upon attitudes and inclination, which are distinctly visible, yet hard to see distinctly." Kuriyama's idea of gazing is related to the methods of a seasoned Chinese practitioner which are developed in Chapter 9 of this volume.

17. Scattered references to various types of tongues and their significance exist in all early Chinese medical writings. The *Nei Jing* mentions many types of tongues but presents them in no orderly fashion. Zhang Zhong-jing in his Discussion on Cold-Induced Disorders [27] and Essential Prescriptions of the Golden Chest [29] (which were originally one book written in 219 C.E.) mentions many additional types of tongue. In some cases he bases entire treatments on tongue changes. (See Appendix A for a discussion of Zhang Zhong-jing.) Subsequent medical authorities such as Chao Yuan-fang (c. 600 C.E.) and the great physician Sun Si-miao (590–682 C.E.) discussed tongue examinations more completely. The first system-

atic presentation of tongues was Ao's Golden Reflections of Cold-Induced Disorders (*Ao-shi Shang-han Jin-jing Lu*), which appeared in 1341 C.E. and recorded thirty-six types of tongues with illustrations. All the subsequent literature on tongues is an elaboration of Ao's work. One of the more important of these texts is Zhang Deng's Mirror of the Tongue for Cold-Induced Disorders (*Shang-han She-jian*), a volume from 1668 C.E. that has 120 illustrations of different tongues. For a discussion of the development of Chinese tongue examination and a fuller presentation of the examination itself, see Beijing Institute, Traditional Chinese Tongue Examination [70]. Also see a similar work with the same title and also by the Beijing Institute [69]. The standard English reference text for tongue examination is Giovanni Maciocia, *Tongue Diagnosis in Chinese Medicine,* Seattle: Eastland Press, 1987.

18. It is possible to ask an almost endless number of questions concerning any aspect of a person's health and illness. Any detail can be dissected into further Yin and Yang aspects. In the Ming dynasty a minimum of "ten questions" was considered necessary for a beginner to obtain pattern discernment. The first list of ten questions seems to have been drawn up by the great codifier Zhang Jie-bing in his Complete Book (*Jing-yue Quan-shu,* 1624 C.E.). His list included (1) cold and hot, (2) perspiration, (3) head and body, (4) urination and stool, (5) food and drink, (6) chest, (7) deafness, (8) thirst, (9) cause, pulse, and color, (10) smell, Spirit, and sight (numbers 9 and 10 include Touching, Looking, and Smelling). Later, Chen Shou-yuan in his Practical and Easy Medicine (*Yi-xue Shi-yi*), published in 1804 C.E., listed his own ten questions, including Zhang's questions 1–8 and then (9) old illnesses and (10) cause. The modern text used as a primary source for this book, Shanghai Institute, Foundations[53], lists the following ten questions: (1) cold and hot, (2) perspiration, (3) head and body, (4) stool and urination, (5) food, drink, and tastes, (6) chest and abdomen, (7) ears and eyes, (8) sleep, (9) old illnesses and history, (10) thought, emotions, lifestyle, habits, and work. For further information, see the listing for "ten questions" in Traditional Chinese Medical Research Institute, *Concise Dictionary of Traditional Chinese Medicine* [34], p. 3.

19. Women's health, sexism, and gender issues are necessarily intimately interwoven in China as elsewhere. For important pioneering discussions, see Charlotte Furth, *A Flourishing Yin: Gender in China's Medical History, 960–1665,* Francesca Bray, "A Deathly Disorder: Understanding Women's Health in Late Imperial China," in D. Bates (ed.), *Knowledge and the Scholarly Medical Traditions,* and Lisa Raphals, "The Treatment of Women in a Second-Century Medical Casebook," *Chinese Science,* 1998; 15: 7–28.

20. It should also be mentioned that another method of pulse taking is featured in the *Nei Jing* alongside the system of palpation of the radial artery. An entire chapter (*Su Wen,* sec. 6, chap. 20) is devoted to this other method, which involves palpation of various arteries over the entire body, each of which is said to correspond

to an internal Organ or to a particular part of the body. It was only in the *Nan Jing* period that the taking of the radial artery pulse clearly became the dominant method. See Appendix C, Note 1.

21. The *Nei Jing* mentions over twenty types of pulses, but the meaning of some pulse names is unclear. Despite this, it is the source of the later, more highly developed theories of pulse examination. The earliest text devoted exclusively to pulse examination is Wang Shu-he, Classic of the Pulse, which appeared about 280 C.E. and which describes twenty-four basic pulse types. This volume combined Wang Shu-he's own clinical experience with information on pulses found in the *Nei Jing*, the *Nan Jing*, and the writings of such clinicians as Zhang Zhong-jing and Hua Tuo. Li Shi-zhen, in his Pulse Studies of the Lakeside Master (first published in 1564 C.E.), lists twenty-seven pulse types. In Essential Readings in Medicine (*Yi-zhong Bi-du*), published in 1637 C.E., Li Zhong-zi discusses twenty-eight "classic" pulses. Other texts mention more pulse types. Modern texts, however, usually refer to twenty-eight pulses.

All the descriptions of pulses in this book are based on those in Li's Pulse Studies [16]; Shanghai Institute, *Foundations* [53]; Shanghai City Traditional Chinese Medical Archives Research Committee, Selections from Pulse Examination [17]; and Wang Shu-he, Classic of the Pulse [22].

It should be noted that pulse examination plays a crucial role in all literate traditional medical systems. In the Egyptian *Edwin Smith Surgical Papyrus* (before 1600 B.C.E.), pulse examination was already an established practice. Galen of Pargamum (129–200 C.E.) completed eighteen treatises on pulse that include finer details of perception than those found in Wang Shu-he's Classic of the Pulse. Galen elaborated over 100 pulse types by distinguishing size, strength, speed, duration of diastole and/or systole, frequency, and hardness and softness. His attention to rhythm and quality generated such famous pulse categories as the gazelling, ant-crawling, worming, and mouse-tailed pulses that continued to be used in the West until the eighteenth century.

22. Most of the diagrams of pulses are based on those found in Liu Guan-jun, Pulse Examinations [61].

7

THE EIGHT PRINCIPAL PATTERNS: THE FACES OF YIN AND YANG

the patterns' basic texture and composition

Up to this point, the reader has been presented with two kinds of information: an abstract description of the human being oriented around the theory of Yin and Yang, and a detailed listing of various signs of disharmony. In this chapter, these two categories of information begin to merge, for each individual is defined by a unique relationship between his or her own bodily signs and the overall movement of Yin and Yang.

The Eight Principal Patterns are the fundamental model for mediating between these two realms: they are the primary faces of Yin and Yang. They allow the physician to penetrate the abstract principles of Yin and Yang, principles that are so simple, yet so hard to grasp because they presume to be the general laws of totality, of everything around us and inside us, in our bodies, our minds, and our spirits. The Eight Principal Patterns serve, then, as a conceptual matrix that enables the training physician to organize the relationship between particular clinical signs and Yin and Yang.

Conceptualizing and distinguishing the Eight Principal Patterns is the first step toward discerning the basic composition and shading of the clinical landscape. For the beginning physician, before the various signs and symptoms gathered by the Four Examinations can be fully understood, they must be perceived within this schema. These patterns are the pencil sketch outlines of the human landscape. These principles also serve as a clinical guideline and teaching device to enable a novice to learn how Yin and Yang, as complementary opposites, interact, combine, and mutually transform each other.

The translation of the expression *ba-gang* as "Eight Principal Patterns" must be explained. *Ba* means eight. *Gang*, originally a term for the head rope of a fishing net, can also mean guiding principles, essentials, or parameters. In the medical tradition, *gang* connotes the primary matrix that guides all clinical discernment.

Bian-zheng, translated here as "distinguishing patterns," is one of the commonest terms in Chinese medical literature. *Bian* means to distinguish, recognize, or clarify, while *zheng* can mean evidence, proof, or emblem and, in a different form, symptom or ailment.

From a modern Western perspective, it is tempting to translate the Chinese words as "differentiating syndromes," but that rendering would distort the uniqueness and potential validity of the Chinese idea.[1] "Syndrome" is a purely descriptive term, suggesting an arbitrary grouping of signs and symptoms that is meaningless without an underlying cause. "Syndrome" implies that something is missing. For the West, "the knowledge of the cause [is] needed to elevate a clinical entity or a syndrome to the rank of a disease."[2]

But the Chinese physician never leaves the realm of signs and symptoms to seek an independent, *a priori* cause or mechanism susceptible to isolation and treatment. During the course of the Four Examinations, the physician simultaneously collects, interprets, and organizes signs—a complex, subtle perception that leads to an understanding of the physiological events taking place in the patient's body.

The work of the Chinese physician, therefore, is to distinguish patterns, not syndromes, by recognizing the state of bodily disharmony within the domain of signs and symptoms. The process of Chinese medicine is the process of weaving together the elements and recognizing a pattern in myriad signs. For the Chinese, patterns are sufficient and are the ultimate guiding conception for diagnosis and treatment.

The construct of the Eight Principal Patterns allows the physician to begin to recognize how the Yin and Yang tendencies of the body may be in disharmony.[3] It enables the physician to distinguish patterns of the broadest, most general type. Occasionally, these are all that are needed to proceed with treatment. In most cases, however, further refinement of the pattern is required in order to discover the unique features of a particular disorder and so determine an appropriate treatment.

Because Chinese medicine never leaves symptoms, never searches behind the phenomena for cause, but seeks only a configuration, much of this chapter and the next is a series of lists or compilations of signs and symptoms. As with any skill, training the mind to see patterns requires frequent repetition. But the reward of patience and perseverance is the discovery of the artistic and poetic effort of Chinese medicine as it attempts to capture the essence of a human organism in disharmony. The casual reader, however, is encouraged to skim and not worry about details. He or she will be able to follow subsequent chapters.

⊣ DISTINGUISHING THE EIGHT PRINCIPAL PATTERNS [*ba-gang bian-zheng* 八 纲 辨 辨]

To discern the Eight Principal Patterns within the signs and symptoms presented by the patient is one of the training physician's major tasks.

The Eight Principal Patterns are composed of four pairs of polar opposites: Yin/Yang, Interior/Exterior, Deficiency/Excess, and Cold/Hot. These Eight Principal Patterns are actually a concrete subdivision of Yin and Yang into six subcategories. This division allows a clearer, more systematic approach to Yin-Yang theory and practice in Chinese medicine. Yin and Yang retain their primacy because of their broad, all-encompassing nature, while the other six patterns are finally subsumed in Yin-Yang patterns.

Patterns of Interior [*li-zheng* 里 证] and Exterior [*biao-zheng* 表 证] Disharmony

The Interior/Exterior distinction is a relatively simple one, preliminary to the other principles. It gives the Yin/Yang clinical picture a basic spatial location by designating the site of a disharmony.

Interior patterns are generated primarily by Internal disharmonies; Exterior patterns by External Influences. These terms will remind the reader of the discussion of Pernicious Influences in Chapter 5, in which illnesses associated with Internal Yin/Yang disharmonies were differentiated from those characterized by the conflict of External Influences and Normal Qi. However, "Interior" and "Exterior" are used here to describe the location and characteristics of a disharmony, rather than its generation.

The weaving together of some of the following signs suggests a pattern of Exterior disharmony: acute illness with sudden onset of chills and fever, head or body ache often accompanied by a thin tongue moss, and a floating pulse. Exterior conditions are often related to what biomedicine would consider an infectious or contagious disease.

Interior disharmonies are all those not considered Exterior. Interior disharmonies are often associated with chronic conditions and often concern a person's constitutional tendencies or basic emotional life.

Because External Pernicious Influences (Exterior Dampness, Wind, Cold, etc.) are both "causes" and also emblems or names for patterns, the pattern of Exterior disharmony has identical signs as the Influence. Interior Pernicious Influences also share a congruence with the signs of an Interior Pernicious Influence.

Patterns of Deficiency [*xu-zheng* 虚 证] and Excess [*shi-zheng* 实 证]

If an illness is characterized by insufficient Qi, Blood, or other textures, or by the underactivity of any of the Yin or Yang aspects of the Organs, the pattern is likely to be one of Deficiency. General signs of Deficiency are: frail and weak movement; ashen, pale, or sallow face; partial and incomplete engagement with life; shallow breathing; pain that is relieved by pressure; spontaneous sweating; copious urination or incontinence; pale tongue material with little or no moss; and an empty, thin, or otherwise weak pulse. Deficiency patterns are usually chronic in nature, and may be thought of as a clinical landscape that is sparsely composed, bleak and desolate.

Broadly speaking, a pattern is likely to be one of Excess when a Pernicious Influence attacks the body, when some bodily function becomes overactive, or when an obstruction causes an inappropriate accumulation of substances such as Qi and Blood. The pattern of Excess is suggested when some of the following signs are woven together: ponderous and forceful movement; a robust encounter with life; a particularly loud and full voice; heavy breathing; chest or abdominal pains that are aggravated by pressure; scanty urination; thick tongue moss; strong (wiry, slippery, or full) pulse. Patterns of Excess can be either chronic or acute and may be seen in the mind's eye as a cluttered clinical landscape.

Patterns of Cold [*han-zheng* 寒 证] and Heat [*re-zheng* 热 证]

The pattern of Cold disharmony generally manifests itself when the body's Yang Qi is insufficient, or when Cold Pernicious Influences are present. A combination of the following signs describes a Cold pattern: slow, deliberate movement; withdrawn manner; white face; fear of cold; cold limbs; a passive, introverted manner; pain lessened by warmth; watery stool; clear urine; thin and clear white secretions and excretions; no thirst or a desire for hot liquids; pale and swollen tongue material with white or moist moss; and a slow pulse. Cold signs indicate that the basic shade of the bodily disharmony is "cloudy," like an overcast, frozen winter.

The pattern of Heat disharmony is associated with either a heat Pernicious Influence, hyperactivity of the body's Yang functions, or insufficient Yin or Fluids, leading to a relative preponderance of Yang. A Heat disharmony is revealed by the following signs: quick, agitated movement; delirium; a talkative, extroverted manner; red face and eyes; whole or part of the body hot to the touch (or it feels hot to the patient); high fever (which may or may not be related to the fever of expelling a Pernicious Influence); irritability; thirst and desire for cold liquids; constipation; dark urine; dark, thick, and putrid secretions and excretions; red tongue material with yellow moss; and rapid pulse. Heat signs suggest that the basic shading of the body disharmony is "bright," and its mood is "jumpy." Table 4 summarizes the signs associated with Deficiency and Excess and the signs associated with Cold and Heat disharmonies.

TABLE 4 *Summary of Main Excess/Deficiency and Heat/Cold Signs*

EXCESS PATTERNS	
General Sign	Ponderous, heavy movement; heavy, coarse respiration; pressure and touch increase discomfort
Tongue	thick moss
Pulse	strong (full, wiry, slippery, etc.)

continued

TABLE 4 *Summary of Main Excess/Deficiency and Heat/Cold Signs (continued)*

DEFICIENCY PATTERNS	
General Sign	Frail, weak movement; tiredness; shortness of breath; pressure relieves discomfort; inactive, passive appearance; low voice; dizziness; little appetite
Tongue	pale material; thin moss
Pulse	weak (empty, frail, minute, etc.)

HEAT PATTERNS	
General Sign	Red face; feel hot; dislike of heat; cold reduces discomfort; rapid movement; outgoing manner; thirst or desire for cold drinks; dark urine; constipation
Tongue	red material; yellow moss
Pulse	rapid

COLD PATTERNS	
General Sign	Pale, white face; limbs cold; fear of cold; heat reduces discomfort; slow movement; withdrawn manner; no thirst, or a desire for hot drinks; clear urine; watery stool
Tongue	pale material; white moss
Pulse	slow

Patterns of Yin [*yin-zheng* 阴 证] *and Yang* [*yang-zheng* 阳 证] *Disharmonies*

Yin and Yang disharmonies are the most general, all-inclusive patterns in Chinese medicine. Indeed, all questions may ultimately be reduced to whether an individual pattern is Yin or Yang.

Yin patterns are combinations of signs associated with Interior, Deficiency, and Cold, while Yang patterns are woven from signs appropriate to Exterior, Excess, and Heat. These relationships are enumerated in Tables 5 and 6.

TABLE 5   *Yin and Yang Used to Summarize the Six Other Principles*

Yin	Interior	+	Deficient	+	Cold
Yang	Exterior	+	Excess	+	Hot

Of course, very few human illnesses can be characterized as pure Yin or pure Yang. If diagnosis were that simple, the task of the Chinese physician would be merely to catalog symptoms, an exercise that would produce a clinical landscape resembling a Cubist painting. Most patients exhibit a complex mixture of Yin and Yang signs and symptoms. For example, an extroverted, agitated personality (Yang) can also be frail, nervous, and easily pushed around (Yin). A slow, obsessive, calculating, and meticulous personality (Yin) can also be aggressive and belligerent (Yang). An individual with a severe contracting abdominal pain worsened by pressure (Excess and Yang) may, at the same time, get relief from a hot bath (Cold and Yin) and may have a slow pulse (Cold and Yin). Moreover, a single symptom might have varying significations because aspects of more than one pattern may be present. For instance, menstrual cramps relieved by Heat (Cold and Yin) may respond uncomfortably to touching (Excess and Yang), or a pulse may be both rapid (Heat and Yang) and thin (Deficient and Yin).

Therefore, the Eight Principal Patterns in their pure form are usually inadequate descriptions of clinical reality. They provide preliminary guidance for further perceptual refinement.

The first level of refinement is combining the Eight Principal Patterns to allow a closer approximation of clinical reality and a finer shading of the picture of disharmony. The way in which the Eight

TABLE 6 *Signs of Yin and Yang Patterns*

EXAMINATION: LOOKING

Yin Signs	quiet; withdrawn; slow, frail manner; patient is tired and weak, likes to lie down curled up; excretions and secretions are watery and thin; tongue material is pale, puffy, and moist; tongue moss is thin and white
Yang Signs	agitated, restless, active manner; rapid, forceful movement; red face; patient likes to stretch when lying down; tongue material is red or scarlet, and dry; tongue moss is yellow and thick

EXAMINATION: LISTENING AND SMELLING

Yin Signs	voice is low and without strength; few words; respiration is shallow and weak; shortness of breath; acrid odor
Yang Signs	voice is coarse, rough, and strong; patient is talkative; respiration is full and deep; putrid odor

EXAMINATION: ASKING

Yin Signs	feels cold; no taste in mouth; desires warmth and touch; copious and clear urine; pressure relieves discomfort; scanty, pale menses
Yang Signs	patient feels hot; dislikes heat or touch; constipation; scanty, dark urine; dry mouth; thirst

EXAMINATION: TOUCHING

Yin Signs	frail, minute, thin, empty, or otherwise weak pulse
Yang Signs	full, rapid, slippery, wiry, floating, or otherwise strong pulse

Principal Patterns are combined, reinforced, or modified illustrates how complex patterns are developed from simple ones. The method is basic to the process by which Yin and Yang combine to embrace reality.

─┤ COMBINATIONS OF THE EIGHT PRINCIPAL PATTERNS

The Pattern of Excess/Heat [shi-re-zheng 实 热 证]

When the patterns of Excess and Heat combine, two Yang patterns are merged, creating a distinct pure Yang Pattern. A typical configuration of the signs of this new pattern might be as follows.

Signs	Excess (Yang)	+	Heat (Yang)
Movement	forceful	+	fast
Pain	intensified by pressure	+	relieved by cold
Tongue	thick moss	+	red with yellow moss
Pulse	full and strong	+	rapid

The Pattern of Deficiency/Heat [xu-re-zheng 虚 热 证]

If patterns of Deficiency and Heat are merged, the resulting combination has both Yin (Deficiency) and Yang (Heat) aspects, which modify each other. The patient will most likely manifest the following signs.

Signs	Deficiency (Yin)	+	Heat (Yang)
Movement	weak and fragile	but	fast
Pain	relieved by pressure	but	relieved by cold
Tongue	little or no coating	but	red
Pulse	thin	but	rapid

The idealized normal Yin/Yang balance of the body, as well as the patterns of Excess/Heat (Excess Yang) and Deficiency/Heat (Deficient Yin), are schematically diagrammed in Figures 37, 38, and

39. (Because they are charts, these diagrams are based on a linearity foreign to the information they are used to present. Nonetheless, given this one qualification, they may be helpful.)

FIGURE 37 *Normal Yin/Yang Balance*

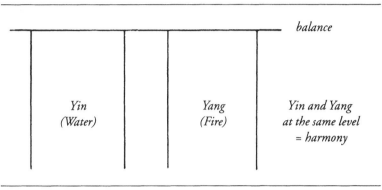

The pattern of Excess/Heat (also called Excess Yang, Figure 38) actually has too much Fire (Yang). Since this is a pure Yang pattern, all the signs will be Yang signs. For example, the movement of the patient may be fast and forceful like that of a prizefighter, the pulse full and rapid, and the tongue would likely be red, with a thick yellow coating.

FIGURE 38 *Pattern of Excess/Heat or Excess Yang*

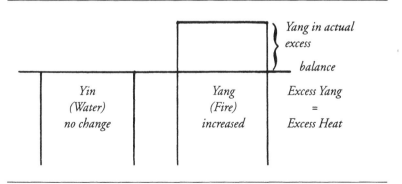

The pattern of Deficiency/Heat (Figure 39) has some qualities of Yang (Fire), but the symptoms actually appear because of insufficient Yin (Water).* The fire signs are "the appearance of Heat," also called "empty Fire" (*xu-huo*), and constitute a combination of Yin and Yang. This pattern of Deficiency/Heat is also known as Deficient Yin.

FIGURE 39 *Pattern of Deficiency/Heat or Deficient Yin*

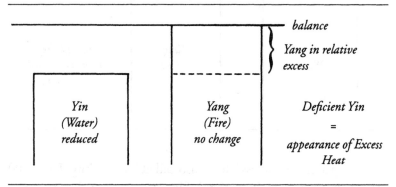

The patient may exhibit movement and activity less forceful than that associated with Excess/Heat, here taking the form of insomnia; restlessness; high, nervous laughter; or jumpy anxiety. There may be sensations of heat, but unlike the fevers of Excess, only the palms of the hands and soles of the feet become warm, or the fever is low, or it occurs only in the afternoon. The tongue is red (Yang), the moss thin (Yin), and the pulse rapid (Yang) but thin (Yin). These signs are often described as "the Yin unable to embrace the Yang": that is, there is insufficient Water to control the normal Fire, and the normal Yang gets out of control.

---

*Fire or Heat is the aspect of life that is activity. It is Yang. Cold would normally be the opposing Yin aspect to Fire, but Cold implies the cessation of life. Therefore, Water is thought to be the Yin aspect that balances Fire in life.

Understanding this process of assessing a place between pure Yin and pure Yang is the first glimpse of how clinical complexity is perceived.

The Pattern of Excess/Cold [*shi-han-zheng* 实 寒 证]

The patterns of Excess and Cold also combine Yin and Yang aspects. A patient with this pattern might manifest the following configuration of signs:

Signs	Excess (Yang)	+	Cold (Yin)
Movement	forceful	*but*	slow
Pain	unrelieved by pressure	*but*	responds to heat
Tongue	thick moss	*but*	pale
Pulse	tight, wiry, full, or otherwise strong	*but*	slow

The signs of Excess/Cold are modifications of the signs of its two primary aspects. The movement and emotions of the patient will be slow but forceful, perhaps robotlike; the patient may experience cramping pain and will not want to move; the painful area dislikes touch but will be relieved by a heating pad; the pulse will be slow and full; and urine will be clear but scanty. Because the pattern of Excess/Cold describes the presence of too much Cold, it is also called the pattern of Excess Yin (see Figure 40, page 228).

The Pattern of Deficiency/Cold [*xu-han-zheng* 虚 寒 证]

Like the Excess/Heat pattern, the Deficiency/Cold pattern is relatively simple because two sets of Yin signs reinforce one another to produce a pure Yin pattern. This might yield the following signs.

Signs	Deficiency (Yin)	+	Cold (Yin)
Movement	frail/weak	+	slow
Pain	relieved by pressure	+	responds to heat
Tongue	little or no moss	+	pale
Pulse	empty, thin, or otherwise weak	+	slow

FIGURE 40 *Pattern of Cold/Excess or Excess Yin*

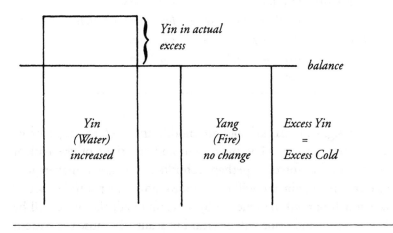

Both Yin aspects in Deficiency/Cold patterns reinforce each other so that the patient's movements and emotions are slow and frail, like those of an old, weak, chronically ill person, and the pulse is both slow and empty. Other signs would also be distinctively Yin, such as clear and copious urine or inability to be assertive.

The pattern of Deficiency/Cold is generated by a relative deficiency of Fire, so that the cold is only the "appearance of Cold" rather than a genuine excess of Cold. Hence, this pattern is also known as one of Deficient Yang (see Figure 41).

The basic combinations of Deficiency and Excess patterns with Cold and Heat patterns are summarized in Table 7.[4]

When a pattern is pure Yin (Deficiency and Cold, Yin within Yin) or pure Yang (Excess and Heat, Yang within Yang), the various signs merge and reinforce each other. When a pattern has aspects of both Yin and Yang (Excess and Cold or Deficiency and Heat), the physician must distinguish whether the Yang aspect predominates— that is, whether the pattern is one of Yin within Yang, or whether the Yin predominates and the pattern is Yang within Yin.[5]

The nature of these patterns can be clarified if we consider why Deficient Yin patterns and their signs (insomnia and night sweats) occur during the night, and Deficient Yang patterns and their signs (constant sleepiness and daytime sweats) happen during the day. Night is the time of inactivity and quiescence, but if a patient has a Deficient Yin pattern, he or she will have difficulty winding down because there is not enough Yin to control the Yang. This relatively excessive activity may not be noticeable during the day when it is normal to be active. At night, however, excess activity would be obviously inappropriate and would manifest itself as a disharmony state. A patient with a Deficient Yang pattern will tend to be under-active, and although this underactivity is appropriate to the normal quiescence of the night, it would be easily noticed during the day.

FIGURE 41 *Pattern of Cold/Deficiency or Deficient Yang*

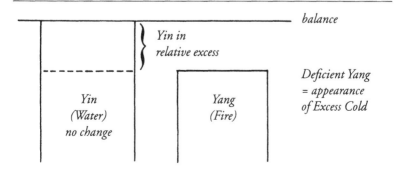

TABLE 7 *Combination of Deficiency and Excess Patterns with Cold and Heat Patterns*

EXCESS HEAT

Yin-Yang Designation	Excess Yang
Generative Factor	Heat Pernicious Influence collects
Common Signs	feel hot; fast, strong movements; assertive; pressure intensifies discomfort; patient desires cold; dark, scanty urine; constipation
Tongue	thick, yellow moss; red material
Pulse	rapid and full

DEFICIENT HEAT

Yin-Yang Designation	Deficient Yin
Generative Factor	Yin fluids depleted, Yin does not embrace Yang, insufficient Yin produces appearance of "empty Fire"
Common Signs	afternoon or evening heat flushes; weak, rapid, nervous movement; night sweats; warm palms and soles; insomnia; dizziness; dark urine
Tongue	little moss; tongue is reddish
Pulse	rapid and thin

EXCESS COLD

Yin-Yang Designation	Excess Yin
Generative Factor	Cold Pernicious Influence collects
Common Signs	ponderous, forceful, slow movement; infrequently change direction; aversion to cold; limbs are cold; heat reduces discomfort, but pressure intensifies it; clear, scanty urine
Tongue	thick, white moist moss; pale material
Pulse	slow and strong (tight, wiry, etc.)

continued

TABLE 7 *Combination of Deficiency and Excess Patterns*
with Cold and Heat Patterns (continued)

DEFICIENT COLD

Yin-Yang Designation	Deficient Yang
Generative Factor	insufficient Yang produces appearance of Cold
Common Signs	frail, weak, slow movement; little commitment, easily changes mind; aversion to cold; heat and pressure relieve discomfort; copious, clear urine; flat affect, no Spirit
Tongue	thin moss; pale, puffy material
Pulse	slow and weak (thin, minute, frail, etc.)

Patterns of True Heat/Illusionary Cold
[*zhen-re jia-han-zheng* 真 热 假 寒 证]
True Cold/Illusionary Heat
[*zhen-han jia-re-zheng* 真 寒 假 热 证]

Sometimes, and commonly in very extreme disharmonies, some signs will appear that are actually illusionary. For example, in the course of a severe Heat disharmony (that is, a disharmony in which the patient is affected by signs associated with Heat), the patient may experience delirium, a burning sensation in the chest and abdomen, and great thirst for cold liquids. The tongue moss will be yellow and dry, and the pulse very rapid and full. Suddenly the patient's limbs turn cold, while other signs remain the same. (In shock, which this is not, other signs would also change.) This sign of cold limbs is termed Illusionary Cold. It is also said to be Illusionary Yin because it is the result of extreme Yang energy forcing Yin to the extremities. The pattern it indicates is called True Heat/Illusionary Cold.

On the other hand, in a very severe Cold disharmony in which the limbs are cold, the pulse is minute, and the stool full of undigested food, the patient might become agitated instead of remaining quiet and withdrawn, as would be expected. The agitation gives the appearance of Heat, although the pattern is one of genuine Cold. This pattern is termed True Cold/Illusionary Heat. It arises because the Yang is so weak that it floats to the surface of the body "like the last flicker of a dying candle." Figures 42 and 43 (pages 246 and 247) illustrate the dynamics of these illusionary sign phenomena.

FIGURE 42 *Pattern of True Heat/Illusionary Cold*

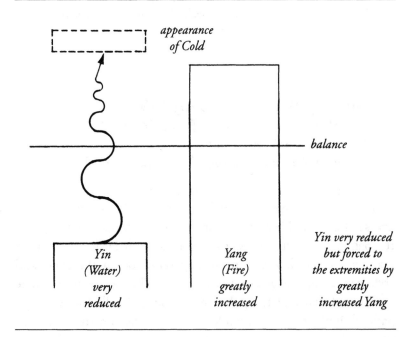

Patterns of Internal/External, Deficient/Excess, Cold/Hot

It is possible for opposite patterns to exist simultaneously. For example, a person may have a chronic Deficiency/Cold pattern, with such signs as cold limbs, watery stool, and pale, puffy tongue. Suddenly, a Heat/Wind Pernicious Influence invades the body and produces a fever, fear of drafts, headache, red, sore throat, and thirst and dry tongue, while the earlier signs remain. This is a case of an Interior/Deficiency/Cold disharmony existing simultaneously with an Exterior/Heat disharmony. Other possible signs in the total pattern can vary greatly, depending on which pattern is dominant at a given moment.

FIGURE 43 *Pattern of True Cold/Illusionary Heat*

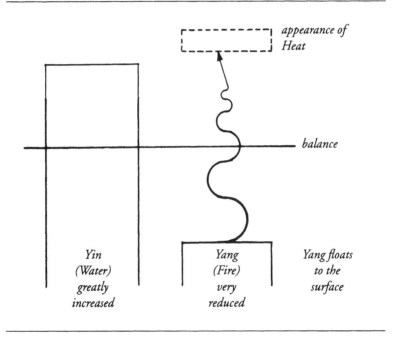

In addition, one pattern of disharmony can often change into another pattern. For instance, a weak Spleen may be unable to vaporize water. A pattern of Deficiency affecting the Spleen can then cause Dampness. But a buildup of Dampness, with symptoms such as edema or accumulated indecision and corresponding changes in pulse and tongue, can then create a pattern of Excess. Or as is more common, a pattern of simultaneously occurring Deficiency and Excess with many possible variations and combinations of symptoms can result. Similarly, Heat can turn into Cold, or vice versa. An Excess/Heat illness of high fever can change into a pattern of Cold/Deficiency. This may be manifested in cold limbs, a very pallid face, deep, weak pulse, or even shock. Or a Deficiency/Heat pattern of irritability, dry mouth, and rapid, thin pulse may appear. A patient could also begin with an Exterior/Cold pattern of a Cold Pernicious Influence with signs like chills, fever, body aches, thin, white tongue moss, and floating and tight pulse. The chills may then disappear and the other signs change to high fever, thirst, irritability, yellow tongue moss, and rapid pulse—that is, a change from a Cold pattern to a Heat pattern. The Chinese clinician constantly sees such continuously changing multiple patterns.

The Eight Principal Patterns are the major categories into which all patterns of disharmony are grouped. For the Chinese, they are the guidelines, the nets that help to capture human reality. They define a disharmony in the most general way, but, as has been shown, they can also be endlessly combined and refined to describe a disharmony more precisely.[6]

NOTES

1. This translation is now common. For example, *A Chinese English Dictionary* (printed by Beijing Foreign Languages Institute [Beijing: Commercial Press, 1978], p. 9) defines *ba-gang* as the "eight principal syndromes."

2. Owsei Temkin, "Health and Disease," in *The Double Face of Janus and Other Essays in the History of Medicine* (Baltimore: Johns Hopkins University Press, 1977), p. 436. Dr. Temkin also points out that the impetus to define a disease by a cause, in its modern form, was partly due to the influence of Robert Koch's monumental discovery of the tubercle bacillus in 1882 and the dramatic effect of bacteriology and germ theory on modern concepts of disease in general.

   Of course, this modern notion of causality is very different from the Aristotelian metaphysical idea of *final* and *formal* causes. In the scientific system, an explanation means a reduction of things into their elementary parts, and the concept of change in terms of *efficient* causality alone.

3. The effort to concretize and clarify Yin and Yang into Eight Principal Patterns is the history of Chinese medicine systematizing itself. Combinations of paired patterns are frequently mentioned and emphasized as the key aspects of disease and treatment in all early texts. The *Nei Jing*, for example, has many references such as: "Yang is Heavenly Qi and rules the Exterior, Yin is Earthly Qi and rules the Interior. Therefore, the Yang way is Excess and the Yin way is Deficiency" (*Su Wen*, sec. 8, chap. 29, p. 179); "The occurrence of the hundred illnesses is in their Excess or Deficiency" (*Su Wen*, sec. 17, chap. 62, p. 334); or "Yin rules Cold, Yang rules Heat" (*Ling Shu*, sec. 11, chap. 74, p. 505). Many other concepts, all of them aspects of Yin and Yang, are also mentioned—Blood, Qi, Chronic, Acute, Falling, Rising, Damp, Dry, Thin, Thick, Soft, Hard, Lower, Upper, Mucus, Fire, Quiescent, Moving, etc. Throughout the history of Chinese medicine, attempts have been made to give the myriad movements of Yin and Yang a less abstract and more systematic form. For example, Kou Zhong-shi, in his Elaborate Pharmacopoeia (*Ben-cao Yan-yi*) of 1116 C.E., codifies the Eight Essentials, which he calls Excess, Deficiency, Cold, Heat, Pernicious Influence, Normal Qi, Interior, and Exterior. For him these are the primary aspects of Yin and Yang that need adjustment when there is disharmony. In 1565 C.E., Lou Ying, in his Outline of Medicine (*Yi-xue Gang-mu*), stated that in order to reharmonize the Yin and Yang of the body, the physician must first determine whether the disharmony is of the Qi or the Blood, Exterior or Interior, Upper or Lower regions of the body, and then in which Yin or Yang Organ. Then one must ascertain whether the imbalance is Deficiency, Excess, Cold, or Heat. The great codifier of the Ming dynasty, Zhang Jie-bing, in his Complete Book, 1624 C.E., states that Yin and Yang are the general principles and that Exterior/Interior, Excess/Deficiency, Heat/Cold are the main aspects. For the Chinese, the actual form of the organization of Yin/Yang is less important than the underlying ability to see Yin/Yang as having many possible aspects and movements. For a full discussion of the historic development of the systematization of Yin/Yang theory, see Jia De-dao, Concise History [95], pp. 231–234.

4. The basic matrix of this table is delineated in the *Nei Jing*: "Deficient Yang then outer Cold, Deficient Yin then inner Heat [identified with empty Fire], Excess Yang then outer Heat, and Excess Yin then inner Cold" (*Su Wen*, sec. 17, chap. 62, p. 341). The symptomology of the charts, and indeed of this entire chapter and the next one, is ultimately based on the *Nei Jing* as systematized by the tradition. The *Nei Jing* is not always consistent in its presentation, but occasionally such sentences appear: "Abundant pulse, hot skin, abdominal distention, lack of urine and stool, and stuffiness with pressure are called the Five Excesses. A thin pulse, cold

skin, lack of Qi, diarrhea or frequent urination, and inability to eat are called the Five Deficiencies" (*Su Wen*, sec. 6, chap. 19, pp. 128–129).

5. For example, in a Deficient Yin pattern (Deficiency/Heat), the matrix of signs may emphasize Heat more than Deficiency (e.g., if the pulse is very rapid but only somewhat thin, or the patient's movement is very quick but only slightly weak). In this case, the Yang predominates and the pattern is Yin within Yang. In another Deficient Yin pattern, the pulse may be somewhat rapid but very thin, and the patient's movement very frail but only slightly quick. In this case, the pattern would be one of Yang within Yin. An evaluation process would take place to determine whether an Excess/Cold (Excess Yin) pattern were Yin within Yang or Yang within Yin. Pure Yin is also called Yin within Yin, and pure Yang is called Yang within Yang. These patterns and their combinations are summarized in the following table.

Designations of Yin-Yang

EXCESS YANG

Pattern Combination	Heat/Excess		
Yin-Yang Combination	Yang within Yang (pure Yang)		
Pulse as Sample Sign	rapid and full		

DEFICIENT YANG

Pattern Combination	Cold/Deficient		
Yin-Yang Combination	Yin within Yin (pure Yin)		
Pulse as Sample Sign	slow and weak		

EXCESS YIN

Pattern Combination	mostly Cold with some Excess	or	mostly Excess with some Cold
Yin-Yang Combination	Yang within Yin	or	Yin within Yang
Pulse as Sample Sign	slow and slightly tight	or	tight, strong, and slightly slow

DEFICIENT YIN

Pattern Combination	mostly Heat with some Deficiency	or	mostly Deficiency with some Heat
Yin-Yang Combination	Yin within Yang	or	Yang within Yin
Pulse as Sample Sign	rapid and slightly thin	or	thin and slightly rapid

In clinical practice, patients fit into the spaces between the pure categories described. Most patients simultaneously have Deficient Cold (Deficient Yang) with some Excess Cold (Excess Yin), or some Excess Heat (Excess Yang) with Deficient Heat (Deficient Yin). The process of evaluation is the same—an appraisal of the predominating proportions. For an example, see Chapter 8, page 275.

6. The Song dynasty (960–1279 C.E.) codification of Yin-Yang theory into the categories that became the Eight Principal Patterns bears a marked resemblance to a similar systematization of Greek medicine developed in Islamic civilization. These two clarifications of the earlier medical tradition coincided in time, and the form and content of the two are strikingly similar.

The Greco-Arab synthesis, like the Chinese, was bipolar. Its Hot and Cold temperaments were the active primary poles, while Dry and Moist were the passive secondary poles. The four humors, tastes, predominant organs, times of year, etc., fit into a dynamic schema of correspondence with the four temperaments. Avicenna (Ibn Sina, 980–1037 C.E.), the "prince and chief of physicians," wrote descriptions of the signs for each of four temperaments, which are roughly equivalent to the Eight Principal Patterns.

For Avicenna, an abundance of Heat had some of the following signs: feeling uncomfortably hot; bitter taste in mouth; rapid gestures; excitability; liveliness; excessive thirst; sense of burning in epigastric region; quick pulse; intolerance of hot food; cold relieves symptoms; symptoms are worse in summer. This is notably like the Chinese Excess Heat pattern. Avicenna's Cold temperament has some of these signs: lack of desire for fluids; deficient digestive power; lack of excitability; slow gestures; flaccid joints; fever, if present, is of the phlegmatic type; cold things easily upset and hot things are beneficial; small, slow, sluggish pulse; symptoms are worse in winter. This easily compares to the Chinese Deficient Cold pattern. Avicenna's abundance of Moisture resembles Dampness or Excess Cold: puffiness; excessive mucoid salivation and nasal secretion; diarrhea; swollen eyelids; difficult digestion; lassitude; moist articles of diets are harmful; soft and wide pulse. And finally, Avicenna's abundance of Dryness resembles Deficient Yin: insomnia; wakefulness; rough, dry skin; hot water and oils are easily absorbed in the skin; symptoms are worse in autumn. See O. Cameron Gruner, *The Canon of Medicine of Avicenna*, part 1, thesis 3, par. 452–500, pp. 257–278, esp. p. 273.

Avicenna was concerned with causality in an Aristotelian sense and would often go so far as to find an entire array of material, efficient, formal, and final causes of an illness. Yet despite this radical difference from the Chinese style, Greco-Arab medicine (like all humoral medicine) correlates all the observable phenomena of a human being into an image derived from the natural environment. This image portrays a human microcosm resembling a universal macrocosm. The net result of this methodology will often produce a striking confluence of ideas.

Similarities to the Chinese model are found even in nonbipolar systems, as in the Hindu Ayurvedic system. For example, *pitha*, responsible for heat production, resembles China's Fire; *vata*, whose presence is indicated by such phenomena as respiration, circulation, and excretion, resembles China's Qi; and *kapha*, which protects the tissues from being consumed by the internal fires of *pitha*, very much resembles the Chinese Yin or Fluids. In pathology, this image configuration method carries over. For example, the Pitha-type headache is "associated with burning sensation in various parts of the head and bleeding from the nose. It is generally aggravated during midday and summer and autumn seasons." The Vata-type headache is "associated with a giddiness, sleeplessness, dryness and roughness of the eyes and various types of pain." Kapha-type headaches have "heaviness of the head, watering of the eyes, inflammation of the middle ear, running of the nose [and] inflammation of the mucus membrane of the nose." Vd. Bhagwan Dash, *Ayurvedic Treatment for Common Diseases*, pp. 94–95. For a general discussion of Ayurvedic medicine, see C. Dwarkanath's *Introduction to Kayachikitsa*. When I worked in an Ayurvedic hospital in India years ago, I found that my Chinese medical background enabled me in a short time to predict the categories that Ayurvedic physicians would use to describe their patients.

The relation and relative importance of causality within Greco-Arab medicine and Ayurvedic medicine are compared by V. K. Venkata-swami, "Humoral Theory and Modern Medicine," in *Theories and Philosophies of Medicine*, comp. by Dept. of Philosophy of Medicine and Science.

8

THE PATTERNS OF THE HUMAN LANDSCAPE

the details of the clinical scene

The Eight Principal Patterns, as we have seen, define the basic picture of human disharmony. Although the general qualities delineated by these patterns sometimes allow the physician to select the proper acupuncture points or herbs, or a combination of the two, that will tend to rebalance the disharmony, more frequently the clinical picture must be refined. By themselves, the Eight Principal Patterns are too crude. This refinement is achieved by using the Eight Principal Patterns as a basic matrix and also seeing or emphasizing signs that relate to the fundamental textures, the Pernicious Influences, or the Organs.

The bulk of this chapter describes the basic clinical patterns commonly seen by practitioners of traditional East Asian medicine. Before this discussion, the chapter has two preliminary sections. The first section deals with general disharmonies of Qi and Blood as common clinical descriptions of the basic polarities of Yin and Yang. The second section reexamines the medical paradigms of East and West. Finally, the reader encounters the first detailed presentation of what an Oriental physician might actually recognize in the human landscape.

⊣ PATTERNS OF QI AND DEFICIENT YANG, PATTERNS OF BLOOD AND DEFICIENT YIN

Qi and Blood are the fundamental textures most often used to describe the first level of refinement in the harmonious and disharmonious states of the human landscape. The Qi's tension and the Blood's repose are the preliminary emblematic categories that most succinctly delineate the Yin-Yang state of a human being. As the *Nei Jing* summarizes, "Disharmonies of the Blood and Qi are the basis of the hundred diseases."[1]

Patterns of Deficient Qi [*qi-xu-zheng* 气 虚 证] *and* Deficient Yang [*yang-su-zheng* 阳 虚 证]

Qi is about dynamic tension, active force, transformation, and creativity. Deficient Qi is inactivity, the absence of tension, and inappropriate stillness. The following signs gleaned from the Four Examinations, when woven together, suggest Deficient Qi: general weakness or lethargy; pale, bright face; shallow respiration; low, soft voice; little desire to speak; dislike of movement; spontaneous sweating; easily lose focus; a passive introverted manner; pale tongue material; and empty, frail, or otherwise weak pulse. The most reliable of these signs are a bright, pale face and a weak pulse.

If the pattern of Deficient Qi is a generalized one in which the entire body's Normal Qi is affected, the physician need not proceed any further with the diagnosis and can start appropriate treatment. The pattern, however, may also be associated with a particular Organ Qi or a particular type of Qi (for example, Protective Qi). In such cases, additional signs specific to a particular type of Qi disharmony will be displayed.

It is important to distinguish the patterns of Deficient Qi from those of Deficient Yang. Deficient Yang includes Deficient Qi. Qi is a Yang phenomenon because it is dynamic. If Qi is deficient, therefore, some aspect of Yang will also be deficient. Furthermore, since Deficient Yang encompasses Deficient Qi, if Yang is deficient, it would follow that Qi, as well as other Yang functions, is deficient. Deficient Yang implies a diminution of Fire, which leads to a relative Excess of Cold or the "appearance of Cold." Therefore, Deficient Yang displays the signs of Deficient Qi as well as signs of Interior Cold, such as cold limbs, slow movement, aversion to cold, puffy tongue, and slow pulse. Often, the shared signs are more severe. Deficient Yang is a broader category of Deficiency than Deficient Qi in two senses: It is more inclusive, and it affects the body at deeper levels. Ultimately, Yang is the more profound dynamic force.

Patterns of Stagnant Qi [*qi-zhi-zheng* 气 滞 证]

Stagnant Qi is a pattern of Excess that occurs when the smooth flow of Qi is stuck in a particular Organ, Meridian, or other part of the body. This pattern usually requires further elaboration to localize it. Stagnant Qi may result from emotional or dietary imbalances, External Pernicious Influences, or trauma. When Qi is Deficient—that is, when there is not enough Qi in a particular part of the body to keep the Qi itself moving—Stagnant Qi may also arise. This is a case of a pattern of Deficiency turning into one of Excess.

A primary symptom of Stagnant Qi is distention and/or soreness and pain. (This does not mean, however, that all soreness and distention result from Stagnant Qi.) The distention or soreness associated with Stagnant Qi characteristically changes in severity and location. If palpable lumps are present, they usually are soft, and they come and go. Psychologically, Stagnant Qi has the feeling of being blocked, frustrated, tense, or moody. A darkish or purplish tongue and a stagnant pulse, such as a wiry or tight pulse, are also salient signs of this pattern.

Patterns of Deficient Blood [xue-xu-zheng 血 虚 证] and Deficient Yin [yin-xu-zheng 阴 虚 证]

Blood is the energetic of repose, receptivity, and relaxation. Blood is the absence of tension; it is rest, nourishment, and cycles of movement; it is absence of goals, the easy acknowledgement of what has already been accomplished. Blood is soft, moistening, and allows for recognition of self-worth. Deficient Blood is the inappropriate presence of tension; it is restlessness, tightness, jumpiness, the absence of responsiveness and receptivity. Deficient Blood may be preceded by loss of Blood, insufficient Spleen Qi to produce new Blood, or Congealed Blood that prevents new Blood from forming. The following signs, when woven together, point to the general pattern of Deficient Blood: dizziness or a sensation of instability; thin, emaciated body; spots in the visual field or otherwise impaired vision; poor memory; weak tremors, tightness, or cramps; numbness in the limbs; dry skin or hair; scanty menses; lusterless, pale face and lips; pale tongue material; and thin pulse. The most decisive of these signs are the restlessness, absence of self-esteem, and the thin pulse. Deficient Blood, like Deficient Qi, may affect a particular Organ, requiring further refinement of the pattern based on additional signs.

Deficient Yin is deeper, more still, and has a deeper sense of tranquillity and stillness. Blood has no goal but still moves in cycles; Yin is pure quiescence and has the sense of arrival. Yin is closer to the Essence (Jing) while Blood is closer to the Qi. Deficient Yin belongs more to the Kidneys while Deficient Blood has a closer relationship to the Liver, Spleen, and Heart. When the Yin is Deficient, it is easily recognized by an inappropriate appearance of movement or heat. Deficient Yin can have "the appearance of Heat"—a relative excess of Yang brought about by a lack of Yin, or Water. Deficient Blood and Deficient Yin often display similar signs, especially emaciated appearance, absence of stillness, dizziness, spots in the visual field, and thin pulse. Deficient Yin, though, will also display Heat signs: agitated manner, red cheeks, warm palms and soles, night sweats, red tongue material, and rapid, thin pulse.[2]

Pattern of Congealed Blood [*xue-yu-zheng* 血 瘀 证]

Blood allows an effortless maintenance and recognition of self. When the Blood loses its easy movement and nurturing presence and accumulates inappropriately, the self generates a "contrary" self. Designated Congealed Blood, one of its primary signs is severe pain. This pain is different from that of Stagnant Qi because it is fixed and stabbing. The self "opposes" itself; there is no respite from pain. Other common signs of Congealed Blood include tumors, lumps, and hard, relatively immobile masses; the body generates its own antithesis. Congealed Blood's sense of the "self splitting from itself" is also recognizable in such signs as the inability to feel safe and feelings of suspiciousness, terror, and paranoia. Also recurring, frequent hemorrhages (because the Blood flow is blocked, causing "spillage"), hemorrhages with clots of a dark, purple tinge (the color of congestion), a dark complexion, dark purple tongue material with red spots, and a choppy pulse all point to the pattern of Congealed Blood. Congealed Blood may be preceded by trauma and abuse, hemorrhage, Stagnant Qi (which cannot move the Blood), or Cold patterns.

Pattern of Hot Blood [*xue-re-zheng* 血 热 证]

The Blood should move smoothly. If Heat affects the Blood it can become "reckless." The major symptom of this Excess/Heat pattern is bleeding. It is often generated by a Heat Pernicious Influence that has invaded deep inside the body, agitating the Blood and making it "reckless"—that is, causing it to leave the normal pathways and to hemorrhage. Symptoms of Hot Blood include: blood in the sputum, vomitus, urine, or feces; bloody nose; excessive menses; and red skin eruptions. Other accompanying Heat signs may include thirst, irritability, scarlet tongue, rapid pulse, and, in extreme cases, delirium.

⊣ EAST AND WEST RECONSIDERED

At this point, the nature of the difference between the perceptions of Eastern medicine and biomedicine needs to be reexamined. In Chapter 1 it was demonstrated in a very simple way that six patients suffering from ulcer could be perceived quite differently by Chinese and Western doctors. This illustrated the fact that a single Western disease entity may become various diagnoses of medical disharmonies within the framework of East Asian medicine.

Now let us take a closer look at the actual study of the sixty-five gastric-ulcer patients from which the six patients were chosen as examples (see Chapter 1, note 7). All of these patients had theoretically identical diseases in the terms of biomedicine.

About half of the sixty-five Chinese diagnoses cited various Spleen disharmonies (Deficiency, Dampness, Cold, etc.), while the rest pointed to Stomach and Liver disharmonies. None of the patients was described as having a Lung or Kidney disharmony. Thus, the diagnoses of the biomedical entity did not yield a totally random sample of Chinese medical disharmonies. From the universe of possible Chinese diagnoses, the single Western diagnosis of gastric ulcer was paralleled by a few specific clusters of disharmony patterns.

If this experiment had been reversed and a number of patients, all diagnosed by a Chinese physician as manifesting the same pattern of disharmony, had been seen by a Western physician, several distinct Western disease entities would be diagnosed. However, a high incidence of certain specific clusters of diseases would emerge. Although there are no one-to-one correspondences between Chinese and Western diagnoses, a type of correlation can indeed be found.

This correlation may be demonstrated by using the pattern of Deficient Spleen Qi as an example. This pattern is associated with such signs as chronic fatigue, lack of motivation and desire, appetite disorder, poor digestion, watery stool, abdominal distention, pale tongue material with thin, white moss, and empty pulse.

If a large group of patients with this disharmony were looked at from a Western perspective, depending on where recruitment occurred, maybe half of them would be diagnosed as having chronic gastrointestinal disorders such as gastroenteritis, ulcers, or nervous stomach. A significant number would be thought to have chronic hepatitis, hemorrhoids, amenorrhea, anemia, and various bleeding disorders. A smaller percentage would be diagnosed as having major depressive disorder, chronic fatigue disorder, and degenerative neuromuscular disorders.[3] It would be unlikely that any of the patients exhibiting Deficient Spleen Qi would be discovered to have acute urinary infections, glaucoma, or pleurisy.[4]

Another example is the pattern of Liver Fire, the signs of which may include red face; red eyes; scanty, dark urine; constipation; severe headaches and/or ringing in the ears; anger and frequent episodes of rage; nausea or vomiting; red tongue material with yellow moss; and wiry, full, and fast pulse. In Western terms, people with this pattern might be diagnosed as having hypertension, migraine, atherosclerosis, acute conjunctivitis, glaucoma and other eye disorders, or acute hepatitis, with a smaller percentage thought to have bleeding disorders and urogenital infections.[5] Some would be considered psychiatric patients. Liver Fire patterns would probably not be associated with such Western diseases as chronic gastrointestinal disorders, tuberculosis, pernicious anemia, or dysentery.

In different Chinese patterns, some of the same Western medical categories can exist. For instance, in both the Deficient Spleen Qi and the Liver Fire patterns, hepatitis and hematolytic disorders would be likely Western diagnoses. It can be seen that a large group of patients with a particular Chinese pattern would frequently encompass a cluster of several biomedical disease entities, producing a statistical correspondence of large groups, rather than any one-to-one correspondences.

This kind of statistical grouping results from large group comparisons because, although the two systems imply different understandings of health, disease, diagnosis, and treatment, they nonetheless deal with the same body. There is an overlap in which some of the bodily functions and locations, as perceived by East and West, are at times comparable, or at least mutually recognizable. And both systems rely on internally consistent frames of reference.

This statistical correlation has been noted in China, especially during the last fifty years, when many patients have been diagnosed by the two systems consecutively or simultaneously.[6] The implications and nature of the diagnosis provided by each system are always different—the Chinese diagnosis is refined by understanding how the disharmony embraces the other Organs and the entire human being, while the Western diagnosis is refined by isolating an exact cause or a precise pathological process.

On the simple level, the correlations between Chinese and biomedicine do not help in formulating correct treatment. You cannot merely look up a disease and its treatment in one system and then find an analog in the other. Nevertheless, amid the strange-sounding formulations of Chinese diagnosis, the correlations, especially of somatic diseases, may help readers familiar with biomedicine to orient themselves. Further explorations of these correlations may open up an avenue for deeper biomedical research into Chinese medicine.

The following discussion of disharmony patterns of the Organs will include statistical correlations with Western diseases that are indicated in clinical reports, studies, and medical texts produced in the People's Republic of China.*

---

*It is interesting to note that some Western diseases, such as epilepsy (*dian-xian*), dysentery (*li-ji*), malaria (*nue-ji*), measles (*ma-zhen*), and consumption (*fei-lao*), exist in the Chinese medical system as well as in the Western one. This correspondence reflects the fact that the two systems ultimately treat the same human body and that certain disease categories are recognized globally by symptoms alone and antedate the rise of modern medicine. Dysentery, for instance, is known by the same symptoms to both

⊣ PATTERNS OF ORGAN DISHARMONY

Describing patterns of disharmony in terms of the Organs that are involved is the next step in refining the understanding of a disharmony. Patterns of disharmony involving particular Organs are primarily an elaboration of the Eight Principal Patterns, the patterns of Qi and Blood disharmonies, and the patterns of Pernicious Influences. These basic patterns are then refined and made specific by the addition of signs and symptoms alluded to in the earlier discussion of Organs.

The patterns of Organ disharmony are not, however, mechanically generated by logical principles, but represent the way in which tradition has modified theory throughout centuries of clinical practice. For example, although the Lungs can have Deficient Yang, such a pattern is not generally discussed in the medical literature. In practice, Deficient Yang of the Lungs is seen as Deficient Lung Qi in combination with Deficient Kidney Yang. Practice determines the "reality" of the clinical category. The patterns of Organ disharmony presented here are the basic, most common patterns of disharmony in clinical Chinese medicine; it is far from being all-inclusive.

Spleen Disharmonies

The Spleen rules transmutation and is the essential focus for the transformative dynamic of Qi in human life. The Spleen allows food

---

East and West. In the modern West, however, the diagnosis of dysentery would be followed by the search for a pathogen—amebic or bacterial—whereas in Chinese medicine, more signs would be collected to categorize the dysentery according to an appropriate pattern. Similarly, Chinese medicine recognizes a pattern similar to the Western entity of pulmonary tuberculosis. A Chinese physician would proceed to classify it as a pattern by synthesizing the accompanying signs and symptoms into a more precise configuration. A modern Western physician would search for the pathogen, identify the disease as tuberculosis, and treat it according to its bacterial origin. This equivalence is approximate. Because the differential criteria are not the same, it is possible for a diagnosis of dysentery or diabetes in Chinese medicine not to be that same entity in biomedicine. (To avoid confusion, all diseases or patterns common to both medical systems will be referred to by their Western nomenclature.)

to become the textures and activities of human life and is responsible for the creative change in life. The Spleen is about engagement, possibilities, and creativity. Li Dong-yuan (1180–1251 C.E.), one of the greatest physicians in Chinese history, described the Spleen's Qi as giving human beings the power to "meet pleasurable affairs, encounter the environment as balmy and suitable, find food agreeable and tasty, see desirable and lovable things, and make a person intelligent and alert."[7] Spleen Qi is the zest that moves life. Spleen disharmonies can have two aspects: Deficient or Excess. Deficiency has to do with insufficient Qi; Excess has to do with the accumulation of Dampness. Sometimes, the Spleen has both Deficiency and Excess together.

Patterns of Deficient Spleen Qi (*pi-qi-xu* 脾气虚) ***and Deficient Spleen Yang*** (*pi-yang-xu* 脾阳虚)   The pattern of Deficient Spleen Qi is associated with such Spleen-specific signs as appetite disorders, slight abdominal pain and distention that are relieved by touching (insufficient Qi to move food), and loose stools (insufficient Qi to complete digestion). If the Consciousness of Potentials (*Yi*) is affected, the person can have poor motivation, lack excitement, be bored, be despondent, or avoid activities that were once pleasurable. He or she is not interested in the world nor engaged in creative transformation. In addition, there are the other signs of Deficient Qi, primarily lethargy, lack of dynamic tension, a pale tongue with thin white moss, and an empty pulse. From this pattern, Western physicians might diagnose gastric or duodenal ulcers, gastritis, hepatitis, chronic dysentery, anemia, or psychiatric disorders including major depressive disorders.[8]

The pattern of Deficient Spleen Yang is a deeper and more serious disharmony than that of Deficient Spleen Qi. It is associated with signs of the appearance of Cold, especially cold limbs; swollen, moist, pale tongue; and slow, frail pulse. Also, certain of the Spleen-specific signs will be more extreme or Cold in nature (for instance, watery stools containing undigested food and abdominal distention or pain that responds favorably to heat as well as pressure). The

Consciousness of Potentials (Yi) might exhibit lack of resolution or defeatism. Deficient Spleen Yang may also affect the movement of water in the body, producing such symptoms as edema, difficulty in urination, and leukorrhea. Patients with Deficient Spleen Yang might be diagnosed in the West as having such chronic diseases as gastric or duodenal ulcers, gastritis, enteritis, hepatitis, dysentery, nephritis,[9] or psychiatric disorders. A Spleen Yang pattern can merge with a Kidney Yang disharmony (see below).

Pattern of Spleen Qi Sinking (*pi-qi-xia-xian* 脾气下陷) The dynamic aspect of Qi is responsible for holding things in place. Stability may require the effort of tension. Deficient Spleen Qi and Deficient Spleen Yang occur when the Qi cannot perform its function of retaining things in their proper place. This pattern is also sometimes called Middle Burner Collapsing. In addition to the signs of Deficient Spleen Qi and Deficient Spleen Yang, this pattern displays signs associated with falling, such as hemorrhoids, prolapse of the uterus, extreme chronic diarrhea, or urinary incontinence. If the Consciousness of Potentials is affected, there can be an exaggerated sense of disability, mislabeled somatic sensation, or converting inconvenience into catastrophe.

Pattern of Spleen Unable to Govern the Blood (*pi-bu-zong-xue* 脾不统血) This is another subcategory of Deficient Spleen Qi or Yang, occurring when the Yang Qi of the Spleen cannot hold the Blood in place. Various kinds of chronic bleeding result: blood in the stool, bloody nose, chronic subcutaneous hemorrhaging, excessive menses, or uterine bleeding. These symptoms are generally accompanied by other signs of Deficiency. (If hemorrhaging were accompanied by signs of Excess or Heat, it would of course be interpreted differently, probably as Hot Blood.)

In biomedicine, the pattern of Spleen Unable to Govern the Blood would commonly appear as functional uterine bleeding, bleeding hemorrhoids, hemophilia, or Henoch-Schönlein purpura.[10]

Pattern of Dampness Distressing the Spleen (*shi-kun-pi* 湿 困 脾) Dampness is accumulations that the Spleen has not successfully moved from one state of being to another. One can say that Dampness is an incomplete transformation, the unfinished creation of the Spleen. Dampness is the possibility of change and creativity that, instead of going from one state to another, has instead piled up and created a kind of "stagnant or swampy pool." Food that is incompletely transformed "sits" and becomes the physical aspect of Dampness, causing distention and bloat. Ideas get stuck and become the worry aspect of Dampness. The Spleen is said to like "dryness" and dislike "dampness." The Spleen likes clarity, definition, and a distinct movement from one state of being to another. Dampness has unclear borders and imprecise boundaries. Dampness is what happens when the possibility of transmutation becomes the burden of unfinished business.

Dampness Distressing the Spleen produces signs and characteristics that can resemble Deficient Spleen. The main difference is that they are marked by a sense of "heaviness" and clutter. On a physical level, Dampness may be indicated by such signs as appetite disorders, sticky-watery stool, nausea, and a feeling of fullness in the abdomen or head, or skin eruptions containing fluids. On a psychological level, Dampness is indicated by excessive worry, ruminations, feelings of being trapped by multiple good possibilities, indecision, having many unfinished projects, procrastination, inability to make clear distinctions (or even clean one's room), excessively taking care of others without the ability to take care of the self. If fatigue is present in a Damp pattern, it often does not hinder the performance of work (especially for others), but it has a sense of heaviness and weariness.

Dampness often results from Deficient Spleen being unable to perform its transformative work. If this happens, it is an example of Deficiency turning into Excess. Because the signs can sometimes be similar, the pulse and tongue may be critical in discerning the difference. A slippery or soggy pulse and a thick, greasy tongue moss are then important signs of Dampness. Sometimes both Deficient and Excess Spleen exist at the same time. This can present a diagnostic challenge that requires skill, experience, and attention to detail to decide whether Yin (Deficiency) or Yang (Dampness) dominates.

In Western terms, this pattern might translate into chronic gastroenteritis, chronic dysentery, chronic hepatitis, or various obsessive-compulsive disorders.[11]

External Dampness Obstructing (*wai-shi-zu* 外 湿 湿) This pattern is similar to the preceding one, although much less common, and occurs when Dampness is an External Pernicious Influence. The Spleen is affected, and the same signs of Dampness Distress are present. In addition, this pattern tends to be relatively acute, characterized by sudden onset and, occasionally, a low fever.

Damp Heat Collecting in the Spleen (*pi-yun-shi-re* 脾 蕴 湿 热) Dampness and Cold are both Yin, and so Dampness patterns are likely to manifest signs of Cold. However, Dampness can also be Hot, and if Heat signs are present, a distinct, common pattern may be perceived. Although Damp Heat Collecting in the Spleen is usually the result of an External Pernicious Influence,[12] this pattern is also associated with eating fatty foods and excessive alcohol consumption. The signs of Dampness will be present as well as the signs of Heat, and the movement of bile can be obstructed, causing jaundice and a bitter taste in the mouth.

A Western physician examining a patient with the pattern of Damp Heat Collecting in the Spleen might diagnose acute gastric inflammation, acute hepatitic infection, cholecystitis, or cirrhosis of the liver.[13]

Because Dampness is Yin and Heat is Yang, one would have to determine in a clinical situation whether the pattern were Yin within Yang or Yang within Yin—that is, which element is dominant. Table 8 suggests some criteria and is presented as an example of the need to make nuanced shades in a clinical perception.

TABLE 8 *Damp Heat Collecting in the Spleen*

SIGNS	MORE DAMPNESS YANG WITHIN YIN
Chest/Abdomen	feeling of fullness
Thirst	no thirst, or thirst without desire for fluids
Urine	scanty and slightly yellowish
Tongue	slightly red material, with yellow and very greasy moss
Pulse	soggy, not too rapid

SIGNS	MORE HEAT YIN WITHIN YANG
Chest/Abdomen	relatively more pain, with some distention
Thirst	thirst
Urine	scanty and very dark yellow
Tongue	red material, with yellow and somewhat greasy moss
Pulse	rapid and slippery

Patterns of Mucus (*tan-zheng* 痰·证) The Spleen is said to be "the mother of Mucus." Mucus is a kind of concentrated "cooked" Dampness. Mucus is heavier and more obstructive than Dampness. Mucus resembles Dampness but its symptomology is more severe and more likely to have a fixed location. Mucus in the stool, relatively soft, mobile swellings, lumps, or tumors (such as goiter, lymphadenopathy, and sebaceous cysts) and a phlegm cough can all be signs of Mucus. Mucus in the Consciousness of Potential makes a person feel deeply confused and mentally blocked. Ruminations get fixed on particular ideas and, in the extreme, a person becomes unconnected to reality. A greasy, thick tongue moss and very slippery pulse are often important signs of Mucus.

Turbid Mucus Disturbing the Head (*tan-zhuo-shang-rao*) is a common Mucus pattern that especially affects the head. Rather than a feeling of heaviness in the head, the patient suffers from severe dizziness—the room can be spinning or the person feel like falling. In Western terms, this pattern is often part of such disorders as hypertension and Ménière's disease.[14]

CLINICAL SKETCH *A patient in the author's practice complained of chronic abdominal distention and discomfort, tiredness, and a feeling of heaviness. He had a sallow complexion and a slow, friendly, phlegmatic ambience. He was comfortable in his work and relationships. His tongue was slightly pale with a very thick, greasy moss, and his pulse was very empty. The Western doctors this patient had consulted diagnosed his condition as a nervous stomach. The signs of distention and heaviness pointed to the pattern of Dampness Distressing the Spleen, which was confirmed by the greasy coating on the tongue. The empty pulse, on the other hand, pointed to the pattern of Deficient Spleen Qi. The pattern of Dampness Distressing the Spleen and the pattern of Deficient Qi are part of a continuum between two textbook points. This patient fell somewhere in between—he manifested aspects of both. He could be described as having the pattern of Deficient Qi turning into Dampness Distressing the Spleen (a Deficiency turning into an Excess, or vice versa). The treatment was to strengthen the Spleen Qi, supplementing the Deficiency, and to expel and disperse Dampness, removing the Pernicious Influence.*

The relative amount of tonification and dispersion that needs to be done in any one case by herbs or acupuncture needles depends on the relative amount of Deficiency and Excess present; that is, on the exact proportions of the patient's unique signs. In fact, the most precise description of the patient's patterns is the exact combination of acupuncture points and herbs used. The "cause"—the Deficient Qi that leads to Dampness—is not treated. Instead, the physician treats the approximate pattern generated at the moment by the particular configuration of manifesting signs. There is no "diagnosis," only the patient-physician encounter and therapeutic response. Hopefully, the patient is helped.

In this case, a series of ten acupuncture treatments and the use of herbs led to complete relief of the symptoms. The tongue greasiness disappeared, but the pulse remained somewhat empty, pointing to a constitutional tendency toward this disharmony.

Liver Disharmonies

The Liver stores the Blood and is responsible for the smooth movement of Qi. The Liver's Blood tempers and relaxes. The Liver's Qi is assertive but flexible. The Liver is sensitive to boundaries; it likes softness. The Liver is exquisitely reactive to being blocked and obstructed and sensitive to the distinction of self and other. Disharmonies of the Liver are associated with stagnation, confrontation, and distortions in boundaries between self and other.

Pattern of Constrained Liver Qi (*gan-qi-yu-jie* 肝气郁结)
The Liver likes the unimpeded but gentle movement of Qi, a "free and easy" environment. The Pattern of Constrained Liver Qi, which is the most common form of Stagnant Qi, is probably the most common pattern of Liver disharmony. The sensation of pain is its most common physical characteristic, and the feeling of frustration or being blocked is its most common psychological sign. Constrained Liver Qi is like feeling a wall in the pathway of movement. The Qi "builds up" and generates pressure and pain or a sense of restriction and inappropriate tension.

Constrained Liver Qi, especially in relationship to the Liver's storing the Blood, can lead to menstrual pain, irregular menses, and swelling of the breasts during menses. If Constrained Liver Qi involves the throat, the patient may feel a lump in the throat, a sensation the Chinese call the "plum-pit" feeling. In the Liver Meridians along the groin, breasts, or flank, Constrained Liver Qi is associated with distention, pain, or lumps; in the neck, there may also be lumps.

Constrained Liver Qi can affect the Spleen, creating a subpattern known as Liver Invading the Spleen (*gan-fan-pi*) which has such signs as nausea, vomiting, sour belching, abdominal pain, and diarrhea. Since these digestive signs also characterize patterns of Spleen disharmony, one must distinguish the pattern of Liver Invading the Spleen by the landscape context of the symptoms. The Spleen pattern would have more tiredness, confusion, and worry; the tongue might be paler and the pulse either empty or slippery. The Liver pattern would be accompanied with more tension and frustration, and the tongue might be darkish or purple (or even normal, if the disharmony is not too chronic), and the pulse manifests as wiry or tight.

Constrained Liver Qi can present as mainly emotional tension and stress. A person who usually feels hampered (while other people in the same situation might not) or easily annoyed, a person who is grumpy and easily becomes a curmudgeon, or a person who sees problems as mainly being the obstacle "others" put in the way, is often exhibiting a Constrained Liver Qi pattern.

Patients with Constrained Liver Qi could be diagnosed in Western terms as suffering from an extremely wide range of disorders, including mastitis, scrofula, digestive disorders, psychological problems, various menstrual problems, and even the stress of ordinary living.[15]

Pattern of Deficient Liver Blood (*gan-xue-xu* 肝血虚) The Liver stores the Blood. The Liver's Blood is responsible for basic repose, unhurried cyclical movements, a gentle milieu, the absence of a need to go anywhere, and the easy sense of self-acknowledgement. The Liver's Blood softens, moistens, and relaxes.

When the Liver's Blood is deficient, a person will be inappropriately tense, feel confined, nervously fidget, have tight tendons, stiff joints, or spasmodic movement. If the Blood does not moderate the Qi, Stagnant Qi can accompany the Deficient Blood and produce many of the signs mentioned in the section above. Menstrual problems such as scanty menses, amenorrhea, irregular periods, and painful menstruation can be due to Deficient Blood. Deficient Liver Blood may also manifest as hazy vision or spots in the field of vision (the Liver opens into the eyes) or pale fingernails (since the Liver manifests in the nails).

Deficient Blood, through the Non-Corporeal Soul (*Hun*), might hinder a person from having an easy sense of self-acceptance, self-worth, and self-esteem. Deficient Blood may be recognized by a person who is always kind to others but fails to be compassionate toward self.

The Liver's Blood provides for the capacity to feel and experience pain. Pain is an unavoidable and necessary ingredient of life. Blood allows for acceptance; the Liver's Blood creates tolerance and "more room" for the limitations and boundaries imposed on human existence. Increased capacity to feel pain means less "negative awareness" of pain—pain can be integrated into a sense of self. Insufficient Blood wants to make things different and causes a person to tense up or excessively resist or react to inevitable pain. (Paradoxically, increasing the avoidance component of pain only increases the total experience of pain.) Insufficient Blood may also make a person physically numb to pain (e.g., numbness in the limbs) or psychologically incapable of tolerating or being compassionate toward his or her own personal suffering.

Deficient Blood will also tend to manifest general Deficient Blood signs such as pale, lusterless face, poor memory, thin pulse, and dizziness. In the world of biomedicine, this pattern might be seen as anemia, menstrual problems, emotional conflicts, chronic muscular skeletal problems, chronic pain syndromes, or various chronic eye problems such as retinitis.[16]

Pattern of Liver Fire Blazing Upward (*gan-huo-shang-yan* 肝火上炎) When the Liver's Blood loses its softening quality and/or the Liver's Qi is obstructed, it easily gets constrained, pent up, and the landscape can finally "explode." The agitated and pressured movement is often upward and outward and called the Pattern of Liver Fire Blazing. (This Pattern also can exist without this previous history.) The Fire of this pattern can be recognized by such signs as splitting headaches, dizziness, red face and eyes, dry mouth, deafness, or sudden ringing in the ears. Inability to control anger, outbursts of hostility and vitriolic abhorrence, explosive, belligerent, and aggressive behavior can also characterize this pattern. The pattern would also have general signs of Excess/Heat (constipation; dark, scanty urine; red tongue with rough yellow moss; and a rapid and full as well as wiry pulse). Liver Fire often injures the Blood Vessels, causing various bleeding symptoms. Patients manifesting this pattern might be diagnosed in the West as suffering from essential hypertension, migraine headaches, bleeding of the upper digestive tract, menopausal complaints, eye diseases such as acute conjunctivitis and glaucoma, or ear disturbances such as labyrinthitis, Ménière's disease, or serious psychological problems.[17]

Pattern of Deficient Liver Yin (*gan-yin-xu* 肝 阴 虚)   The Liver's Blood concerns cycles of movement and a rambling ambience. It moistens and softens. Blood depends on Yin. Usually, the ultimate Water of a person is located in the Kidney, the root of Yin. But when a Chinese physician detects Liver Organ disharmony signs that appear in the context of issues related to stillness, quiescence, and moisture (Yin signs), the category is designated as a Liver Yin pattern. The category often overlaps with Deficient Liver Blood but also has distinct signs and is said to be "deeper." (It can also overlap with Deficient Kidney Yin; see below.)

The pattern of Deficient Liver Yin is an Empty Fire pattern (the appearance of Heat in a Deficient Yin pattern; see Figure 39), woven from the usual symptoms of Deficient Yin such as red cheeks, hot flashes, hot palms and soles, nervousness, reddish tongue, and thin, fast pulse. It has the signs of Yin not being able to embrace the Yang that are characterized by weakness, agitation, and uncontrolled heat signs. This Liver pattern also has Liver-specific signs such as dizziness (a general Deficient Yin symptom, but especially associated with the Liver), muddled vision, dry eyes and other eye problems, fidgety nervousness, restlessness, poor self-esteem, and self-deprecation. The pulse is likely to be wiry. A Western physician confronting patients with this pattern may diagnose essential hypertension, nervous disorders, chronic eye ailments, and menopausal complaints.[18]

The pattern of Turbid Mucus Disturbing the Head, which is a Damp Spleen pattern, often accompanies Liver Fire, Liver Yang, and Liver Yin patterns. It may be discerned by such additional signs as extreme dizziness, a thick, greasy tongue moss, and slippery aspects of the pulse.

Pattern of Arrogant Liver Yang Ascending (*gan-yang-shang-kang* 肝 阳 上 亢)   This pattern is a label for a place that is recognized between Liver Fire Blazing Upward and Deficient Liver

Yin. It exists between Excess Fire (Excess Yang) and Empty Fire (Deficient Yin). In fact, most real clinical situations exist among two or more patterns. People resist being put into categories. We have chosen to discuss this "intermediate" pattern and systematically compare it to the two patterns on each side, partly because Arrogant Liver Yang is common, but also because it further illustrates Chinese medical perception.

The three patterns—Arrogant Yang, Liver Blazing, and Deficient Liver Yin—as well as Constrained Liver Qi and Deficient Blood, can be seen as generatively interrelated. For example, the stagnation of Liver Qi easily transforms into Liver Fire. This Fire, over a period of time, can damage Liver Yin and produce Arrogant Liver Yang Ascending or Deficient Liver Yin. Although our language is that of causality, in a patient these patterns may follow or intersect one another, or may even appear simultaneously.

In fact, even identifying a particular pattern is problematic, since every textbook pattern is only a theoretical image and is seldom found unambiguously in an actual patient. Thus, Excess Fire and Deficient Yin patterns are theoretically quite distinguishable, but one often faces clinical situations in which the distinction is hardly clear at all, since the signs seem to point to a pattern somewhere in between the two. Such an admixture of signs is so common in Liver disharmonies that Chinese medical tradition has designated a separate pattern to describe it—Arrogant Liver Yang Ascending. Figure 44 illustrates the continuum of Liver Heat Patterns from Excess Fire (Excess Yang) to Empty Fire (Deficient Yin). Chinese medical tradition theoretically defines three points on this continuum as three separate patterns in order to teach students how to organize signs, weave patterns, and prescribe treatment. In actuality, the level of Fire and Water in a patient can vary infinitely, and the specific clinical pattern woven for a particular patient will involve shadings that suggest aspects of all three Liver Heat patterns. For example, it would be possible to have the pulse characteristic of Liver Fire, the eye signs of Deficient Liver Yin, and the emotions characteristic of

Arrogant Liver Yang Ascending. The physician must use skill, experience, and sensitivity to evaluate the relative importance of the various signs and prescribe the correct treatment.

In clinical practice, most Organ disharmonies present this type of admixture of signs suggesting several patterns. In the case of these three Liver disharmonies, however, this clinical reality has become a common theoretical consideration because of its commonness, its value as a guide to therapeutics, and its usefulness as a teaching device. It is a good example of the fact that paired opposites of the Eight Principal Patterns (e.g., Excess Yang and Deficient Yin) are not mutually exclusive. Instead, they define the ranges of continuums that the skilled physician learns to appreciate. The absolute separation of complementary opposites is self-contradicting.

Pattern of Liver Wind Moving Internally (*gan-feng-nei-dong* 肝 风 内 动) This pattern occurs when Liver Fire or Liver Yang precipitates uncontrollable and/or sudden movement or rigidity in the body. Its signs include those of other Liver disharmonies, with the addition of Wind signs such as trembling, difficulty in speaking, extreme stiff neck or tetany, spasms and convulsions, pulsating headaches, extreme dizziness, ringing in the ears, sudden facial rigidity or twitching, and unconsciousness (as in apoplexy). Liver Wind usually develops out of an extreme form of some other Liver pattern. Thus, if the Liver Wind were a result of Constrained Liver Qi, there would be a dark or purplish tongue; if it resulted from Liver Fire Blazing Upward or Arrogant Liver Yang Ascending, a reddish tongue would be seen.

Pattern of Cold Stagnating in the Liver Meridian (*han-zhi-gan-mai* 寒 滞 肝 脉) This pattern arises when Cold obstructs the Liver Meridian in the area of the groin. Signs include pain and distention in the lower side and groin; a swollen scrotum, which feels as if it were being pulled downward; moist tongue with white moss; deep, wiry, slow pulse; and discomfort relieved by heat. In

FIGURE 44 *Continuum of Liver Heat Patterns*

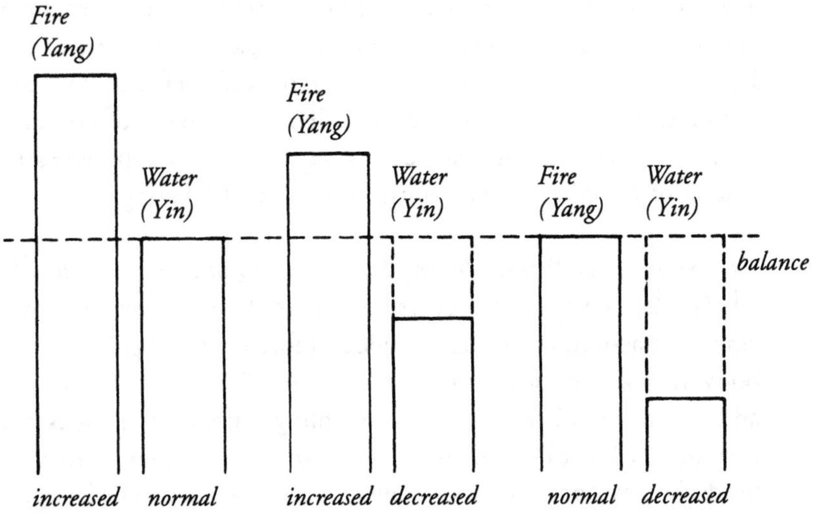

LIVER FIRE BLAZING UPWARD (EXCESS FIRE)	ARROGANT LIVER YANG ASCENDING, EXCESS FIRE, AND DEFICIENT YIN (EMPTY FIRE) SIMULTANEOUSLY	DEFICIENT LIVER YIN (EMPTY FIRE— APPEARANCE OF HEAT)

Fire (Yang)	Water (Yin)	Fire (Yang)	Water (Yin)	Fire (Yang)	Water (Yin)	balance
increased	normal	increased	decreased	normal	decreased	

HEAT

whole body constantly hot	periodic hot flushes in head and face	palms and soles hot; slight afternoon fever

HEADACHE

severe, splitting	throbbing	mild

EYES

red, swollen, painful	reddish; some pain	spots in field of vision; dryness

DIZZINESS

severe	moderate	mild

continued

FIGURE 44 *Continuum of Liver Heat Patterns (continued)*

LIVER FIRE BLAZING UPWARD (EXCESS FIRE)	ARROGANT LIVER YANG ASCENDING, EXCESS FIRE, AND DEFICIENT YIN (EMPTY FIRE) SIMULTANEOUSLY	DEFICIENT LIVER YIN (EMPTY FIRE—APPEARANCE OF HEAT)
EMOTIONS		
violent fits of anger	anger or depression	nervous irritability or depression
PULSE		
full, rapid, and wiry	rapid and wiry	thin, rapid, and wiry

the West, this pattern would be seen as one type of hernia (a term used in both Western and Chinese medicine) or as a urogenital disorder such as pelvic inflammatory disease.[19]

Cold Stagnating the Liver Meridian can affect the head and emotions. The most common signs are headache, vomiting, inability to express anger, and hostility turned inward on the self. The outward appearance of such a person tends to be absolutely without aggression and classical sources mention suicidal ideation.[20]

CLINICAL SKETCH *This example is taken from the collected case histories of Dr. Wu, a famous traditional physician in China.[21]*

The patient, a male aged forty-two, first visited on February 3, 1964. His complaints included throbbing temples and soreness at the top of the head.

From the Four Examinations, it was learned that the patient had dark yellow urine, difficulty in defecating, a poor appetite, painful teeth, painful right flank, painful eyeballs, and excessive dreaming. He was easily annoyed and often could not control his anger. His tongue was red; the moss was thick, greasy, and white; and the pulse was sinking and wiry. A Western medical examination at the same hospital diagnosed hypertension (blood pressure 180/130 mm Hg) and the beginnings of coronary heart disease.

Dr. Wu's diagnosis was Constrained Liver Qi accompanied by Liver Fire Ascending to Disturb the Head. His treatment called for harmonizing the Liver, cooling Liver Fire, and transforming Mucus.

An analysis of the process leading to this diagnosis is interesting. The yellow urine and difficult stools point to Heat, as does the red tongue. The flank pain and wiry pulse point to Constrained Liver Qi. The headaches, pounding temples, and eye pain suggest Liver Excess, because of the wiry pulse. The lack of appetite and the greasy moss point to Mucus and to Liver Invading the Spleen.

One question that could be raised is why the patient has a sinking rather than a rapid pulse. Dr. Wu's interpretation was that some signs point to Heat, while others point to Constrained Liver Qi and Mucus. The Fire is only affecting the Head and tongue material, while the tongue moss and sinking pulse indicate the Constrained qualities. The Constrained Liver Qi is interpreted as invading the Spleen because of the digestive symptoms. The Mucus may in fact be Cold, although Dr. Wu's diagnosis did not mention this. His treatment, however, while mainly using Fire-cooling herbs, also used two warm herbs to transform Mucus.

The entire treatment was herbal. A prescription of twelve herbs, including Gardenia jasminoides, Gentiana scabra, *and* Heliotis diversicolor *(abalone shell), was given to the patient. After he had taken the decoction for three days, a noticeable improvement was reported (blood pressure 130/90 mm Hg). A similar prescription was then given for nine more days, after which the patient reported that he felt much better. On the third visit, the physician prescribed an herbal pill to be taken for a longer period of time to make the treatment's effect continue.*

There is no traditional Chinese understanding of blood pressure, as the concept was first noted by French scientists during the eighteenth century. And in medicine it was not routinely used until 1912, when the Massachusetts General Hospital began measuring it on all entering patients. It should be mentioned, however, that the Chinese pharmacopoeia has many herbs that modern research has demonstrated can lower blood pressure.[22] This fact was irrelevant to the physician, though, who achieved excellent results by basing his treatment on reharmonizing the entire body. Using only those Chinese herbs that Western research has linked to reducing blood pressure (i.e., using a Western paradigm to select Oriental herbs) would have probably produced poorer results.[23] The rapid response of this patient seems extremely unusual. In most cases, Chinese herbs would be much slower, less reliable, and more inconvenient than Western medications for hypertension.

It should be clear that the Western entity known as hypertension can be found in various types of patterns and that this example of Liver Fire is but one common type. Other common patterns could include Liver and Kidney Yin both Deficient, and Kidney Yin and Yang both Deficient.[24]

Kidney Disharmonies

The Kidneys are the root of Water (Yin) and Fire (Yang). The Kidneys store the Essence (Jing) and are responsible for profound beginning and ultimate endings. The Kidneys allow for the inexorable unfolding of the life cycle. If Blood and Qi are the fundamental polarity of ordinary human activities, the Kidneys' Water and Fire are the foundation of the deep substratum that ultimately shapes the stages of human life. Depletion in the Kidneys is often linked to disruptions in other Organs, either preliminary to those disharmonies or as a final consequence of them. The Kidneys rarely are described as Excess; the Organs connected to Kidney disharmony can be either Deficiency or Excess.

Pattern of Deficient Kidney Essence (*shen-jing-bu-zu* 肾精不足) The Essence is the source of the inevitable and almost imperceptible movement of human life through birth, development, maturation, decline, and death. The Essence is the source of the Yin and Yang. The Jing is "juicy," still, effortless, and moistening. Yet the Jing moves with a dynamic that is relentless and is compelling as the movement of time itself. The Essence guides toward what is both unknown and uncertain and inevitable and absolute. Essence embodies the mystery of life.

Deficient Kidney Essence tends to display signs relating to development, maturation, or reproduction. Any distortions in the gracefulness of these processes often relate to Deficient Kidney Essence. In a child, signs pointing to such a pattern include slow physical or mental development, late or incomplete fontanel closure, or poor general skeletal development. Sexual dysfunction such as sexual anxiety and pain or discomfort with intercourse often belongs to Essence Deficiency. Premature aging or senility, bad teeth, poor long-term memory, and brittle bones are common signs of Essence depletion. Anguished fear of death, not being able to experience old age as a "ripening" into self-awareness, or the absence of a sense of trustful recognition are important signs that the Kidneys' Essence has not enabled the Will to find an ultimate Wisdom in life.

Deficient Kidney Essence is not described as either Yin or Yang (it includes both). Clinically, Yin and Yang are rarely equally diminished, and a Deficient Essence pattern will tend slightly toward either the Yin or the Yang side, with appropriate tongue and pulse signs reflecting the tendency. Such a tendency can also be read in the nuances of other signs. For example, in the area of sexual problems, a pattern of Deficient Essence somewhat more Deficient on the Yang side might lead to impotence in a man and a lack of sexual interest in a woman because there is a lack of the Fire that arouses. Deficient Essence weighted toward the side of Deficient Yin, however, might lead to premature ejaculation or insufficient vaginal secretions since the Yin cannot properly embrace the Yang.

Pattern of Deficient Kidney Yin (*shen-yin-xu* 肾阴虚） The Yin of the Kidney is the source of the quiescence and deepest tranquillity in a person's long-term being and behavior. The Yin's Water, presence, and stillness is "deeper" than the Blood's repose. The Yin precedes any activity. The Yin is the ultimate stillness.

The pattern of Deficient Kidney Yin (also called Kidney Water Exhausted) is a condition of Empty Fire. The Water cannot embrace the Fire, so Fire inappropriately flutters. The stillness is reduced, and there is a relative excess of movement, but the agitation is weak. Kidney-specific signs might include ringing in the ears or loss of hearing (the Kidneys open to the ears); weak, sore back; premature ejaculation; long-term forgetfulness; and vertigo. As a long-term constitutional tendency, a person prefers a cooler room, few extra clothes, and winter to the summer. This pattern also shares the general signs of Deficient Yin such as thin or shriveled constitution, dry throat, dry skin, hot palms and soles, red cheeks, heat flashes, night sweats, reddish tongue with little moss, and a thin, rapid pulse.

A Kidney Yin person can be riddled with fear, existential angst, and dread of death. The fear produces a frantic movement of flight and a restless assertion against the inevitable. A person begins to "will" what is impossible and runs around in a kind of existential frenzy and dizziness that makes a caricature of the timelessness and wisdom that old age can offer a person.

Western doctors might correlate Deficient Kidney Yin with essential hypertension, lumbago, chronic ear problems, diabetes, chronic urogenital infections or dysfunction, menopausal complaints, or the general physical or psychological debilities people can have with aging.[25]

Pattern of Deficient Kidney Yang (*shen-yang-xu* 肾 阳 虚) The Kidney Yang is the Fire in human life. It is the ultimate resolution and the most powerful assertion of will. If the Qi is about the dynamic tension that allows dynamic activity in ordinary human life, the Kidney's Yang is the deep resolution that propels and targets the major episodes in the life cycle.

The pattern of Deficient Kidney Yang, also called Weak Life Gate Fire (*ming-men-huo-ruo*), manifests signs of Deficiency and the "appearance of Cold" (that is, a Deficiency/Cold pattern). Thus, its signs include a bright white or darkish face; wet skin; subdued, quiet manner; fear of cold; and cold limbs. As a constitutional long-term tendency, such people turn the thermostat up, wear extra clothes, and prefer the summer to the winter. Kidney-specific signs could include a cold and sore lower back, lack of libido, sexual anxiety, sterility, loose teeth, and deafness or loss of hearing. In addition, there might be copious, clear urine; night urination; or dripping urine. (If the Fire ruling Water function is affected in the opposite way, signs of edema and problems of insufficient urination might develop.)

A Kidney Yang Deficient person can be paralyzed by fear. The unknown incapacitates his or her ability to move and mobilize. Such a person will tend toward passivity and lack an ability to assert himself or herself. He or she can be controlled by other people or institutions, easily take blame, and feel guilty. He or she experiences a disproportionately large sense of responsibility for a comparatively small amount of volition.

The pulse of a Kidney Yang pattern will generally be frail and slow or minute, and will often be particularly frail and sinking in the third pulse position. The various patterns involving Deficient Kidney Yang would be diagnosed in the West as a very wide range of disorders, including chronic nephritis, lumbago, sexual dysfunction, chronic urinary and prostate problems, chronic ear disorders, adrenal gland hypoactivity, hypothyroidism, or the general physical or psychological problems associated with aging.[26]

CLINICAL SKETCH *Some interesting examples come from two case series that explored the efficacy of Chinese medicine in treating the Western medical entity known as systemic lupus erythematosus (SLE), a serious and often fatal autoimmune disease.*

Two studies, the first dealing with 120 cases of lupus, the second with 22 cases, both concluded that traditional herbal treatments reduced the mortality rates from lupus more effectively than Western therapy, and that in a high proportion of cases, Chinese medicine is helpful in treating the disorder.[27] Obviously, for scientific validity to be attached to such assertions, the treatments would need to be performed under experimental conditions in the context of a randomized controlled trial (see Appendix E).

The first study found that several distinct disharmony patterns arise when diagnosing SLE. Here is a case history from the second study, which emphasized Kidney patterns.

On May 23, 1960, a woman, aged thirty-two, came to the hospital complaining that her facial skin, especially her cheeks, seemed to have injuries similar to frostbite. The condition had gradually gotten worse over the previous six months. She also complained of sore joints and back pain, dizziness, palpitations, insomnia, night sweats, and an occasional low fever. She was often thirsty, but had no desire to drink. Since the illness began, her hair had been falling out and her menstrual blood had diminished.

The Chinese examination noted a depleted Will, thinness of the whole body, low voice, and dark complexion. Her cheeks had a purple-red rash, the center of which was gray and scaled. Her eyes were sunken and darkish in the sockets; her hair was thin; the tongue moss was thin and white; the tongue material was cracked and bright red; and the pulse was thin and slightly rapid, with the third position especially weak.

Following the Chinese clinical examination, the patient was given a battery of Western medical tests. Some of the lab findings include: white blood cell count 2,400/mm³; red blood count 3.06 × 10⁶/mm³; total protein 8.6 grams percent; platelets 54,000/mm³; sedimentation rate 32 mm/hour (Cutler). An electrocardiogram showed arrhythmia, LE *prep negative.*

The dizziness, night sweats, heart palpitations, recurring low fevers, cracked and red tongue, and thin and rapid pulse all pointed to Deficient Yin. The backache, the weak third position on the pulse, the darkened eye sockets, and the loss of hair suggested that the Deficiency was in the Kidneys. The joint soreness was interpreted as Wind Invading the surface Meridians, obstructing the Qi and Blood. The rash on the face was thought to be the Heat of Deficient Yin Affecting the Blood, thus resulting in skin eruptions. (See Appendix C.)

The Chinese physician chose an herbal treatment that combined fourteen herbs to nourish the Kidney Yin and Blood, cool the Blood, and expel Wind. The herbs used included Rehmannia glutinosa, Polygonum multiflorum, *and* Paeonia lactiflora. *The patient was given a prescription to be taken daily for eighteen days. When she returned for the next examination, the rash had somewhat subsided. She was given a slightly different prescription. By the time she returned in five days, the rash had been very visibly reduced, her appetite had improved, and her joints were less sore. The backache, palpitation, and night sweats were all gone. White blood cell count was 4,500/mm³, red blood cell count was 3.84 × 10⁶/mm³, and platelets were 98,000/mm³. The patient continued to show improvement with additional treatment.*

Heart Disharmonies

The Heart is responsible for a human being's timely interaction in time and place. It allows for manners, ceremony, and propriety. The Heart is about appropriate connection in terms of place, person, or project. The Heart stores the Heart Spirit and also rules the Blood and is responsible for the evenness of the pulse. Because the Heart Organ operates in a short time frame, when its patterns become chronic they are usually perceived as linking with other Organs that can sustain them for longer durations of time.

Patterns of Deficient Heart Blood (*xin-xue-xu* 心 血 虛) and Deficient Heart Yin (*xin-yin-xu* 心 陰 虛) The Heart's Blood is the responsive and relaxed component of the link to time and place. The Heart's Yin has a deeper quiescence and stillness. Both disharmony patterns share overlapping signs: heart palpitation, sweating, forgetfulness, insomnia, anxiety with situations and people. These signs are thought of as the Blood or Yin unable to embrace the Qi or Yang.

Heart Blood and Heart Yin both have discomfort and a feeling of unease that is related to particular situations. Heart Blood patterns are likely to have shyness and a sense of vulnerability or a wanting to withdraw; Heart Yin patterns are likely to be a person who is visibly jumpy or chatty or who makes a determined effort to conceal anxiety.

Both patterns can have signs of inappropriate behavior. But Deficient Blood is closer to awkwardness; Deficient Yin is more flighty and restless. Both patterns can have signs of insomnia. But Deficient Blood tends to have trouble falling asleep; Deficient Yin will often awake in the night. Both patterns will have trouble with speaking in public; but Blood patterns may tend to forget the words while a person with Deficient Yin in haste may say unintended words. Both patterns tend to forget. But Heart Blood forgets routine things like the keys while Heart Yin forgets the name of a place or person.

Of course, other signs and the tongue and pulse will help separate the two patterns. The Blood pattern will have a pale face and a thin pulse; while the Yin pattern will have a reddish face, a thin, rapid pulse, and other signs of Heat.

Sometimes the Blood and Yin patterns overlap and are hard to distinguish. If the problem is chronic, the associated "deeper"

Organs help to determine the diagnosis. Deficient Heart Blood is often associated with Deficient Spleen Qi because the Spleen produces the Blood, while Deficient Heart Yin is usually related to Deficient Kidney Yin because the Kidneys are the source of the Yin of the Organs.

When Western doctors examine patients exhibiting Deficient Blood or Yin of the Heart, they often find cardiovascular disorders characterized by tachycardia, arrhythmia or anemia, hypertension, hyperthyroidism, and anxiety disorders.[28]

Patterns of Deficient Heart Qi (*xin-qi-xu* 心气虚) ***and Deficient Heart Yang*** (*xin-yang-xu* 心阳虚) Patterns of Deficiency of the Heart Qi or Heart Yang have to do with the effort needed to ensure the evenness of the pulse. The signs of either are associated with irregular pulse types such as knotted or intermittent. Qi and Yang have the usual other signs that accompany their pattern.

These patterns can be associated with the absence of the tension or assertion needed to make a connection with people. In this situation, signs may include lacking warmth in connecting to people, being unable to sustain a conversation, being unable to communicate one's meaning or intention, or being too slow to express oneself. An absence of joy may also be a sign of Heart Qi or Yang being depleted.

Most commonly, Deficient Heart Qi or Yang is an associated pattern with Deficient Kidney Yang (the Kidney are the root of Yang) or Deficient Lung Qi (because there is a link to the "sea of the Qi" in the chest). Western doctors who examine patients displaying Deficient Heart Qi or Yang (usually with a Kidney or Lung pattern) often observe cardiac insufficiency, coronary atherosclerosis, angina pectoris, or anxiety disorders.[29]

Patterns of Congealed Heart Blood (*xin-xue-yu* 心血瘀) Insufficient Heart Qi or Heart Yang to move the Blood in the chest often precedes and accompanies the pattern of Congealed Heart

Blood.[30] This extremely serious condition is an instance in which a Yin condition produces a partial Yang condition. The resulting pattern may be Yin within Yang, indicated by a strong pulse, or Yang within Yin, indicated by a weak pulse. In either case, Congealed Heart Blood will manifest Yang signs of stabbing pain and purple face and tongue, along with such Yin signs as lassitude, palpitations, and shortness of breath. The pulse is likely to be in between Yin and Yang, for example, choppy or wiry.

Mucus may also contribute to the obstruction of Blood. The resulting Mucus Obstructing the Heart and Congealed Blood pattern would have accompanying Mucus signs, such as thick, greasy tongue moss, woven into the clinical picture.

Patients manifesting the pattern of Congealed Blood are often diagnosed in Western terms as suffering from angina pectoris, pericarditis, or coronary artery disease.[31] A Western doctor would, after this diagnosis, further examine the heart to investigate possibilities for surgery. A Chinese doctor, after diagnosing the pattern Congealed Heart Blood, would need to determine whether the pattern was one of relative Excess or Deficiency, what aspects of Heat or Cold were present, and what other Organs were involved.

Patterns of Cold Mucus Confusing the Heart Openings (han-tan-mi-xin-qiao 寒痰迷心窍) *and Mucus Fire Agitating the Heart* (tan-huo-rao-xin 痰火扰心) Mucus affecting the Heart implies that the Heart's connection to time and space is occluded and seriously disrupted. The person is disoriented and not relating to ordinary reality. From a Western perspective, these mucus patterns imply serious mental disease.

Cold Mucus Confusing the Heart Orifice is often a seriously mentally ill person who cannot function in a normal social environment. A "bag lady" or a mentally handicapped homeless person belongs here. Since Cold Mucus is Yin, the behavioral signs might include an inward, restrained, foolish manner; muttering to oneself, delusions, staring at walls; and sudden blackouts. Delusions are common and the person is often friendly and not threatening. Potential harm is usually unintentionally self-inflicted. Other signs such as coldness, passivity, fixations, a white, thickly coated tongue, and a slippery pulse are likely to be present. If the person drools phlegm, it is white or watery. The condition can also be less serious and be delineated by such signs as disorientation, lack of logical thinking, confused thoughts, or thoughtless or just sloppy behavior.

Mucus Fire Agitating the Heart is Yang. The person is assertive, agitated and aggressive, and may incessantly talk. Harm can easily be inflicted on others as the delusions have a quality of persistent resentment or belligerent hostility. Restraints may be needed. All the Mucus Heart patterns are generally linked to other Organs, but Mucus Fire is most often connected to the Liver Organ, which is partially the origin of the aggression. If the person drools phlegm, it tends to be yellow.

Often Mucus disharmonies of the Heart may be seen to correspond to Western categories of mental illness. At other times, these disharmonies correlate with such Western disease entities as gram-negative sepsis and encephalitis, when they affect cerebral functions, or apoplexy, or epilepsy.[32]

CLINICAL SKETCH *A clinical report published in a Chinese journal of traditional medicine[33] detailed the course of thirty-one patients with premature ventricular contractions (PVCs) who were treated by Chinese traditional medicine. Western scientists evaluated the patients by electrocardiography and blood chemistry before and after treatment, and reported that traditional Chinese therapy led to complete recovery in 38.7 percent of the patients, brought improvement to 38.7 percent, and had no effect on the remaining 22.6 percent. No patient in this study suffered any side effects from the treatment.*

In general, the Chinese physicians distinguished two broad types of disharmony: Excess (Congealed Blood) and Deficiency (Deficient Qi and/or Blood). Each patient was treated with herbal prescriptions to correspond with the exact variation of the pattern the patient exhibited. Here are the details of one particular case.

The patient, a male bookkeeper aged fifty-three, was first examined on January 5, 1978. His chief complaint was heart palpitations. His chest had felt distended and full for the past nine months, with the discomfort especially severe after exertion. He had a long history of coughing up sticky white phlegm, especially in the winter. His tongue material was dark purple and reddish with a white, greasy moss. His pulse was primarily knotted.

The Western evaluation by electrocardiogram showed a heart rate of eighty-eight beats a minute with five PVCs *per minute. Blood chemistry data included readings of 286 mg/ml cholesterol and 196 mg/ml triglycerides. An x-ray examination revealed a normal heart with changes consistent with emphysema.*

The traditional Chinese physician found several patterns existing simultaneously. The pattern of Congealed Heart Blood was predominant, revealed by the darkish tongue, chest pressure, knotted pulse, and heart palpitations. Secondary aspects of Mucus Obstructing the Heart were seen in the signs of phlegm and greasy tongue moss. In addition, the symptoms of coughing, phlegm, sensitivity to winter cold, and white, greasy moss pointed to Cold Damp/Mucus Obstructing the Lungs. In addition, the reddish tongue and rapid pulse were associated with Deficient Heart Yin.

The patient received a seven-day herbal prescription that contained eleven ingredients including Pueraria, Trichosanthes, *and* Salvia miltiorrhiza. *The purpose of the herbs was mainly to move Blood and also to transform Mucus and slightly nourish the Heart Yin. After taking the herbs for seven days, the patient reported a reduction in palpitations and reduced feeling of heaviness in the chest. He also coughed less and the* PVCs *were reduced to three to four beats per minute.*

The patient was then given a similar prescription for a period of thirty-five days. After this, most symptoms disappeared. Upon reexamination by Western scientists, the patient's electrocardiogram showed no evidence of premature ventricular contractions or of any other abnormality. Blood evaluation showed 255 mg/ml cholesterol and 95 mg/ml triglycerides. The patient was discharged with an additional herbal prescription to maintain his improvement.

It is interesting to note that several of the herbs used in this patient's prescription have been studied by pharmacologists and demonstrated to dilate the coronary arteries, thus increasing the supply of blood and oxygen to the heart.[34]

Obviously, this report does not prove that Chinese medicine works according to criteria acceptable for biomedicine. It is a case report, and the entire discussion lacks such safeguards of modern research methodology as concurrent controls and blind assessment.

Nonetheless, it gives a flavor of the contemporary intersection of Chinese and biomedicine in China and pattern thinking. For a discussion of acceptable evidence for the determination of efficacy in the modern West, see Appendix E.

Lung Disharmonies

The Lungs are the "tender Organ" and most susceptible to External Pernicious Influences. The Lungs are also the Organ concerned with activity in moment-to-moment units of time. They rule respiration and animated reactivity. The Lungs easily feel lack of completion. Disturbances in inhalation and exhalation (such as cough or asthma) and excessive grief (inability to experience the preciousness of a complete event) are salient characteristics of Lung disharmonies. Acute Lung disharmonies are dealt with extensively in Appendix A and Appendix E. They will be briefly discussed here. Chronic Lung disharmonies are often connected to other Organs, which facilitates their extension in time. Sometimes the other Organ can make it more difficult to detect the Lung component of the disharmony.

The Pattern of Cold Violating the Lungs (*han-xie-fan-fei* 寒邪犯肺) This is an External Cold Pernicious Influence pattern that especially affects the Lungs. It is likely to be woven together by such signs of External Cold as chills, a slight fever, head and body aches, and, since the pores are blocked by Cold, a lack of perspiration. Also expected would be a thin, white tongue moss, and a floating, tight pulse. These signs will be accompanied by Lung disharmony symptoms such as stuffy or runny nose, asthma, or a cough with a thin, watery sputum. Occasionally, this pattern can be chronic. In the West, patients with this pattern would often be diagnosed as suffering from the common cold, acute or chronic bronchitis, bronchial asthma, or emphysema.[35]

The Pattern of Heat Clogging the Lungs (*re-xie-yong-fei* 热邪壅肺) This pattern manifests the usual signs of an External Heat

Pernicious Influence such as fever, slight chills, perspiration, thirst, constipation, dark urine, red tongue with dry, yellow moss, and fast pulse. In addition, there will be Lung-specific signs such as a red, sore, swollen throat, asthmatic breathing, or a full cough with a yellow, sticky expectorant. There may be a runny nose with thick yellow phlegm or, since Heat can injure fluids and cause Blood to move recklessly, a dry or bleeding nose.

A Western doctor, looking at patients with this pattern, might diagnose the common cold, acute or chronic bronchitis, pneumonia, tonsillitis, or pulmonary abscess.[36]

The Pattern of Mucus Dampness Hindering the Lungs (*tan-shi-zu-fei* 痰湿阻肺) This pattern usually runs a longer course than the previous two patterns. While it can be generated by an External Damp Pernicious Influence, more often it is the result of any External Influence invading the body and encountering a preexisting chronic disharmony with tendencies toward Mucus accumulation. Chronically Deficient Spleen or Kidney Qi, for example, may lead to Dampness and Mucus buildup, predisposing the body to this pattern of disharmony. Common signs include full, high-pitched coughing, wheezing, or asthma with copious phlegm; chest and flank distention and soreness; increased difficulty in breathing when lying down (since it is even harder for Lung Qi to descend when the body is horizontal); thick, greasy tongue moss that is either white or yellow depending on whether the obstructing Mucus is Cold or Hot; and a slippery pulse (the major sign of Mucus Dampness). In the West this pattern would be perceived most often as chronic bronchitis or bronchial asthma.[37]

The Pattern of Deficient Lung Yin (*fei-yin-xu* 肺阴虚) This pattern can occur when chronically Deficient Yin, usually of the Kidneys, affects the Yin of the Lungs. It may also be a consequence of Heat Invading the Lungs and remaining within the body for so long that the Heat injures the Lung Yin. Signs include a dry cough with little or no phlegm, bloody sputum (if Heat has injured the

Blood Vessels), and such general signs as an emaciated appearance, low voice, red cheeks, afternoon fever, night sweats, reddish tongue with a small amount of dry moss, and a thin, rapid pulse. In Western terms these conditions might be diagnosed as pulmonary tuberculosis, chronic pharyngitis, bronchiectasis, or chronic bronchitis.[38]

Deficient Lungs can accompany and be hidden within any chronic Yin disharmony. If it accompanies a Deficient Liver Yin pattern, a person can be a high-performance person yet feel sad, disappointed, unsatisfied, and restless with a tendency to be easily annoyed. If it accompanies a Deficient Kidney Yin pattern, the person can have longstanding unresolved grief accompanied by fear and angst.

Deficient Lung Qi (*fei-qi-xu* 肺气虚) This pattern usually occurs either as the result of an External Pernicious Influence remaining in the Lungs for a long period and injuring the Qi (an Excess condition turning into one of Deficiency) or because of various Internal disharmonies that affect the Lungs. The signs of this pattern are exhausted appearance and Spirit, low voice and lack of desire to talk, and weak respiration. If a cough is present, it is weak. A sad affect may be present. If the Protective Qi has also been weakened, there are other signs such as daytime sweats and lowered resistance to colds. In Western terms such symptoms might point to emphysema, chronic bronchitis, pulmonary tuberculosis, allergies, longstanding depression, or chronic bereavement.[39]

CLINICAL SKETCH *The following example is taken from the author's private practice. A woman, aged twenty-six, complained of wheezing, difficulty in breathing, and coughing, especially in the middle of the night. Sleeping was very difficult. The pattern had begun suddenly when the patient was sixteen years old and had gotten steadily worse. The patient constantly felt tightness in her chest, unrelated to seasonal changes, and when an attack started, there was much sneezing and coughing. Phlegm with a thick and yellow quality was produced. The patient's medical history was otherwise insignificant. She was very thin, with dark rings under her eyes. Her energy level was good except during an attack, and she did not report any emotional stress but seemed a little pressured and anxious. She was an accomplished banking executive despite her young age and claimed that relationships were not a priority in her life. She thought her greatest virtue was efficiency and "not taking nonsense." Nonetheless, she cried when she responded to the sad tone in my question about sorrowful times in her life. Her tongue was red and cracked in the middle and had scattered red dots. Her pulse was rapid (ninety-six beats per minute) and also slippery and slightly thin.*

When she first came for treatment, she was taking Western medication but wanted an alternative because the drugs made her dizzy, tired, and nauseated.

Many of the signs pointed to the pattern of Heat in the Lungs: yellow phlegm, rapid pulse, red tongue, and thirst. Other signs, such as the thin body, the chronic nature of the disorder, the peeled and cracked tongue, and thin pulse, pointed to Deficient Yin. The wheezing, thick phlegm, and slippery pulse indicated that Mucus was present. The affect of sadness pointed to an underlying long-term Lung disharmony. A combination of acupuncture and herbal treatments was administered to cool the Lung Heat, nourish the Yin of the Lungs, and eliminate Mucus. This therapy brought many of the symptoms under control within two weeks.

Although the patient is still subject to occasional attacks, they are less frequent and intense. When needed, she uses an inhalator containing Western medications. She also claimed that the treatments helped her to "kick back," be less pressured to perform, and generally be more receptive.

This chapter has focused on those major patterns of disharmony that are most common in the Chinese medical tradition—disharmonies involving Qi, Blood, and the individual Organs.[40] Appendix B describes the common patterns associated with the disturbances of the Yang Organs.

Beyond this point, the discernment of patterns becomes much more complex and cannot easily be continued without clinical experience and extensive discussion of classical texts. In the next chapter, therefore, we will leave behind the discussion of particular patterns of disharmony and will return to the theory and fundamental perspectives of traditional East Asian medicine.

NOTES

1. *Su Wen* [1], sec. 17, chap. 62, p. 335.
2. It should be noted that it is possible for there to be a Qi-Blood continuum very different from a Blood-Yin continuum. Because "Qi is the commander of Blood" and "Blood is the mother of Qi," very often Deficient Blood and Deficient Qi exist simultaneously and merge together. This situation gives rise to a very common clinical situation in which the patient has signs of both Deficient Qi and Deficient Blood. Sometimes this situation gives a Cold appearance (for instance, cold limbs) because the Deficient Qi aspect develops signs of Deficient Yang.
3. This example is based on the author's impression of a population in China. If the sample of patients was drawn from a clinic in the West the proportions would undoubtedly be different. For an interesting discussion of treating Western medical categories with methods that tonify Spleen Qi, see Shanghai Institute, *Study of Prescriptions* [87], pp. 227–230.
4. It is possible for a person with a particular Chinese medical disharmony to be considered healthy or a hypochondriac after a Western physician's examination. The opposite could also be true: a Chinese medical practitioner might see no disharmony in a situation where a Western medical disease is diagnosed. Each system has blind spots from the perspective of the other.
5. For a discussion of the treatment of Western medical categories with methods that cool Liver Fire, see Shanghai Institute, *Study of Prescriptions* [87], pp. 47–48.
6. In China, people often go from a Western practitioner to a traditional practitioner and vice versa, or are treated in a hospital where both medical systems are used simultaneously.
7. Li Dong-yuan, *Discussion of the Spleen and Stomach with Commentary* (*Pi-wei Lun Zhu-shi*). Commentary by Henan Province Academy of Chinese Medicine. Beijing: People's Press, 1976, p. 260.
8. *Selected Explanations of Traditional Chinese Medical Terms* [33], p. 135; Zhejiang Committee, *Foundations* [91], p. 84. The Chinese text often omits psychological correlates for many patterns. There is a tendency to avoid psychological labels in the medical culture (see Arthur Kleinman, *Patients and Healers in the Context of Culture*, 1980). The author has added some psychological labels to the correlated biomedical entities to correct for this tendency in Chinese texts. See Chapter 5, note 16.
9. Ibid.; Shanghai Institute, Distinguishing Patterns and Dispensing Treatments [52], p. 223.
10. Zhejiang Committee, *Foundations*, p. 84.
11. Guangzhou Ministry, *Essentials of Traditional Chinese Medicine* [75], p. 98.

12. Because the Yang Organs are generally more affected by External Pernicious Influences, this pattern is often considered Damp Heat in the Stomach and Intestines. See Appendix B.

13. Guangzhou Ministry, *Essentials*, p. 98.

14. Shanghai Institute, *Foundations*, p. 218.

15. Ibid., p. 185.

16. Guangzhou Ministry, *Essentials*, p. 95; *Selected Explanations*, p. 132.

17. Guangzhou Ministry, *Essentials*, p. 94; *Selected Explanations*, p. 133. By Five Phase correspondence, it would seem that ear problems should be mainly a disharmony of the Kidney. In clinical practice, however, Kidney disharmony is generally associated with Deficiency patterns involving the ear, whereas Liver or Gall Bladder disharmony is associated with Excess patterns. Acute eye problems are often associated with the Lungs.

18. Zhejiang Committee, *Foundations*, p. 79.

19. Beijing Institute, *Foundations*, p. 121; Zhejiang Provincial Committee, *Clinical Study of Traditional Chinese Medicine* [90], p. 356.

20. Zhang Zhong-jing, *Discussion on Cold-Induced Disorders* [28]. This discussion is in several sections concerning the herbal formula called Evodia Decoction (*Wu-zhu-yu Tang*) See Section 8 on Yang Ming diseases.

21. Clinical Cases of Wu Shao-huai (*Wu Shao-huai Yi-an*) [78], pp. 57–59. Dr. Wu, at the time his clinical reports were published, had over sixty years of clinical practice and was principal of the Jinan City Institute of Traditional Chinese Medicine.

22. Chen Xin-qian, *Pharmacology* [71], pp. 381–383, Tang and Eisenbrand, *Chinese Drugs of Plant Origins*, 1992, and Chang and But, *Pharmacology and Applications of Chinese Materia Medica*, 1987. In practical terms, conventional biomedical medications are more reliable and convenient for the treatment of hypertension.

23. Eleventh People's Hospital of Shanghai Institute, *Theory and Treatment of Hypertension* [72]. See entire study.

24. Zhejiang Committee, *Clinical Studies*, pp. 241–244.

25. Shanghai Institute, *Foundations*, p. 192; *Selected Explanations*, p. 145; Zhejiang Committee, *Foundations*, p. 17.

26. Ibid., p. 193; Guangzhou Ministry, *Essentials*, p. 105. On the issue of guilt in China see Wolfram Eberhard, *Guilt and Sin in Traditional China*, Berkeley: University of California Press, 1967.

27. "Treatment of Systemic Lupus Erythematosus with Combined Traditional Chinese and Western Medicine," SJTCM, September 1979; Shanghai First Medical Hospital, *Studies on the Kidneys* [84], pp. 22–26. A somewhat similar case has recently been published in the scientific literature. See H. K. Yap et al., "Improvement in Lupus Nephritis Following Treatment with a Chinese Preparation," *Archives of Pediatrics*, 1999; 153: 850–852.

28. Shanghai Institute, *Foundations* [53], p. 172; Zhejiang Provincial Committee, *Foundations of Traditional Chinese Medicine* [91].

29. Ibid., p. 171; Zhejiang Committee, *Foundations* [91], p. 72.

30. This pattern is called Heart Blockage (*xin-bi*) in the *Su Wen* (sec. 20, chap. 43).

31. Zhejiang Committee, *Foundations* [91], p. 73; Shanghai Institute, *Foundations*, p. 173.

32. Ibid., p. 74. Many parallels to the pathology of classic Greek humoral medicine and Chinese concepts can be found. Here the parallel is striking. Hippocrates describes epilepsy, paraplegia, apoplexy, and convulsions as humidity of the brain with excess phlegm often accompanied by dryness causing overexcitability. The humoral origin is similar to the Chinese, but the Greek attention to morphology "correctly" puts the disturbance in the brain rather than the Heart.

33. "Clinical Observations of Effectiveness of Traditional Chinese Medicine in Treating Thirty-One Cases of Premature Ventricular Contractions," sjtcm, March 1979.

34. "Forty-Nine Cases of Coronary Heart Disease Treated by Heart-Comforting Decoction of *Pueraria lobata* and *Trichosanthes kirilowii*," sjtcm, July 1979, p. 19; Zhongshan Institute, *Clinical Uses of Chinese Medicines* [92], pp. 36, 273, 485.

35. Zhejiang Committee, *Foundations*, p. 89; *Selected Explanations of Traditional Chinese Medical Terms* [33], p. 140.

36. Ibid., p. 90.

37. Selected Explanations [92], p. 141.

38. Zhejiang Committee, *Foundations*, p. 91; *Selected Explanations*, p. 142.

39. Ibid., p. 91.

40. Chapter 8 has mainly described patterns of single Organ disharmony. A brief summary of a few patterns involving two Yin Organs simultaneously is presented in Table 9 for readers interested in this level of detail.

TABLE 9 *Patterns Involving Two Yin Organs Simultaneously*

DEFICIENT HEART QI AND DEFICIENT LUNG QI

Signs	palpitations; sadness; absence of joy; shortness of breath; weak cough; asthma; sweating
Tongue	pale
Pulse	frail

DEFICIENT HEART BLOOD AND DEFICIENT SPLEEN QI

Signs	palpitations; insomnia; worry at the wrong time and wrong place; inability to concentrate; abdominal distention; loose stools; lethargy; pale, sallow complexion
Tongue	pale
Pulse	empty or thin

continued

TABLE 9 *Patterns Involving Two Yin Organs Simultaneously (continued)*

HEART AND KIDNEY LOSE COMMUNICATION (HEART YIN AND KIDNEY YIN BOTH DEFICIENT)

Signs	palpitations; insomnia; irritability; unstable expression of will; forgetfulness; guilt; vertigo; tinnitus; dry throat; sore back; sexual anxiety; night sweats
Tongue	reddish, dry material; little moss
Pulse	thin, rapid, sinking

HEART YANG AND KIDNEY YANG BOTH DEFICIENT

Signs	palpitations; inability to express feelings or assert will; passive; cold appearance; edema; scanty urine
Tongue	pale, swollen, moist material; white moss
Pulse	sinking and minute

LUNG YIN AND KIDNEY YIN BOTH DEFICIENT

Signs	cough with little mucus; mouth dry; voice low; inability to feel satiated; always wanting something; restless; lower back sore and weak; night sweats; red cheeks; afternoon fever; sterility
Tongue	red material; little moss
Pulse	thin and rapid

DEFICIENT LUNG QI AND DEFICIENT KIDNEY YANG (KIDNEY UNABLE TO GRASP QI)

Signs	asthma; shortness of breath; exertion worsens condition; difficulty crying; sadness and fear dominate; low voice; sweating; cold limbs
Tongue	pale, moist, swollen material
Pulse	frail or empty

DEFICIENT SPLEEN QI AND DEFICIENT LUNG QI

Signs	shortness of breath; cough; tired; weak; poor digestion; bored; sadness and worry; asthma accompanied by copious, thin, white phlegm; loose stools; edema
Tongue	pale, with white moss
Pulse	empty

continued

TABLE 9 *Patterns Involving Two Yin Organs Simultaneously (continued)*

DEFICIENT SPLEEN QI AND DEFICIENT KIDNEY YANG

Signs	cold; bright white complexion; lower back cold and sore; passive; worry; fear; guilt; loose stools; edema; diffculty of urination
Tongue	pale, moist, swollen, with white moss
Pulse	frail and especially sinking

LIVER INVADING SPLEEN

Signs	tense; moody; frustrated; distended abdomen; loose stools; passing gas
Tongue	dark or normal material; white moss
Pulse	wiry

LIVER FIRE INVADING LUNGS

Signs	quick and excessive anger; vertigo; red eyes; bitter taste in mouth; serial coughing; coughing blood
Tongue	red, with thin yellow moss
Pulse	wiry and rapid

DEFICIENT LIVER YIN AND DEFICIENT KIDNEY YIN

Signs	vertigo; headaches; spots before eyes; forgetfulness; tinnitus; dry mouth and throat; lower back sore and weak; hot palms and soles; red cheeks; menses irregular or reduced; self-deprecation; irritable; fear that makes a person jumpy
Tongue	red, with little moss
Pulse	thin and rapid

9

CHINESE
MEDICINE
AS AN ART

or on the Penetrating Divine Illumination

So far, this book has presented the basic step-by-step logic of Chinese medicine. We have examined the process of perceiving patterns in the myriad of events, feelings, sensibilities, needs, and intentions that make up a human life. Bits and pieces have been put together in an ever-refined image of Yin and Yang. This method—putting the stones, mountains, mist, and pebbles of human life into a clinical image—is the learning method that the tradition uses to train novice physicians. The tradition expects a new physician to become proficient in this method with the commitment and effort of a lifetime of practice, study, and reflection.

But, in fact, underneath this method is a counterprocess—a Yin opposition to a Yang method. This process has to do with the dialectic between *whole* and *part*, another level of Yin and Yang. This parallel undercurrent is the artistry of Chinese medicine as opposed to its knowledge. It is the method that allows the clinical landscape to be more than a metaphor and for the Chinese physician to claim that his or her work imitates that of the artist.

For both the Chinese artist and the clinician, the landscape is "dedicated to the expression of the inner spirit instead of the physical verisimilitude [and the] that painting should reflect a . . . spontaneous and instantaneous flow of the brush."[1] A landscape needs to capture an essence, "to suggest more than the merely visible and open . . . up to the life of the spirit."[2] This artistic method of East Asian medicine manifests on multiple and continuous levels. (For convenience, the chapter divides this artistry into three stages.) Each progressive level of the dialectic between *whole* and *part* reveals a deeper layer of an ancient art whose mastery is one of the ultimate goals of the dedicated East Asian physician. Each level of the dialectic also embodies a unique aspect of the physician's response in the clinical encounter.

We have already touched on the first level of the dialectic. Chinese medicine is never *addition*—gathering the parts (i.e., complaints, signs, and symptoms) to make a whole. The parts never constitute a whole. In fact, the whole determines the components; context governs. In the clinical landscape, "the reality of things only exists—and thus only manifests itself—in a totality, through the force of propensity [the inherent Yin-Yang dynamic] that links its various elements in a whole."[3] No component of the pattern can be isolated; no piece has an ontological significance independent of the entire environment.

A simple example may be helpful. Consider a patient with dry eyes. In Chapter 6 and Chapter 8, we have said that this sign or complaint is usually part of a Deficient Liver Blood or Yin condition. The reason for the association is in part the appearance of the symptom (lack of moisture) and in part because, in the accumulated clinical experience of Chinese physicians, dry eyes often are accompanied by the signs of Deficient Blood (e.g., thin pulse, pale tongue, poor self-esteem) or Deficient Yin (e.g., thin, rapid pulse, reddish tongue, self-deprecation).

This common association, however, is not always accurate. If the signs accompanying dry eyes were to point to aspects of Excess (e.g., a strong pulse and hostility), the complaint would probably be seen as part of a pattern of Liver Fire or Arrogant Liver Yang Ascending. Dry eyes could also be part of a Deficient Kidney Yin pattern if a different set of signs (rapid, frail pulse and inordinate fear) were present. It is possible for dry eyes to be understood as part of a pattern of Heat Violating the Lungs if accompanying signs included acute onset, cough, and rapid, floating pulse. Less typical possibilities would be various Deficient Qi or Deficient Yang patterns, which "should" have "wet" complaints. In these cases, "atypical" dryness in the eyes would be interpreted as the Qi or Yang unable to raise Water. The configuration stamps the fragment. Sometimes aspects of multiple patterns merge. In fact, any pattern (or combination) could have the complaint of "dry eyes." The energetic significance of dry eyes is ultimately infused by the landscape. Earlier chapters have already taken this level of artistry into account. Without it, a diagnosis or clinical assessment of the human landscape would not be possible.

The second level of the East Asian dialectic of *whole* and *part* has to do with the fact that there is no ultimate separation between whole and part. The whole imprints on each single unit of the clinical landscape. What the sinologist François Jullien has said about Chinese painting also applies to the clinical landscape: "it should be remembered that, according to Chinese 'physics,' every element in the landscape, from the great mountain ridges to the individual tree or rock, owes its creation solely to the accumulation of cosmic energy and is constantly flooded by that same energy."[4] In the clinical landscape, the Chinese physician can see the *whole in any part*. At this level of artistry, the concern is particularity. A truly adept physician can diagnose from almost any single piece in the human configuration. In the finest shadings of a particular emotional ambience, or tongue, or manner of walking, or pulse, the master physician can discern a pattern, because the whole leaves its characteristic mark on each part.

Again, a simple example may be helpful. A particular pattern should produce a distinct cough. A pattern of Cold Wind Invading the Lungs, for example, would probably be associated with a round, full cough. A Hot Wind pattern would manifest as an agitated cough with a drier sound, and there would be difficulty in coughing up sputum. Mucus Obstructing the Lungs would produce a full, high-pitched, watery sound (less forceful than Cold Wind) with a lot of sputum. The cough of a Deficient Lung Yin pattern would be raspy, weak, and frail. The Kidneys Not Grasping the Qi would produce a short, weak cough with some gurgling or wheezing. A Liver Invading the Lungs cough would have a spurting, projective quality, with many coughs in a series and then a rest. The cough of Congealed Blood Obstructing the Chest would be weak and have a slushy texture.[5] One could similarly diagnose the pattern of a cough from other single signs such as pulse or tongue.[6]

This same sense of any detail being a reflection of the whole is true for any aspect of a person, even a single emotion. For example, fear is generally associated with the Kidneys. But the whole configuration impacts and refines any detail. A fear from Kidney Yang might be associated with an inability to be decisive in relationships while the fear of Kidney Yin might be linked with a pattern of not being able to form stable relationships. Fear can be attached to other Organs. The emotion of fear connected to the Liver may hide behind an aggressive veneer, while Spleen fear would be entwined in worry and ruminations. A Heart fear might be connected to clumsiness and confusion. (The fear itself would probably, but not necessarily, be connected to the Kidneys.)

The ability to detect such refined impressions takes a high level of skill—beyond the skill required by the first level. It was epitomized for me by an elderly Chinese doctor who was my first teacher of the tradition.[7] After a new patient would call to make an appointment (there was no secretary), Dr. Hong would often tell me what acupuncture points or herb formula he was likely to use. (The patient would not have necessarily even mentioned the problem.) He gave me a look of patience when I stared quizzically. Only later did he tell me he could guess the energetic of the person by how he or she accepted, negotiated, or fussed during the exchange concerning appointment time.

This second level of artistry, however, is not meant for the performance of impressive diagnostic feats, although sometimes it is helpful in a complex case. Its value lies in the way it sharpens the therapeutic response. The artistry of the first level, seeing how the whole shapes the part, is crude, even with its artistry; it simplifies as it discerns. Its artistry is generic. The particularity of the second level (the pieces reflect the whole) allows for additional refinement. Any fragment of the terrain actually needs a distinct assortment of herbs (in various dosages) and acupuncture points (with various methods of stimulation). A treatment for Wind Cold with a scratchy nose is slightly different from the treatment for Wind Cold with a hoarse throat or Wind Cold with a stiff neck. Indecisive fear, unstable fear, aggressive fear, ruminating fear, and confused fear may all relate to the Kidneys, but each requires its own unique set of herbs and acupuncture points. (The herbal pharmacopoeias and acupuncture manuals provide the information needed to select the appropriate treatment. Also, depending on the pattern and its details, the physician may have to deliberately modulate the quality of the therapeutic relationship.) The particularity of the second level allows a matching of individual and very precise signs with specific and exact interventions in the context of an overall pattern (level one). The details of level two can be diagnostic, but, more critically, they guide the therapeutic response to the clinical landscape. The particularity of level two permits a concrete and nuanced treatment.

The artistry of level two, which reflects the details of pieces of the landscape in an acupuncture or herbal treatment, can be very sophisticated and actually renders a portrait of a person. A good physician can read the herbal formula written for a patient by another experienced physician and easily describe the patient with a surprising amount of detail. If the diagnosis of level one is the title, the therapeutics is the short story. It encodes the person's complaint, the relative prominence of other signs and symptoms, the timing of events, the general emotional ambience of the person, and possibly even a glimpse of the person's biography.[8]

The third level of the dialectic of *whole* and *part* is the most profound; words are often inadequate to describe the process. The medical classics say that mastery takes a lifetime. The issues here are *totality* and *immediacy*. Level one (which concerns how the whole shapes the parts and allows a diagnosis) and level two (which concerns how the whole can be seen in the parts and permits a unique combination of herbs or acupuncture points) are actually preludes. Level three is the ultimate refinement of the physician's art. It involves the possibility to "intimately . . . [and] intuitively apprehend the landscape in its entirety . . . opening it up to the infinity and the breath [Qi] that gives life."9

This third level of artistry has to do with an intimate, intuitive, and immediate encounter of humanity. In the medical tradition, this level of artistry is called the "Penetrating Divine Illumination" (*tong shen ming*).10 It is the Chinese medical tradition's attempt to mimic the artist and "rid the landscape of all the weight of inessentials and restore it to the simple movement that gives it form and existence."11 It is the alchemical core of Yin-Yang medicine.

The Penetrating Divine Illumination is a prominent feature in the classical texts of the East Asian medical tradition. (Modern books tend to gloss over its role because of a resemblance to mystical or placebo-like phenomena.) In the *Nei Jing*, Qi Bo, the physician who teaches the Yellow Emperor, uses the Penetrating Divine Illumination to "penetrate [the essense] of the myriad of things" and perceive as if the "wind has blown the clouds away."12 Qi Bo tells the Emperor that his own teacher (who by implication is the "genuine" master) exclusively relied on the Penetrating Divine Illumination.13 In other places, the *Nei Jing* reverentially insists that this method is superior (is the "Spirit" of medicine) compared with the more linear and primitive forms of examining a patient.14 Other early texts echoed this refrain.15 In fact, the method is extensively praised in the few Chinese books that describe medicine that predate the *Nei Jing*. For example, Bian Que, the legendary physician, says that although he knows of four methods of assessment and the method of taking the pulse, he does not bother with them. "Your way of using techniques [questioning and pulse taking] is like peeping through a tube to see the sky or looking for the pattern in things by peering through a crack."16 His art, it seems, is to discern the pattern instantaneously; he "intuitively apprehended its general movement."[17] So the physician, like the painter, "must be inspired, must possess a particularly sensitive consciousness, so that he can 'unite in spirit' with his landscape and, by exposing himself to it and communicating with it, grasp in a stroke how the whole scene functions."[18]

In fact, Qi Bo and Bian Que are expressing the necessary hidden implication of the Chinese medicine method and the dialectic of *whole* and *part*. If level one is true (one needs to apprehend the whole to interpret the pieces) and if level two is true (the whole infuses the parts), then level three must also be true—the whole is always a palpable presence in the immediate encounter of patient-physician. In fact, the whole is the only thing that is fundamentally present.

The Penetrating Divine Illumination is the "secret" method buried within the Four Examinations and pattern discernment that easily eludes the novice physician; it can only be consciously grasped by the seasoned veteran. The Penetrating Divine Illumination cannot be taught; it grows within the physician as the craft is honed. After a lifetime of practice, using the simpler levels of knowing and artistry in Chinese medicine, it automatically and autonomously reveals that it was always present. The poetic wholeness alone is real; everything else was minor. Zhu Dan-xi (1280–1358 C.E.), the "Cinnabar Creek Master," says that this vision is "the capacity of the sage."[19] For the wizened practitioner, everything else is preliminary. All knowledge and art leads here. I first learned about this kind of vision from Dr. Hong, my first teacher, who would routinely gain his patients' confidence by casually bringing up details of their life that they had not even mentioned before! He just knew. His intuition had been refined in a crucible of experience that gave him capacities beyond what is ordinarily thought possible.

But the point of the Penetrating Divine Illumination has nothing to do with impressing patients or clinical theatrics. And it is much more than a knowledge that infuses the preliminary levels of art. While the encounter of level one allows for a diagnosis and level two allows for a nuanced formulation of herbs and acupuncture, it is level three (the Penetrating Divine Illumination) which allows for the mysterious transmutation at the core of the healing encounter. The Penetrating Divine Illumination (even if it is hidden from the beginner's consciousness of a novice physician) is the very basis for the success of any treatment and clinical engagement. The Penetrating Divine Illumination is not merely an intuitive knowing; it is "a secret treatment," what *Wu Kun* (1551–c. 1620 C.E.) called "the medicine without form."[20] The Penetrating Divine Illumination is akin to the moment in the landscape painting that is "the secret, particular point where the success or failure of the painting is decided. In other words . . . [it] is what every landscape painting depends on for its life."[21] The Illumination is the core dialectic of healing—the point where receptivity (Yin) automatically and instantaneously becomes transformation (Yang). The moment of the Penetrating Divine Illumination is the resonance of Qi between the patient and the physician. Intimate knowing and profound witnessing effortlessly become the elixir for profound transmutation. Assessment and treatment, patient and doctor, Yin and Yang merge. Healing manifests.

The Penetrating Divine Illumination starts as an assessment and instantaneously becomes intervention. The Penetrating Divine Illumination is the magic of soul meeting soul, Spirit reflecting Spirit. The instantaneous recognition necessarily initiates profound treatment. The immediate responses of the physician in the clinical encounter—the words, posture, gestures, questions, attention, intention, genuineness, empathy, compassion, belief, and vision—deeply affect and resonate with the Spirit of another human being. The Divine Penetrating Illumination is the ultimate basis of healing. Qi Bo, the medical teacher in the *Nei Jing*, admits that his sage teacher not only was not dependent on normal diagnostic methods, but also had no use for routine therapeutic interventions such as herbs or acupuncture. His teacher, the symbolic archetypal master that all physicians aspire toward, both knew *and treated* exclusively by the Penetrating Divine Illumination. The discernment of the Penetrating Divine Illumination automatically "moves the Essence (Jing) and transforms the Qi."[22] Intense communication and intimate recognition automatically resonate and affirm the integrity of a patient's Qi and Spirit.[23]

For the physician, using the Penetrating Divine Illumination was the elusive and highest artistic goal. Each generation of East Asian practitioners spoke of it.[24] Xu Shu-wei (1080–1154 C.E.), author of a major Song dynasty medical compilation, cautioned his students that ultimately "to make the patient feel better before taking the medicine is the most direct method."[25] Sun Zhun, the leader of the seventeenth-century Korean medical delegation to China, said that the Chinese used a "method of healing that begins even before the medicine reaches the mouth."[26] Wu Ju-tong (1758–1836 C.E.), the famous Qing-dynasty physician, said he relied on the method of Qi Bo's teacher when he encountered "internal and complex illnesses."[27] The Divine Penetrating Illumination is the Essence (Jing) and Wisdom of healing. Future generations of East Asian healers will undoubtedly aspire to practice this deepest mystery of their healing tradition.

The Penetrating Divine Illumination is the highest form of the Yin and Yang of healing. I used to watch it when I worked with my first teacher. Just from being and talking with Dr. Hong, most patients encountered within themselves a depth of humanity deeper than the difficulty or tragedy of any illness. Authenticity and integrity were experienced. The Qi shifted. The Spirit was touched. No matter how broken or isolated a person felt before the appointment, a meeting with Dr. Hong was an opportunity for both an expression and a recognition of his or her most genuine humanity.

NOTES

1. Chan, *Chinese Philosophy*, p. 210.
2. Jullien, *The Propensity of Things*, p. 174.
3. Ibid., p. 99.
4. Ibid., p. 137.
5. Chapter 38 of the *Su Wen* is titled "Discussion on Coughing" and is devoted to distinguishing coughs produced by the various Organs. Its method is to rely primar-

ily on variations of accompanying symptoms. For instance, a cough that is part of a Liver disharmony is said to induce flank pain, making it difficult to twist the trunk (*Su Wen*, sec. 10, chap. 38, pp. 214–217). Coughing itself, however, also indicates that at least the Lungs are affected, for coughing is the sound of the Lungs. (*Su Wen*, sec. 7, chap. 23, p. 150).

6. The pulse is usually emphasized in Chinese medicine. Table 10 shows the correlation between pulse disharmonies that are likely to involve cough.

TABLE 10 *Correlation of Pulses and Disharmonies with Cough*

PULSE	PATTERN OF DISHARMONY
Floating and tight	Exterior/Cold/Wind
Floating and rapid	Exterior/Hot/Wind
Slippery	Mucus Obstructing
Thin and rapid	Deficient Yin
Empty	Deficient Qi
Frail and slow	Kidneys not Grasping Qi (affecting Lung Qi)
Wiry	Liver Invading Lungs
Choppy and intermittent	Congealed Heart Blood Obstructing Qi of Chest

7. The doctor was Hong Yuan-bain, who was the author's first teacher of Chinese medicine. After his education, Dr. Hong lived as an apprentice-student with Cheng Dan-an (1899–1957) in Wuxi, China. Dr. Hong died in 1975. Dr. Cheng was one of the most noted traditional Chinese physicians of the twentieth century, and when he died he was chairman of the Chinese Academy of Medicine.

8. At this second level, the treatment response is creative and detailed. But it always remains embedded in the general principle explained by Lao Tsu ages ago:

> When [the string] is high, bring it down
> > When it is low, raise it up.
> When it is excessive, reduce it.
> > When it is insufficient, supplement it.

Chan, *Chinese Philosophy*, p. 174. Sun Si-maio (618–907 C.E.) put this therapeutic principle in a famous negative formulation: "If Excess is added to, Deficiency is reduced, flow drained, obstruction blocked, Cold chilled, Heart warmed, then illnesses increase and instead of viewing a patient's life, I see his death." *Thousand Ducat Prescriptions* [19], sec.1, chap. 2, p. 1.

9. Jullien, *The Propensity of Things*, p. 102.

10. This translation of *tong shen ming* comes from Martha Li Chiu. See Chiu, *Mind, Body, and Illness in a Chinese Medical Tradition*, pp. 109–111. Her translation of *Shen* (Divine) is usually translated as Spirit in this text. Shigehisa Kuriyama trans-

lates *tong shen ming* as "penetrating insight" or "divine enlightenment." See *The Expressiveness of the Body*, 1999, pp. 153–155.

11. Jullien, *The Propensity of Things*, p. 95.

12. Quoted in Chiu, *Mind, Body, and Illness in a Chinese Medical Tradition*, p. 110.

13. *Inner Classic of the Yellow Emperor: Simple Questions Translated into the Vernacular. (Huang-di Nei-jing Su-wen Yi-shi)*, Nanjing College of Chinese Medicine (ed). Shanghai: Shanghai Science and Technology Press, 1981, sec.1, chap. 13, p. 111.

14. There are many discussions of the Penetrating Divine Illumination. Most often they are in the context of dividing diagnosis into three (or two) gradations of skill. The Penetrating Divine Illumination is invariably the "Spirit" level while pulse taking or asking questions is relegated to "workmanlike" (*gong*). For example, see *Su Wen* [1] chap. 8; *Ling Shu* [2] chap. 1, p. 2; and *Ling Shu* [2] chap. 4, p. 80.

15. *Classic of Difficulties* [3], chap. 61, p. 134. An English translation and commentary on this section can be found in Paul U. Unschuld, *Nan-Ching: The Classic of Difficult Issues*, Berkeley: University of California Press, 1986, pp. 539–544.

16. Yang Zhang-xian and Chi Zhi-da (eds.) *Comparative Vernacular Translation of the Historical Records* (Shi Ji), vol. 5. [Wen-bai Dui-zhao Quan-yi Shi ji (Beijing: Shi-hua Shu-dian, 1992) p. 37.] The *Shi Ji* (Historical Records) was written in the early Han dynasty. It includes a biography of Bian Que, probably part fact and part fiction, which takes place during the Warring States period of the fifth century B.C.E. It is a critical early literate source of information on the early medicine of China.

17. Jullien, *The Propensity of Things*, p. 101.

18. Ibid.

19. Zhu Dan-xi described this method as "the living noose" (*huo tao*). The discussion can be found in Complete Medical Section: Collection of Ancient and Modern Books (*Yi-bu Quan-lu: Gu-jin Tu-shu Ji-cheng*), collected under imperial order by Chen Meng-lei, et al. Volume 7. (Hong Kong: Yuguang Press, 1962 [1726 C.E.]) p. 1610. Also see Zhu Dan-xi, *Secrets of the Cinnabar Creek Master (Dan-xi Xin-fa)*. Beijing: Beijing City Zhongguo Shudian, 1986 [1347 C.E.]).

20. Wu Kun. *Verified Medical Prescriptions (Yi fang yao)*, Jiangsu: Jiangsu Science and Technology Press, 1985 [1584 C.E.]), p. 9.

21. Jullien, *The Propensity of Things*, p. 102.

22. At this point, the *Su Wen* is speaking of the Penetrating Divine Illumination and says that this nonphysical component of intervention is a form of incantation (*zhu*). *Su Wen* [1] chap. 10, p. 73.

23. There is a roughly analogous topic in the biomedical literature that raises similar issues. This discussion of the placebo effect, the impact of diagnosis, and the therapeutic relationship on clinical outcomes is unfortunately often marginalized instead of being seen as a critical core of medicine. For a flavor of such discussion in the biomedical literature, see Howard Brody, "Diagnosis Is Treatment," *Journal*

of Family Practice, 1980; 10: 445–449; Harold C. Sox, et al., "Psychologically Mediated Effects of Diagnostic Tests," *Annals of Internal Medicine*, 1981; 95: 680–685; Howard Brody, "Placebo Response, Sustained Partnership, and Emotional Resilience in Practice," *Journal of the American Board of Family Practice*, 1997; 10: 72–74; K. B. Thomas, "General Practice Consultations: Is There Any Point in Being Positive?" *British Medical Journal* 1987; 294: 1200– 1202; Sherrie H. Kaplan, et al., "Assessing the Effects of Physician-Patient Interactions on the Outcomes of Chronic Disease," *Medical Care* 1989; 27: S110–S127; Moira Stewart, "Effective Physician-Patient Communication and Health Outcomes: A Review," *Canadian Medical Association Journal* 1995; 152: 1423–1433; Ted J. Kaptchuk, "Powerful Placebo: The Dark Side of the Randomised Controlled Trial," *Lancet* 1998; 351: 1722–1725.

24. The East Asian medical literature has an important genre of writings that describe medical treatment and cures taking place without the use of herbs or acupuncture. They relied solely on the skill of the physician in shifting the Qi during the clinical encounter. They are actually clinical descriptions of cases using the Penetrating Divine Illumination. For a summary of such writings, see Preface in Hugh MacPherson and Ted J. Kaptchuk (eds.), *Acupuncture in Practice: Case History Insights from the West* (New York: Churchill Livingstone, 1997). Also see Vivien W. Ng, *Madness in Late Imperial China: From Illness to Deviance*, Norman, OK: University of Oklahoma Press, 1990, pp. 38–43.

25. Xu Shu-wei, *Prescriptions of Universal Benefit from My Own Practice (Pu-ji Ben-shi Fang)*, Shanghai: Shanghai Science and Technology Press, 1978 [1132 C.E.].

26. Quoted in Zhong Jian-hua and Man Ming-ren (eds.), *Practical Chinese Medical Psychology (Shi-yong Zhong-yi Xin-li Xue)*, Beijing: Beijing Publishers, 1987, p. 127.

27. Quoted in Wang Ke-zhong, *Spiritual Dimensions of Chinese Medicine (Zhong-yi Shen-ju Sue-shou)*, Beijing: Zhongyi Guiji, 1988, p. 132.

10

THE WEB THAT
HAS NO WEAVER—
AND MOUNT SINAI

or on the location of truth

This book has presented an overview of the Chinese perceptions of the human landscape. Both the basic knowledge and the artistry has been considered. The patterns of disharmony are the framework of this investigation, and so, in a sense, they comprise a theory. The Western mind, however, requires that a theory sum up phenomena and formulate a general principle to explain their nature and relationship. A theory implies a truth. Are patterns of disharmony true? This is a tricky question that brings us to the abyss that separates Chinese and Western thought.

The Chinese worldview is circular and self-contained. It imagines that the universe is a whole, a macrocosm, made up of the constant unfolding and flux of Yin and Yang. Chinese medicine, like Chinese thought in general, begins and ends with this notion of a whole, within which all the parts are related to each other and also to the whole. The Chinese physician begins with a knowledge of the whole, made up of the countless details codified in traditional medical texts. Through clinical experience, he or she develops a sensitivity. The physician aspires, through an effort of years, to capture the tradition's artistry. The physician learns to embrace the microcosm of another person. He or she learns to feel his or her own microcosm. But is any of this real? Is it more than the imagination? Are these patterns of harmony and disharmony real?

The concept of patterns describes the movement of Yin and Yang in the human being, but also exemplifies the way in which Yin and Yang unfold in the universe. The Eight Principal Patterns— Interior/Exterior, Deficiency/Excess, Cold/Hot, and Yin/Yang— interrelate in the person as they do in the universe. Any pattern of disharmony that emerges when these aspects of Yin and Yang intertwine with a patient's specific signs is thus a particular manifestation of the universal movement of Yin and Yang. All phenomena partake of the whole.

Patterns of disharmony are real and true in the sense that they provide a way to perceive the Chinese notion of what has been called "the web that has no weaver."[1] The web is the macrocosm—the universe—that is considered to be uncreated, but to exist through the dictates of its own inner nature: that is, through the constant unfolding of Yin and Yang. There is no "truth" behind or above the things we see; there is no creator or first cause; yet the things we see continue, and their continuing is the eternal process of the universe.

Perhaps only the words of a Taoist philosopher can take us any closer to this paradoxical reality:

The operations of Heaven are profoundly mysterious. It has water-levels for levelling, but it does not use them; it has plumb lines for setting things upright, but it does not use them. It works in deep stillness. . . .

Thus it is said, Heaven has no form and yet the myriad things are brought to perfection. It is like the most impalpable of featureless essences, and yet the myriad changes are all brought about by it. So also the sage is busied about nothing, and yet the thousand executives of State are effective in the highest degrees.

This may be called the untaught teaching, and the wordless edict.[2]

The Chinese description of reality does not penetrate to a truth; it can only be a poetic description of a truth that cannot be grasped. The Heart, Lung, and Kidneys of this volume are not a physical heart, lung, or kidneys; instead they are personae in a descriptive drama of health and illness. For the Chinese, this description of the eternal process of Yin and Yang is the only way to try to explain either the workings of the universe or the workings of the human being. And it is enough, because the process is all there is; no underlying truth is ever within reach. The truth is immanent in everything and is the process itself.

Can a system of knowledge rooted in such a "metaphysics" have anything to communicate to Western medicine? By now, Chinese medicine, especially acupuncture, has achieved some acceptance in the biomedical enterprise (see Appendix E). Acupuncture is the object of widespread interest, and attempts are being made to integrate certain of its techniques into the mainstream of biomedical practice. In some areas of society, the practitioner of Chinese medicine is even enjoying a kind of vogue. People have always had inflated expectations about medicine, and the Chinese doctor can all too easily become a focus for those who hope for a cure-all, an infallible elixir, a sideshow potion that the medical establishment either doesn't know or conspires to suppress.

The current turning away from biomedicine, however, cannot be explained solely on the basis of unrealistic expectations. It is more likely that many people have begun to see that too often biomedicine is simply not concerned with general well-being because it can only assess very small, discrete bits of information. Also it is rooted in a society whose routine processes not only provoke stress but contaminate the environment to such an extent that every new comfort may conceal a new threat to life. Our medicine parallels our society. New cures often produce side effects of unexpected virulence. Moreover, our central medical institution, the hospital, is structured like nothing so much as a health factory—a contradiction in terms. And probably most important, people feel that there is no place for their feelings, intentions, beliefs, and values in the biomedical perspective. Biomedicine often leaves the "person" in the waiting room.

Chinese medicine offers a different vision of health and disease, one that is implicitly critical of biomedicine because it refuses to see a complaint or disease as separable from the rest of a person. Most important, Chinese medicine attempts to locate illness within the unbroken context or field of an individual's total physical and psychological being. It aims to heal through treatments that encompass the whole of the individual as closely as possible. In contrast, the ideal of biomedicine is to probe with laserlike accuracy, penetrating to the microscopic agent of disease in the tissue, the cell, and ultimately the DNA molecule. The chief weakness of biomedicine, in short, is that it tends not to see the whole.

Chinese medicine has other notable strengths. Chinese remedies are sometimes effective, and they are generally gentler and safer (see Appendix E). Chinese medicine, in addition, is better able than biomedicine to conceptualize illnesses arising from the complex interrelationships of physical and mental phenomena. (Indeed, the very idea of the unity of body, mind, and spirit is one of biomedicine's blind spots.) Chinese medicine, because it emphasizes balance and relationship more than measurable quantity, can also frequently discover and treat a disorder before it is perceptible by the most sophisticated Western diagnostic techniques. Chinese medicine is capable of touching many places that evade the microscope and that, after all, constitute human reality.

Chinese medicine has an ability to measure quality. Labels such as Dampness or Deficient Blood are ultimately metaphoric brushstroke images of the texture of human life. Modern biomedicine, following on the heels of the scientific revolution, broke the living continuity of experience, the actual texture of human reality, into measurable units. Reality becomes perceptible only in relationship to a projection of units of space, time, motion, and matter. For many modern doctors, the idiosyncratic and personal response to illness—

e.g., the patient's desire to use many blankets, feelings, thoughts concerning work, sense of values and meaning—has become buried in the transition from the traditional to the scientific. This may have been appropriate at one point in history and led to many monumental achievements in health care, but problems have arisen. Much that is human and medically effective may have been lost or remains to be discovered because modern health care too often avoids seeing human beings as self-conscious human beings with feelings, intentions, and self-created meaning. It can easily fail to recognize that the illness of real people are not simply isolatable events reducible to mechanical and experimental models.

On the other hand, no honest Chinese physician can fail to be awed by the achievements of biomedicine, by the ease with which a drug such as streptomycin, or a technique such as open heart surgery, can penetrate to the core of disorders that Chinese medicine finds complex and intractable.

Because Chinese medicine collects only external signs to perceive an overall form, it has blind spots of its own. And one of its greatest strengths—its perception of the body as a whole—can be its greatest weakness. For Chinese medicine can never separate the part from the whole, even when a clinical situation demands that the overall relationships be ignored and a particular part be treated directly. A tumor or a large gallstone must sometimes be identified, isolated, and removed. Chinese medicine rarely does this—it lacks both the theory and the technique.

And, because it stresses quality and proportion, and sees quantity as secondary, Chinese medicine can be weak on prognosis. For example, most tumors that are fixed in location are thought to result from Congealed Blood and are treated by appropriate reharmonizing techniques. But Chinese medicine cannot easily focus on the tumor itself to determine whether it is malignant or benign. A good Chinese doctor can often sense that a disharmony is life-threatening, but this is not a central issue in the Chinese medical method. He or she cannot attempt to offer a quantifiable prognosis the way biomedicine can.

Modern biomedicine is clear, precise, and definite. It has the sure stroke of exact measurement as opposed to the more fallible stroke of artistic judgment. Its precision and technology allow swift intervention that can be crucial in life-threatening situations.

Modern biomedicine and traditional Chinese medicine are two discrete systems of theory and practice that have complementary strengths and weaknesses. They seem to need each other very much. Obviously, on a practical level, each system needs to share. If something helps the patient, it should be used. And, in both Asia and the West, the two systems are learning how to clinically coexist. But on the theoretical level, can either system absorb anything of genuine consequence from the other? On the level of thinking about health and illness, can there be mutual learning?

On the Chinese side, such hope may be unreasonable. Although Chinese medicine has developed considerably in its history, this progress is a long spiral that moves forever around its point of origin, the ancient texts. Since this point of origin is assumed to contain the seed of everything that can be known, all development is a form of slow exegesis within a broad conceptual framework. The ancient books are the language of Chinese medicine, and while the vocabulary can be expanded and enriched, the grammar and syntax are fixed. Complete and self-contained, traditional Chinese medicine is incapable of assimilating anything that challenges its fundamental assumptions. New ideas and substances can be identified and even incorporated, but they can never expand or transform the fundamental matrix. So, vitamin B_{12} is very Yang, penicillin is very Yin, but there is nothing beyond Yin and Yang.

Perhaps it is precisely because Chinese thought is uninterested in cause, is circular, and sees the universe as being in a state of spontaneous cooperation without a creator or regulator, that it lacks an impulse to go beyond its own organization of observations. There is no desire to discover an ultimate reality transcending phenomena, no need to go beyond the immanent. Chinese thought cannot expand or transcend its own limitations. Its concept of the unity of opposition calls for sharpened clarity and one-pointed vision, and it precludes the idea that humankind can ever attain higher levels of truth. Ultimately, "returning is the movement of the Tao."[3] This vision has abided through the millennia and, undoubtedly, it will endure and remain relevant.

At first glance, biomedicine seems equally impervious to alternate modes of perception. Given its current bureaucratic entrenchment, its disposition toward technological solutions, and its arrogant faith in its own destiny, a strong argument can be made that biomedicine will never see anything more in the Chinese system than a curious bag of tricks that need the application of the scientific method to separate the wheat from the chaff.

Yet biomedicine has in recent years been increasingly critical of itself. Even within the inner sanctum, rumblings can be heard. An article in the *Journal of the American Medical Association* speaks of the:

> *limitations of a linear, reductionist approach in our attempt to describe natural phenomena. . . . [There is an] acute awareness of the havoc that the modernist worship of science has wrought upon Western popular consciousness. . . . Science can tell us nothing about an individual. Science speaks in terms of probabilities, of means and standard deviations, the behavior of groups . . . of people, not of individual entities.*[4]

Biomedical philosophers have begun calling for the reintroduction of the personal experience into medicine.

> *Objective evidence is valued to the exclusion of subjective evidence. . . . If the shortcomings of modern biomedicine are to be effectively addressed . . . the very canons of medical evidence must be revised. Subjective evidence must be rehabilitated and rejuvenated with better methods of subjective clinical investigation. . . . The connotation of subjective as idiosyncratic, irrational, unreliable. prejudiced, and especially, beyond or beneath truth and falsehood must be exchanged for a view of the subjective which sees it as the personal, the meaningful, the situated, and especially the concrete.*[5]

Some Western physicians have begun to speak of a clinic of "social poetics" where the task

> is to be open to being "arrested" or "moved" by certain fleeting, momentary occurrences in what patients do or say. For sometimes in such moments, in our responding to the unfolding motion of their whole body and voice—as they respond to the circumstances in which they find themselves—we can begin to sense what the unique nature of their inner world of pain and suffering is like for them.[6]

Even the *New England Journal of Medicine* has shown glimpses of this discontent:

> Medicine's traditional concern primarily for the body and for physical disease is well known, as are the widespread effects of the mind-body dichotomy on medical theory and practice. I believe that this dichotomy itself is a source of the paradoxical situation in which doctors cause suffering in their care of the sick. . . . The profession of medicine is being pushed and pulled into new areas, both by its technology and by the demands of its patients. Attempting to understand what suffering is and how physicians might truly be devoted to its relief will require that medicine and its critics overcome the dichotomy between mind and body and the associated dichotomies between subjective and objective and between person and object.[7]

Ecological criticism of modern medicine has also brought forth new ideas:

> Microbial agents, disturbances in essential metabolic processes, deficiencies in growth factors or in hormones, and physiological stress are now regarded as specific causes of disease. . . . Unquestionably the doctrine of specific etiology has been the most constructive force in medical research for almost a century and the theoretical and practical achievements to which it has led constitute the bulk of modern medicine. Yet few are the cases in

which it has provided a complete account of the causation of disease. Despite frantic efforts, the causes of cancer, of arteriosclerosis, of mental disorders, and of the other great medical problems of our times remain undiscovered. It is generally assumed that the cause of all diseases can and will be found in due time by bringing the big guns of science to bear on the problems. In reality, however, search for the causes may be a hopeless pursuit because most disease states are the indirect outcome of a constellation of circumstances rather than the direct result of single determinant factors.[8]

Paradoxically, these new ideas in Western medicine, ideas that point toward an awareness of human experience and the totality of being, have arisen as a direct result of the Western urge to penetrate phenomena and to find the transcendent truth behind them. Western thought, at its most noble and honest, is nourished by the constant tension between unknown and known, imperfect and perfect. Western humanity is quickened by a metaphysical dilemma—on the one hand, it was created in the image of the Almighty, and on the other, it was created from dust. Western humankind is enmeshed in creating and becoming; it labors in growth and development. Perhaps this is a consequence of Judeo-Christian emphasis on an omnipresent, transcendent God making impossible the attainment of human perfection. Perhaps this idea is related to the Greek metaphysical notion that "we are what we are because of what we can become." In any case, it is an idea altogether missing in China, an attitude that contrasts sharply with the Chinese view of truth as inherent in the harmonious arrangement of the given.[9]

Western medicine can be criticized for insensitivity, for arrogance, for storming Heaven—but the fact remains that, at its best, it is humble, and humility is integral to the best scientific thought. For all its misuses, the idea of progress implies that not everything has been achieved, that more is yet to come. In order to remain scientific, medicine must believe that what it discovers, yet tomorrow may undermine and revolutionize everything it believes today. Western science, in its idealized paradigm, unlike traditional Chinese thought, is necessarily receptive to the new. And there is now a new sense of organism, interconnectedness, quality, meaningfulness, and unity emerging on the frontiers of modern medicine. The development of Western thought is creating room for new models and theories. There is a perception that medicine needs art, progress needs wisdom, and precision needs vision.

As science encounters Chinese medicine, Western investigation will inevitably tend to reduce the techniques of acupuncture and herbology to a biochemical Western model (see Chapter 4, notes 10 and 11). Science will seek to test the practical Chinese claims of clinical efficacy (see Appendix E). Besides these concrete investigations, can we hope that the uncanny Taoist spirit of interrelatedness will illuminate those places that evade the Western yardstick so that more than just new techniques are learned? By moving toward a view of human health and illness that is both analytical and synthetic, the West may be able to create a richer paradigm of healing.

While mystery and profundity can be found in both East and West, the more "progressive" insight lies in the West with its idea of creator and creating, being and becoming. In the dynamics of the Judeo-Christian-Islamic transcendent Creator, or of Greek metaphysics, can be found the seeds, hope, and impetus for a constant striving toward progressive maturation, increased knowledge, and ever-deeper recognition of truth. Dynamic revelation and unfolding are implicit in the dialectics of the West.

The story is told that on Mount Sinai, in addition to the Law, Moses was given a list of all diseases and their cures. This Book was later destroyed by a pious king who was anxious to restore humility among his subjects.[10] At its best, Western medicine knows that we can never reconstruct this Book, but it also knows that, in the face of our own incompleteness, we must continue to try. The classical books of traditional East Asian medicine have been written. The Western book, which is always being created, will undoubtedly incorporate Chinese characters.

NOTES

1. "The conception . . . [is] of a vast pattern. There is a web of relationships throughout the universe, the nodes of which are things and events. Nobody wove it, but if you interfere with its texture, you do so at your peril. . . . This web woven by no weaver . . . approach[es] a developed philosophy of organism." Needham, *Science and Civilization*, vol. 2, p. 556.

2. Lü's Spring and Autumn Annals (c. 240 B.C.E.), quoted in Needham, *The Great Titration*, p. 324.

3. *Tao-te Ching*, chap. 40.

4. James S. Goodwin, "Chaos and the Limits of Modern Medicine," *Journal of the American Medical Association*, 1997; 278: 1399–1400, p. 1399.

5. Mark Sullivan, "In What Sense Is Contemporary Medicine Dualistic?" *Culture, Medicine and Psychiatry*, 1986, 10: 331–350, pp. 331, 348.

6. Arlene M. Katz and John Shotter, "Hearing the Patient's 'Voice': Toward a Social Poetics in Diagnostic Interviews," *Social Science and Medicine* 1996; 43: 919–931, p. 919.

7. Eric J. Cassel, "The Nature of Suffering and the Goals of Medicine," *New England Journal of Medicine*, 1982; 306: 639–645, p. 640.

8. René Dubos, *Mirage of Health* (New York: Harper Colophon Books, Harper & Row, 1959, 1979), p. 102.

9. This idea has been strongly articulated by Mote. The Chinese "are apparently unique in having no creation myth; that is, they have regarded the world and man as uncreated, as constituting the central features of a spontaneously self-generating cosmos . . . having no will external to itself." Frederick F. Mote, *Intellectual Foundations of China*. New York: Alfred A. Knopf, 1971; pp. 17–18.

10. Babylonian Talmud, Zeraim, *Berakoth*, 106, and Mo'ed, *Pesachim*, 566. The king was Hezekiah.

THE STAGES
OF DISEASE:
A SERIES OF
CLINICAL SCENES

This appendix on the progression of illness illustrates the evolution and flexibility of Chinese medical thinking and demonstrates its vitality. Chinese medicine is a corpus of knowledge composed of a great many commentaries written during the past twenty centuries. Although there is apparent confusion in its history, it would be a mistake to overlook the fact that Chinese medicine has also undergone a lengthy process of self-modification. Chinese medicine always goes back to its respected and revered sources, but they are continuously scrutinized and supplemented. In short, the living tradition perpetually rediscovers itself.

This process of self-revitalization is exemplified by historical developments in the Chinese approach to febrile diseases. Among the most common clinical pictures observed by physicians East and West are illnesses that involve fever and a sequence of events that includes onset, peak, and recovery. (Until very recently, these illnesses were the major cause of death.) In the modern West, these disorders would probably be described as infectious and contagious diseases. Chinese physicians describe such febrile illnesses as sequential patterns of disharmony.

This appendix is also an important example of East Asian medicine's emphasis on context and ability to simultaneously maintain multiple medical frameworks. While the patterns we have discussed so far are based primarily on synchronicity in the appearance of signs and symptoms, the presentation in this appendix emphasizes "the sequential analysis of stages in the progress of medical disorders."[1] The pattern of longitudinal time is emphasized over the pattern of configuration.

Initially, febrile patterns were thought to occur within a six-stage sequence. Later, a possible four-stage sequence was also developed, to supplement the earlier thinking and to give physicians an alternative theory with which to work. Both the six-stage and the four-stage sequences comprise the basic perceptual framework with which Chinese physicians diagnose and treat febrile illnesses.[2] The concept of pattern sequences in febrile diseases also elaborates on the Exterior patterns of the Eight Principal Patterns, as well as the patterns of Pernicious Influences, but emphasizes time and sequence more.

⊣ THE PATTERN OF SIX STAGES [*liu-jing bian-zheng*]

The idea of a six-stage pattern of disease was first developed by one of the greatest physicians in Chinese history, Zhang Zhong-jing, in his classic *Shang-han Lun* (Discussion of Cold-Induced Disorders), written around 220 C. E. Dr. Zhang studied and synthesized all the medical writings of his time to develop the six-stage pattern. His ideological point of departure was an unclear and obscure passage from the *Nei Jing* that describes six disease stages,[3] and from this he created an elaborate, logical, and practical sequence pattern. The treatment method and prescriptions described in this pattern are still memorized by all practitioners of traditional Chinese medicine.

Dr. Zhang's Discussion of Cold-Induced Disorders became the second most important work in Chinese medical literature and generated at least as many commentaries as the *Nei Jing*, even though it emphasized treatment methods and prescriptions rather than theory. The elegance and subtlety of the Discussion lie in the minimal number of signs it uses to delineate a pattern and in the delicacy and precision of its prescriptions and their permutations.

The six stages presented in the Discussion comprise a series of patterns that map out the course of diseases characterized by Pernicious Influences entering the body and generating fever. Usually, Dr. Zhang suggests, such diseases begin with the first stage and proceed in sequence to the sixth; however, a disease can go straight to any stage, skip stages, or even move in reverse.

The first stage is called *Tai Yang* (Greater Yang). In the Discussion, this stage is characterized by fear of Cold or Wind, fever, headache, and a floating pulse.[4] (Within the rubric of the Eight Principal Patterns, this is a pattern of External Cold Pernicious Influence.) The Discussion mentions many distinctions and variations in the *Tai Yang* stage.[5] This stage marks the onset of illness, after which the Pernicious Influence can enter either the *Yang Ming* or the *Shao Yang* stage.

The *Yang Ming* stage (Yang Brightness) is characterized by "fever, perspiration, no fear of cold, but rather a fear of heat."[6] Irritability, thirst, and rapid, big, and full pulse are the important *Yang Ming* signs. This stage marks the internal development of the disease, and according to the Eight Principal Patterns, this is an Interior/Heat pattern.

The third stage is *Shao Yang* (Lesser Yang). Logically, this category should precede *Yang Ming*. The order of presentation, however, is based on the original *Nei Jing* narrative and therefore was not changed. The signs that designate the *Shao Yang* pattern include "chills and fever coming alternately, chest and flanks distended, bitter taste in the mouth, no appetite, irritability, and urge to vomit."[7] The fever and chills resemble those of malaria, occurring separately and distinctly. *Shao Yang* belongs to a subcategory within the principle of Exterior/Interior and is known as a half-Exterior/half-Interior pattern. Since *Shao Yang* has neither the simultaneous chills and fever of an Exterior pattern nor the Interior signs of fever and no fear of cold, it is considered an in-between. This pattern is intimately tied to the Gall Bladder and Triple Burner Meridian pathways and is therefore associated with flank pain, bitterness in the mouth, blurry vision, and wiry pulse.

The first three stages—*Tai Yang, Yang Ming,* and *Shao Yang*—are patterns of Excess. The fourth and fifth stages are patterns of Deficiency and Interiority, and are not really concerned with Pernicious Influences; the sixth stage is considered a miscellaneous one. A Pernicious Influence can enter the body during the last three stages either by proceeding sequentially through the first three or by going directly inside.[8]

The fourth stage is *Tai Yin* (Greater Yin). It is characterized by a full and distended abdomen, lack of thirst, along with "vomiting, no appetite, great diarrhea, and occasional pain."[9] The commentaries consider this state a pattern of Deficient Spleen Yang.

The fifth stage is *Shao Yin* (Lesser Yin) and is thought to be a step deeper. Many commentaries call this the most serious stage. Its salient signs are "minute pulse and a great desire to sleep."[10] Other signs are aversion to cold, cold limbs, and lack of fever. The commentaries consider this stage a pattern of Deficient Yang, especially of the Kidneys.

The sixth stage is *Jue Yin* (Absolute Yin). Logically, it should be the deepest and most serious stage. The Discussion, however, reveals that this is actually a miscellaneous pattern in which the Yin and Yang of the body act in a complex manner so that some areas are Hot and others are Cold. The text also discusses worms.[11]

The pattern of six stages, along with its many subcategories and great number of prescriptions, was for many hundreds of years the basis for treating febrile diseases of outside origin. (The prescriptions for the last three stages served as the basis for treating Internal disharmonies.) Slowly, however, physicians began to criticize it for its omissions and one-sidedness. Many clinicians and theorists believed that Dr. Zhang's Discussion emphasized Cold Pernicious Influences to the virtual exclusion of Heat Pernicious Influences, focused on Cold Injuring the Yang while forgetting to deal with Heat Injuring the Yin, and dealt with Deficient Yang while ignoring Deficient Yin. (Also, it is possible that the nature of illness changed through the ages, with better sewage, sanitation, social stability, and improvements in nutrition.)

THE PATTERN OF FOUR STAGES [*wei-qi-ying-xue bian-zheng*]

Later Chinese physicians working from the beginning of the Ming dynasty (1368–1644 C.E.) through the Qing dynasty (1644–1911 C.E.) developed what became known as the pattern of four stages.[12] This construct was intended to address the inadequacies of the pattern of six stages. It was not a refutation of the Discussion of Cold-Induced Disorders; rather it was a supplement that provided a more comprehensive method for treating febrile diseases. Depending on the clinical signs, a Chinese doctor could now interpret the disorder by means of either the six- or the four-stage sequence. The pattern of four stages became known as a development of "Warm Disease School" *(wen-re-xue)*. Although this school occurs late in Chinese medical history, it is universally accepted as part of the classical Chinese medical tradition, demonstrating how patterns, theories, and clinical perceptions change and are refined for greater clarity and accuracy.

The Warm Disease School traced its origins to a few scattered sentences in the *Nei Jing* that refer to Heat illnesses, such as "Winter injures with Cold, in Spring there will be Warm illness,"[13] and to a few brief references in the Discussion, such as "Tai Yang illness, fever and thirst, no fear of cold, is Warm illness."[14]

Taking four words from the *Nei Jing* that describe physiological entities, the Warm Disease School went on to develop an alternate series of patterns of Heat illness. They depicted four broad sequential scenes of febrile disharmonies.[15] In this schematic representation, febrile diseases are thought to be able to enter four distinct depths of the body.

The first stage, called the pattern of the Wei Portion *(wei-fen-zheng)* occurs when a Pernicious Influence is in the Wei portion or the first depth of the body. (*Wei* is the Chinese word for Protective Qi.) Disharmonies of this pattern are characterized by fever, a slight fear of cold, headache, coughing, slight thirst with or without perspiration, either the tongue material or the tip of the tongue slightly red, and a floating and rapid pulse. Within the rubric of the Eight Principal Patterns, it is a pattern of Exterior Heat. It is not described in Dr. Zhang's Discussion.

The second pattern of the four stages, the pattern of the Qi Portion *(qi-fen-zheng)*, occurs when the Pernicious Influence enters the Qi portion, or the second depth of the body. This happens if the Pernicious Influence is not dispelled from the Wei portion and manages to penetrate deeper into the body. Its primary sign is fever without fear of cold, which is similar to the *Yang Ming* stage of the six-stage sequence or to an Interior/Heat pattern of the Eight Principal Patterns. Various subpatterns develop, depending on the types of Heat involved and which Organ is invaded. The details of this stage are extensively dealt with in the literature. For example, Heat in the Lungs displays the signs of high fever, wheezing, coughing, yellow tongue moss, and thirst; Heat in the Stomach produces high fever, sweat, dark, scanty urine, constipation, abdominal and epigastric pain, and flooding pulse.

The third stage of the four stages is called the pattern of the Ying Portion (*ying-fen-zheng*). The word *Ying* describes the Nutritive aspect of Qi that is associated with Blood, and the Ying stage is the next depth of the sequence. The main signs include a scarlet red tongue, irritability, restlessness, delirium or coma, fever that is greater at night, thirst (but not so great as that associated with the Qi Portion), slight red skin eruptions, and a thin, rapid pulse. Because the Pernicious Influence is in the deeper Yin portions of the body, the tongue becomes scarlet and the Shen is very easily disturbed, while thirst is reduced because some Fluids vaporize and ascend to the tongue. Because the Ying stage is preliminary to the Blood stage, one often sees the beginning of skin rashes and eruptions, which are signs of Heat in the Blood.

The pattern of the Blood Portion (*xue-fen-zheng*) is the final, deepest, and most serious of the four stages. All signs of the Ying Portion now worsen; the patient succumbs to a high fever, delirium, or coma, is extremely irritable, and has distinct and dramatic skin eruptions and rashes. As the Heat disturbs the Blood, there is reckless movement with such signs as vomiting of blood, nosebleeds, blood in the stool or urine, and skin eruptions. The Shen may also be greatly disturbed. The Heat in this stage can injure the Yin and the Blood, thereby easily allowing Wind to arise with such signs as tremors, stiffness, eyes staring upward, and teeth locked shut. Sometimes this stage has more manifestations of Deficiency, and the Heat can be thought of as injuring the Yin, Fluids, and Blood. The signs accompanying this are low fever (morning cool/evening hot), hot palms and soles, dry teeth, sunken eyes, trembling hands, and a very thin pulse.

The Pericardium is often affected in Warm illnesses. The most common problem is Heat disturbing the Shen during a Warm illness. This phenomenon is usually described as Heat collapsing into the Pericardium. It occurs most often during the Ying or Blood stage. Whenever the Pericardium is so affected, the Shen may become unclear, and coma or delirium can develop. Serious irritability and a trembling tongue are often the first signs of such a collapse. Another common alternative pattern that also influences the Shen and accompanies External Heat illnesses is Mucus Obstructing the Pericardium. Table 11 distinguishes these two patterns.

TABLE II *Heat Patterns Affecting the Pericardium*

SIGN	HEAT PERNICIOUS INFLUENCE COLLAPSING INTO PERICARDIUM
Shen	coma, often with convulsions or nervous activity
Fever	high fever
Stool	often no change, or constipation
Pulse	thin and rapid or wiry and rapid
Tongue	scarlet, dry material; yellow moss

SIGN	TURBID MUCUS OBSTRUCTING PERICARDIUM
Shen	coma, or patient is sometimes awake
Fever	lower fever
Stool	loose stools
Pulse	soggy and rapid or slippery and rapid
Tongue	red material; white, greasy moss or yellow, greasy moss

NOTES

1. Hans Ågren, "Chinese Traditional Medicine: Temporal Order and Synchronous Events" in J. T. Fraser, N. Lawerence, and F. C. Haber (eds.), *Time, Science, and Society in China and the West* (Amherst, MA: University of Massachusetts Press, 1986), p. 212. This essay contains an excellent discussion of multiple versions of time in Chinese medical thought.

2. This topic of Chinese medical theory is called Distinguishing Patterns of External Heat Disorders (*wai-gan re-bing bian-zheng*).

3. The *Nei Jing* states that on the first day of Cold invading the body it injures the *Tai Yang*. On the second day it injures the *Yang Ming*, on the third day the *Shao Yang*, the fourth day the *Tai Yin*, the fifth day the *Shao Yin*, the sixth day the *Jue Yin*. If the disease continues, it repeats this cycle. See *Su Wen*, sec. 9, chap. 31, pp. 183–185. *Tai Yang, Yang Ming, Shao Yang, Tai Yin, Shao Yin*, and *Jue Yin* are also names for the Meridians. But a connection between the six stages and the Meridians was not explicitly stated in Chinese medical literature until a commentary on Dr. Zhang's Discussion was written by Zhu Kong in 1107 C.E. It should also be noted that, although the six stages seem to be based on the *Nei Jing*, many schol-

ars believe, because of syntactical evidence, that the Discussion of Cold-Induced Disorders was written before the bulk of the *Nei Jing* in the southern regions. For an English-language discussion of the history of the text, see Dean C. Epler, "The Concept of Disease in an Ancient Chinese Medical Text: The Discourse on Cold-Damage Disorders (*Shang-han Lun*)," *Journal of the History of Medicine*, 1988; 43: 8–35.

4. Zhang, Discussion [27], sec. 1, p. 1.

5. The most important distinction in this stage is between a situation in which there is no perspiration, which is considered Excess, and a situation where there is perspiration, which is considered Deficiency.

6. Zhang, Discussion, sec. 182, p. 116.

7. Ibid., sec. 96, p. 57.

8. The last three stages are actually of little use in treating febrile illnesses and have little diagnostic value in general. They are important mainly because the recommended prescriptions are the basis for much of the traditional therapy.

9. Zhang, Discussion, sec. 273, p. 161.

10. Ibid., sec. 281, p. 166.

11. Zhang Zhong-jing's Essential Prescriptions of the Golden Chest [29], which originally was part of a single volume that included the Discussion, goes on to discuss various Interior disorders, gynecological disorders, and complex situations.

12. Among the most important of these physicians were Ye Tian-shi, whose major book was Discussion of Warm Diseases (*Wen-re Lun*, 1746 C.E.), and Wu Ju-tong, whose major work is Refined Diagnoses of Warm Diseases [23], 1798 C.E. The most important English discussion of the "Warm Disease School" and how it represents a radical discontinuity from "Cold-Induced Disorders" is Marta E. Hanson, "Inventing a Tradition in Chinese Medicine: From Universal Canon to Local Medical Knowledge in South China, The Seventeenth to the Nineteenth Century" (Ph.D. diss., University of Pennsylvannia, 1997).

13. *Su Wen* [1], sec. 1, chap. 3, p. 21; also sec. 2, chap. 5, p. 35.

14. Zhang, Discussion, sec. 6, p. 3.

15. The discussion of the pattern of four stages is based on that in Nanjing Institute, Lecture Notes on Warm Illnesses [80], pp. 5–10. The discussion on the Pericardium is based on Shanghai Institute, *Foundations* [53], pp. 236–239.

YANG ORGANS
IN DISHARMONY

The main function of the Yang Organs is to receive and digest food, absorbing the useful portion and transmitting and excreting waste. Because Yang Organs are primarily involved with "impure" substances such as untransformed food, urine, and excrement, they are considered less Internal than the Yin Organs, which are concerned with the "pure" or fundamental textures of Qi; Blood, Essence, and Spirit. Yang Organs play a less crucial role than Yin Organs in both theory and practice. In acupuncture, however, the Yang Meridians are at least as important as the Yin Meridians.

Each Yang Organ is coupled with a Yin Organ in what is called an Interior-Exterior relationship (see Table 1 in Chapter 3), and the Meridian pathways of each pair of coupled Organs are connected. Some Yang Organs have an intimate relationship with their corresponding Yin Organ. Other Yang-Yin couplings seem to be merely a mechanical working-out of Five Phase correspondences. (See Appendix F.)

The correspondences between Liver and Gall Bladder, Spleen and Stomach, and Kidney and Bladder have actual physiological significance and are valuable in the practice of Chinese medical pathology. The correspondences between Heart and Small Intestine and between Lungs and Large Intestine are to be found in their Meridians and are of less consequence in the actual practice of medicine.

The Yang Organs are generally more involved with Excess and Heat disharmonies than their Yin counterparts. The most common Bladder disharmony is Damp Heat Pouring Downward (Heat/Excess), while Kidney disharmonies are usually patterns of Deficiency.

The Stomach and Spleen also exhibit these tendencies and show their complementary opposition in relation to Dampness and Dryness. The Stomach likes Dampness and is sensitive to Dryness, while the opposite is true of the Spleen. Thus, Deficient Yin of the Stomach is a common pattern, while Dampness disharmony is typical of the Spleen. The complementary relationship of the Stomach and Spleen is also emphasized by the direction of their Qi: downward from the Stomach and upward from the Spleen. Therefore, a disharmony of the Stomach will display signs of nausea, vomiting, and belching (reversals of the usual direction of movement), while the Spleen's disharmony is associated with loose bowels and hemorrhoids.

Gall Bladder and Liver disharmonies are difficult to distinguish clinically because the Liver, unlike the other Yin Organs, often tends to be associated with Heat and Excess. There is a different distinction, however, in that Gall Bladder disharmonies are often seen to be more Exterior and Liver disharmonies more Interior.

The patterns of Small Intestine and Large Intestine disharmonies are not usually related to their corresponding Yin Organs except in acupuncture, where Meridians of the Yang Organs are used to treat their corresponding Yin Organs. Most commonly, Small and Large Intestine disharmonies are related to the Spleen, with a tendency to involve Excess, Stagnation, or Heat (for instance, Damp Heat in the Large Intestine). Often the symptom of gurgling or rumbling (borborygmus) distinguishes these disharmonies from those of the Stomach and Spleen.

The Triple Burner does not exist apart from other Organs and is rarely involved in patterns that distinguish it from the other Organs. (Again, this is not true of its Meridian, which has a distinct existence and therapeutic use.)

The most common Yang Organ disharmony patterns are summarized in Tables 12–16.[1]

TABLE 12 *Stomach Disharmony Patterns*

Signs	Tongue	Pulse
Stomach Fire Blazing		
thirst; excessive appetite; bad breath; gums swollen and painful; burning sensation in epigastrium; explosive behavior; manic episodes	red material; thick yellow moss	flooding, or rapid and full
Deficient Stomach Yin		
dry mouth and lips; no appetite; dry vomit or belching; constipation; nervousness	peeled, reddish material	thin and rapid
Stagnant Stomach Qi[1]		
epigastrium is distended and painful; pain often extends to sides; pain is often emotionally related; belching; sour taste in mouth; moodiness; frustration	darkish material	wiry
Congealed Blood in Stomach		
stabbing, piercing pain in epigastrium; distention; touch aggravetes pain; black or dark stools; darkish face; suspiciousness; paranoia	darker material with red dots; thin yellow moss	wiry and choppy
Deficient Cold in Stomach[2]		
slight, persistent pain in epigastrium; discomfort relieved by warmth, eating, and touching; shy; easily influenced by others	pale material; most white moss	deep or moderate without strength

1. Often called Liver Invading Stomach.
2. Often called Deficient Spleen Yang.

TABLE 13 *Small Intestine Disharmony Patterns*

Signs	Tongue	Pulse
Deficient Cold of Small Intenstine[1]		
slight, persistent discomfort in lower abdomen; gurgling noises in abdomen; watery stools	pale material; thin white moss	empty
Stagnant Qi of Small Intestine[2]		
groin and hypogastrium have urgent pain, often extending to lower back; one testicle descends more than the other	white moss	deep and wiry or deep and tight
Excess Heat of Small Intestine[3]		
irritability; cold sores in mouth; sore throat; urination is frequent and even painful, with dark urine; lower abdomen feels full; talkative	red material; yellow moss	rapid and slippery
Obstructed Qi of Small Intenstine		
violent pain in abdomen; constipation; no gas passes; possible vomiting of fecal material	greasy yellow moss	wiry and full

1. Often discussed as Deficient Spleen Qi.
2. This pattern often describes hernias and is often discussed as Cold Obstructing the Liver Meridian.
3. This pattern is often called Heart Fire Moving by Meridian to Small Intestine and is an exception in which the Heart and Small Intestine are clinically coupled.

TABLE 14 *Large Intestine Disharmony Patterns*

Signs	Tongue	Pulse
Damp Heat Invading Large Intestine[1]		
urgent need to defecate, intensifies after defecation; stool has pus or blood; burning anus; often accompanied by fever	red material; greasy yellow moss	slippery and rapid
Intestinal Abcess[2]		
urgent pain in lower right abdomen; fever, or no fever; resists touch	red material; yellow moss	rapid
Exhausted Fluid of Large Intestine		
constipation; dry stool; often associated with postpartum condition	red and dry material	thin
Cold Dampness in Large Intestine[3]		
rumbling in intestine; abdomen sometimes painful; diarrhea; clear urine	moist, greasy white moss	deep and slippery
Deficient Qi of Large Intestine[4]		
chronic diarrhea; slight persistent lower abdominal discomfort; rumbling in intestine; pressure relieves discomfort; cold limbs; tired Shen	pale material; white moss	frail

1. Often called Damp Heat Dysentery.
2. This pattern is mentioned in the Ling Shu and discussed in detail by Zhang Zhong-jing. It is analogous to the Western entity of appendicitis.
3. Often called Dampness Distressing the Spleen.
4. Often called Deficient Spleen Yang.

TABLE 15 *Gall Bladder Disharmony Patterns*

SIGNS	TONGUE	PULSE
Excess Gall Bladder Heat		
flank and chest are painful and distended; bitter taste in mouth; vomits bitter fluid; patient angers easily	red material; yellow moss	wiry, rapid, and full
Damp Heat in both Gall Bladder and Liver		
jaundice (Yang type with bright yellow color); painful flanks; scanty, dark urine; fever; nausea; vomiting; resentment; festering belligerence	red material; greasy yellow moss	wiry, rapid, and slippery
Deficient Gall Bladder Heat		
vertigo; frightens easily; timidity; indecision; unclear vision; annoyance at little things	thin white moss	wiry and thin

TABLE 16 *Bladder Disharmony Patterns*

SIGNS	TONGUE	PULSE
Damp Heat Pouring Downward into Bladder		
frequent, urgent, painful urination; fever; thirst; dry mouth; backache	red material; greasy yellow moss	wiry and rapid or slippery and rapid
Damp Heat Accumulating and Crystallizing in Bladder		
urine occasionally contains sandlike pieces; difficult urination or sudden urine obstruction; occasional violent stabbing pain in lower groin or back; occasional blood in urine	reasonably normal	reasonably normal
Turbid Damp Heat Obstructing Bladder		
urine contains coudy or murky substances	red material; greasy moss	soggy and rapid

continued

TABLE 16 *Bladder Disharmony Patterns (continued)*

Signs	Tongue	Pulse
Deficient Bladder Qi[1]		
incontinence or frequent urination or bed wetting	moist white moss	deep and frail

1. Often called Deficient Kidney Yang.

NOTES

1. Tables 12–16 are based on those in Tianjin City, *Traditional Chinese Internal Medicine* [55], pp. 29–45, and in Anhui Institute, *Clinical Handbook* [68], pp. 34–38.

PULSES
REVISITED

Pulse examination can be the most important of the Four Examinations and is crucial to pattern discernment in general. This appendix amplifies the earlier discussion of pulses. It is presented especially for those readers who are practitioners or students of Oriental medicine and are already familiar with rudimentary pulse theory. The general reader may, however, be interested in the ways that significations (or Yin-Yang correspondences) change depending on a complete configuration of signs.

The pulse can be taken at three positions on the radial artery (see Chapter 6). There are correlations between these pulse positions and certain Organs. Authorities within the tradition have various ideas about the exact correlations; the main opinions are presented in Table 17.[1] In the textual sources, these correspondences are mentioned but given little clinical discussion.

It is important to realize that the twenty-eight pulses rarely appear alone. Usually two or more appear in combination. For each pulse type, therefore, there is a list of the other pulses that often combine with it.

A pulse can appear in all three or in only one of the positions on the radial artery. To give a sense of how the tradition deals with different pulse positions, tables have been included for the more important pulses. The "Bilateral" column in each table describes the symptoms or patterns that are associated with the pulse when it appears in only one position, but on both

TABLE 17 *Pulse Position Correlations: Summary of Opinions from Major Authoritative Sources*

	FIRST Superficial	Deep	SECOND Superficial	Deep	THIRD Superficial	Deep
LEFT HAND						
Nei Jing 1st cent. B.C.E.						
	Sternum	Heart	Diaphragm	Liver	Abdomen	Kidney
Nan Jing c. 200 C.E.						
	Arm *Tai-yang*	Arm *Shao-yin*	Leg *Shao-yang*	Leg *Jue-yin*	Leg *Tai-yang*	Leg *Shao-yin*
Wang Shu-he's Classic of Pulse c. 280 c.e.						
	Small Intestine	Heart	Gall Bladder	Liver	Bladder	Kidney
Li Shi-zhen's Pulse Studies 1564 C.E.						
	Heart		Liver		Kidney (Life Gate)	
Zhang Jie-bing's Complete Book 1624 C.E.						
	Pericardium	Heart	Gall Bladder	Liver	Bladder, Large Intestine	Kidney
RIGHT HAND						
Nei Jing 1st cent. B.C.E.						
	Chest	Lungs	Spleen	Stomach	Abdomen	Kidney
Nan Jing c. 200 C.E.						
	Arm *Yang-ming*	Arm *Tai-yin*	Leg *Yang-ming*	Leg *Tai-yin*	(text unclear)	
Wang Shu-he's Classic of Pulse c. 280 C.E.						
	Large Intestine	Lungs	Stomach	Spleen	Triple Burner (Life Gate)	Kidney
Li Shi-zhen's Pulse Studies 1564 C.E.						
	Lungs		Spleen		Kidney (Life Gate)	
Zhang Jie-bing's Complete Book 1624 C.E.						
	Sternum	Lungs	Stomach	Spleen	Triple Burner Life Gate Small Intestine	Kidney

hands. This information is an opinion based on statements of Li Shi-zhen (1518–1593 C.E.) in his classic Pulse Studies of the Lakeside Master. The "Left Side" and "Right Side" columns present a simplification of major early opinions on the significance of the pulse when it appears in only one position and on only one hand. These statements derive from the comprehensive compilation made by the Shanghai City Traditional Chinese Medical Archives Research Committee.[2]

When a Chinese physician takes a pulse, there is a sense of openness—of endless possibility—about what will be found. There is always the chance that any pulse may have a meaning different from the one traditionally assigned to it. The following discussion of the twenty-eight classic pulses is intended to impart something of that sense of possibility.

⊣ FLOATING PULSE

A floating pulse is generally defined as the sign of an Exterior pattern of disharmony or of the presence of an External Pernicious Influence. Yet a floating pulse is also commonly found when there are no other signs of an Exterior pattern (such as sudden onset of fever, headache, chills, etc.). If this floating pulse is weak, it is generally a sign of Deficient Yin (or Deficient Blood), with the Yang in relative Excess so that the pulse rises higher than normal. This is an example of the Yin being unable to embrace the Yang. If the floating pulse is strong, it is generally a sign of Internal Wind Pernicious Influence or of Excess Yang.

Common Pulse Combinations: Floating Pulse

PULSE	ASSOCIATED SYMPTOMS AND/OR PATTERNS
Floating and rapid	External Heat Pernicious Influence
Floating and tight	External Cold Pernicious Influence
Floating and slippery	Wind and Mucus of Internal Origin or Stagnant Food
Floating and long	Excess
Floating and short	Deficiency, especially of Qi
Floating, flooding, big	External Summer Heat Pernicious Influence

TABLE 18 *The Various Positions and a Floating Pulse*

FIRST POSITION	
Bilateral (Li Shi-zhen)	Wind with a headache; Wind and Mucus in chest
Left Side	Heart Yang Ascending; insomnia; irritability
Right Side	External Wind; Rebellious Qi in Lungs; cough; asthma

SECOND POSITION	
Bilateral (Li Shi-zhen)	Deficient Spleen Qi and Excess Liver Qi
Left Side	Constrained Liver Qi; pain
Right Side	Stagnant Spleen Qi; distended abdomen; vomiting

THIRD POSITION	
Bilateral (Li Shi-zhen)	constipation or anuresis
Left Side and Right Side	Deficient Kidney Qi; difficulty in urination; lumbago; vertigo; menstrual irregularities

⊣ SINKING PULSE

This pulse is generally considered the sign of an Interior pattern. When a sinking pulse is weak, it is a sign of Deficient Yang, since it means that the Yang cannot lift the pulse. If the sinking pulse is strong, it is generally a sign of Cold restraining the upward movement of the Yang. Occasionally an individual has signs of an External Pernicious Influence along with the sinking pulse. This is usually interpreted as signifying the existence of an underlying Deficient Yang or Deficient Qi pattern that renders the patient unable effectively to combat the External Pernicious Influence. A sinking pulse is also considered the general pulse of Kidney disharmonies. In the winter or for heavy people, however, it is considered normal for the Qi and Blood to be deeper, producing a sinking pulse.

Common Pulse Combinations: Sinking Pulse

PULSE	ASSOCIATED SYMPTOMS AND/OR PATTERNS
Floating and rapid	External Heat Pernicious Influence
Floating and tight	External Cold Pernicious Influence
Floating and slippery	Wind and Mucus of Internal Origin or Stagnant Food
Floating and long	Excess
Floating and short	Deficiency, especially of Qi
Floating, flooding, big	External Summer Heat Pernicious Influence

TABLE 19 *The Various Positions and a Sinking Pulse*

FIRST POSITION	
Bilateral (Li Shi-zhen)	Mucus Obstructing Chest
Left Side	Deficient Heart Yang; desire for sleep
Right Side	Deficient Lung Qi; cough; shortness of breath; asthma
SECOND POSITION	
Bilateral (Li Shi-zhen)	Cold in Middle Burner; pain
Left Side	Constrained Liver Qi; pain
Right Side	Deficient Spleen Qi; diarrhea
THIRD POSITION	
Bilateral (Li Shi-zhen)	Deficient Kidney Qi; lumbago; diarrhea
Left Side and Right Side	Deficient Kidney Qi; lumbago; sore knees; vertigo; impotence; sterility; painful menses; leukorrhea

⊣ SLOW PULSE

A slow pulse represents Cold. If this pulse is weak, it signifies insufficient Yang to move the Qi and Blood. If this pulse is strong, it is a sign that Excess Cold is restraining the Qi and Blood. (This sign is often associated with pain.) On rare occasions a slow pulse is accompanied by a constellation of signs pointing to a Heat pattern.[3] Often such a Heat pattern has additional aspects of Dampness, which acts to restrain the movement of Qi and Blood and gives the slow pulse a "soft" quality. It is also possible for a slow pulse with great strength to appear in a Heat pattern without Damp aspects as the result of Heat Pernicious Influence getting "stuck." (This is very rare for Heat but occasionally occurs in acute Heat patterns with abdominal distention or constipation.)

Common Pulse Combinations: Slow Pulse

PULSE	ASSOCIATED SYMPTOMS AND/OR PATTERNS
Slow and floating	Exterior Cold
Slow and choppy	Deficient Blood
Slow and slippery	Mucus
Slow and thin	Deficient Yang
Slow and wiry	Cold pain

⊣ RAPID PULSE

This pulse signifies Heat. Heat generally encourages activity so that the movement of the Qi and Blood increases. A rapid pulse with strength signifies Excess Heat; a rapid but weak pulse points to Deficient Heat or Empty Fire. In rare situations, a rapid pulse may accompany a Deficiency/Cold pattern. Such a rapid pulse is an illusionary sign of Heat and is instead a sign of extreme Deficient Yang floating to the outside of the body.[4] (The patient's situation is serious in this case because the pattern and pulse do not match.)

Common Pulse Combinations: Rapid Pulse

PULSE	ASSOCIATED SYMPTOMS AND/OR PATTERNS
Rapid and thin	Deficient Yin (Empty Fire)
Rapid and floating	likely presence of carbuncle or skin ulcers
Rapid and slippery	Mucus Fire
Rapid and hollow	extreme loss of blood
Rapid and wiry	Liver Fire

---| THIN PULSE

A thin pulse can mean that the volume of Blood is reduced, therefore signifying Deficient Blood, often accompanied by Deficient Qi. Occasionally a thin but strong pulse is associated with Dampness Obstructing Qi and Blood.

Clinically, a thin pulse must be distinguished from a minute pulse, which is less clear and distinct than the thin and usually even weaker.

Common Pulse Combinations: Thin Pulse

PULSE	ASSOCIATED SYMPTOMS AND/OR PATTERNS
Thin and wiry	Deficient Liver Blood
Thin and choppy	extreme Deficient Blood
Thin and deep	Dampness Obstructing Qi and Blood, with pain
Thin and minute	Deficient Yang

TABLE 20 *The Various Positions and a Thin Pulse*

FIRST POSITION	
Bilateral (Li Shi-zhen)	Deficiency with vomiting
Left Side	Heart palpitations; insomnia
Right Side	Qi exhausted from vomiting
SECOND POSITION	
Bilateral (Li Shi-zhen)	Deficient Spleen Qi and Deficient Stomach Qi; distended abdomen; emaciation
Left Side	Liver Yin exhausted
Right Side	Deficient Spleen Qi; abdominal distention
THIRD POSITION	
Bilateral (Li Shi-zhen)	"Cinnabar Field" (Original Qi) Cold; Yin collapsed
Left Side	sexual anxiety; diarrhea
Right Side	Kidney Yang Cold and exhausted

⊣ Big Pulse

A big pulse often is not specific enough to have a clear designation, and Li Shi-zhen therefore left it out of his codification of pulses. (He discusses only twenty-seven pulses.) A big pulse is usually either strong, which makes it similar to a full pulse, or weak, which makes it similar to an empty pulse. If a pulse's strength lies between strong and weak (that is, if it is moderate) and still is big, the tendency is to say that it signifies Excess (and also Heat) in the Yang-ming Meridians (the Stomach and Large Intestine Meridians). These Meridians are said to have the most Qi and Blood[5] and to most easily manifest and/or register Excess/Heat. If there are no accompanying signs of Excess, this pulse may be considered the sign of a strong constitution.

Common Pulse Combinations: Big Pulse

PULSE	ASSOCIATED SYMPTOMS AND/OR PATTERNS
Big and floating	Deficiency or Exterior/Heat
Big and sinking	Interior/Heat or Kidney Disharmony
Big and wiry	Shao-yang Disharmony
Big and moderate	Damp Heat
Big and floating	Stomach Excess

TABLE 21 *The Various Positions and a Big Pulse*

FIRST POSITION	
Bilateral (Li Shi-zhen)	(omitted)
Left Side	irritability; epilepsy; Wind Heat
Right Side	Rebellious Qi; swollen face; cough; asthma

SECOND POSITION	
Bilateral (Li Shi-zhen)	(omitted)
Left Side	Wind with vertigo; hernia
Right Side	Stagnant Qi; Excess Stomach Qi; distended abdomen

THIRD POSITION	
Bilateral (Li Shi-zhen)	(omitted)
Left Side	Kidney Qi obstructed
Right Side	dark urine; constipation

⊣ Empty Pulse

Different sources all agree that an empty pulse represents Deficiency, but there is disagreement as to whether this pulse necessarily has a superficial aspect. Some sources seem to relate the empty pulse to Deficient Blood (*Nei Jing*,[6] Li Shi-zhen[7]); others relate it to Deficient Qi (*Mai Jing*[8]). In general, if the empty pulse is especially superficial, it is said to signify Deficient Blood (that is, to have a Deficient Yin aspect); if it is less superficial, then it signifies Deficient Qi (that is, it has a Deficient Yang aspect). Compared with a thin pulse, an empty pulse is more indicative of Deficient Qi; compared with a frail pulse, it is more indicative of Deficient Blood.

Modern texts and clinical practice seem to agree that an empty pulse is more closely related to Deficient Qi than to Deficient Blood. This interpretation results from concentrating on the big or swollen nature of the pulse, which would be a characteristic of Deficient Qi. The bigness of the pulse is thought to signify the Qi not governing or "wrapping" the Blood.

The Organ most associated with an empty pulse is the Spleen. This association further contributes to the identification of an empty pulse with Deficient Qi, because the Spleen, in itself, is frequently associated with Deficient Qi or with a combination of Deficient Qi and Deficient Blood patterns, but rarely with Deficient Blood patterns alone.

An empty pulse can also be associated with the onset of a Summer Heat Pernicious Influence.

Common Pulse Combinations: Empty Pulse

Pulse	Associated Symptoms and/or Patterns
Empty and rapid	Deficient Yin
Empty and slow	Deficient Yang
Empty and very soft	Deficient Protective Qi, with spontaneous sweating

TABLE 22 *The Various Positions and an Empty Pulse*

FIRST POSITION	
Bilateral (Li Shi-zhen)	Blood unable to nourish Heart
Left Side	Heart palpitations
Right Side	spontaneous sweating

SECOND POSITION	
Bilateral (Li Shi-zhen)	Deficient Qi with distended abdomen
Left Side	Blood unable to nourish tendons
Right Side	distended abdomen

THIRD POSITION	
Bilateral (Li Shi-zhen)	Deficient Blood and Deficient Essence; bones feel hot
Left Side	lower back and knees are sore or atrophying
Right Side	Deficient Yang

⊣ FULL PULSE

The opposite of an empty pulse, a full pulse is most often felt at the onset of an Excess/Heat disorder, but it can be part of any Excess pattern. Occasionally, especially if the pulse is also somewhat moderate, it can be a sign of a strong constitution. Clinically, it is possible for a full pulse to be part of a Deficiency pattern if all the other elements of a configuration indicate Deficiency.[9] Such a full pulse is illusionary and is thought to be a sign that the prognosis is poor.

Common Pulse Combinations: Full Pulse

PULSE	ASSOCIATED SYMPTOMS AND/OR PATTERNS
Full and tending to sinking, wiry	Cold Ascending
Full and rapid	Lung abscess
Full and tending to floating	External Wind Cold Damp Pernicious Influence
Full and sinking	Interior pattern of Stagnant Food or unharmonious emotions
Full and wiry	Liver Fire

TABLE 23 *The Various Positions and a Full Pulse*

FIRST POSITION	
Bilateral (Li Shi-zhen)	Wind Heat affecting head; sore throat; stiff tongue; sensation of pressure in chest
Left Side	stiff tongue
Right Side	sore throat

SECOND POSITION	
Bilateral (Li Shi-zhen)	Heat in Middle Burner; distended abdomen
Left Side	Liver Fire; flank pain
Right Side	pain in epigastrium

THIRD POSITION	
Bilateral (Li Shi-zhen)	Heat in Lower Burner; lumbago; constipation; abdominal pain
Left Side	constipation; abdominal pain
Right Side	Rebellious Fire Ascending

┤ SLIPPERY PULSE

This pulse is generally a sign of Excess Mucus, Dampness, or Stagnant Food and is therefore considered Yang (Excess) within Yin (Dampness), or vice versa. Li Shi-zhen and other sources (including sections of the *Nei Jing*) differ slightly, but they all imply that a slippery pulse has aspects of Heat and is a Yang pulse. Clinically, a slippery pulse is often seen along with coughs, heavy expectoration, indigestion from stagnant food, Damp Heat pouring into the Bladder, and Damp Heat in the Intestines. A slippery pulse may also accompany pregnancy and can be a sign of a strong constitution.

Common Pulse Combinations: Slippery Pulse

PULSE	ASSOCIATED SYMPTOMS AND/OR PATTERNS
Slippery and wiry	Stagnant Food, or Mucus with Constrained Liver Qi
Slippery and tight	Cold Mucus Obstructing

TABLE 24 *The Various Positions and a Slippery Pulse*

FIRST POSITION

Bilateral (Li Shi-zhen)	Mucus in chest; vomiting; belching with sour taste; stiff tongue; cough
Left Side	Heart Heat; fitful sleep
Right Side	Mucus with vomiting or nausea

SECOND POSITION

Bilateral (Li Shi-zhen)	Liver Spleen Heat; Stagnant Food
Left Side	Liver Fire; vertigo
Right Side	Spleen Heat; Stagnant Food

THIRD POSITION

Bilateral (Li Shi-zhen)	"wasting and thirsting"; diarrhea; hernia; urinary problems
Left Side	dark urine; difficult urination
Right Side	diarrhea; Fire Ascending

—| CHOPPY PULSE

Although primarily a Yin pulse, a choppy pulse can have aspects of either Deficiency or Excess. If a choppy pulse is also weak or thin, it is a sign of insufficient Blood or Essence to fill the Blood Vessels. If it is strong, resisting the fingers, it is generally a sign of Congealed Blood Obstructing Movement. On rare occasions, a choppy, strong pulse can even point to Dampness Obstructing Movement, which is the same signification carried by its opposite type of pulse (i.e., slippery). Some sources include an irregular pulse, which in any one breath beats a different number of times ("the three and five not adjusted") under this type of pulse. This is important because there is no other pulse category that includes this irregularity. Clinically, a choppy pulse is often seen along with Heart and chest pain (this figures prominently in the *Nei Jing*), with illnesses accompanied by great loss of blood or fluids, and with Kidney exhaustion (great Deficiency), especially when related to sexual functions.

Common Pulse Combinations: Choppy Pulse

PULSE	ASSOCIATED SYMPTOMS AND/OR PATTERNS
Choppy and wiry	Constrained Liver Qi, Congealed Blood
Choppy and frail	Qi exhausted (great Deficiency)
Choppy and minute	Deficient Blood and Deficient Yang
Choppy and thin	Dried Fluids (Deficiency)

TABLE 25 *The Various Positions and a Choppy Pulse*

FIRST POSITION	
Bilateral (Li Shi-zhen)	Deficient Heart Qi; chest pain
Left Side	Heart pain; Heart palpitations
Right Side	Deficient Lung Qi; cough with foamy sputum

SECOND POSITION	
Bilateral (Li Shi-zhen)	Deficient Spleen Qi and Deficient Stomach Qi; painful distended flank
Left Side	Deficient Liver Blood
Right Side	weak Spleen; inability to eat

THIRD POSITION	
Bilateral (Li Shi-zhen)	Essence and Blood are injured; constipation or dribbling urination, or bleeding from anus
Left Side	lower back is weak and sore
Right Side	weak Life Gate Fire; Essence is injured

⊣ WIRY PULSE

A wiry pulse implies that something is restricting the movement of Qi and Blood. This pulse is generally associated with a reduction in the Liver's smooth spreading function, but it can also accompany a Cold pattern or any pattern with pain. Clinically, a wiry pulse may also appear with a Mucus pattern that accompanies a pattern of Liver Invading the Spleen. At other times, a wiry pulse may signify a complex pattern such as one of simultaneous Hot and Cold, or a pattern of half-Interior/half-Exterior.

Common Pulse Combinations: Wiry Pulse

PULSE	ASSOCIATED SYMPTOMS AND/OR PATTERNS
Wiry and slow	Liver Cold
Wiry and rapid	Liver Fire
Wiry, rapid, and thin	Deficient Liver Yin
Wiry, rapid, and big	Liver Fire Blazing
Wiry and sinking	Interior Stagnation with pain

TABLE 26 *The Various Positions and a Wiry Pulse*

FIRST POSITION	
Bilateral (Li Shi-zhen)	Mucus obstructing diaphragm; headache
Left Side	Heart pain
Right Side	headache; chest and flank pain

SECOND POSITION*	
Bilateral (Li Shi-zhen)	(omitted)
Left Side	malaria; palpable masses in abdomen; spasms
Right Side	Deficient Spleen Qi; Cold Stagnant Food

THIRD POSITION	
Bilateral (Li Shi-zhen)	hernia; leg cramps
Left Side	lower back and leg pain; cramps; lower abdominal pain; hernia
Right Side	abdominal pain; diarrhea

*Qin Bo-wei, the famous twentieth-century practitioner, says that a right second pulse position being by itself wiry is a sign of Wood (Liver) Excess Conquering Earth (Spleen) and is often seen in abdominal pain or diarrhea (Medical Lecture Notes [64], p. 90).

⊣ TIGHT PULSE

A tight pulse signifies that movement is restricted because of Cold. When a Cold Pernicious Influence attempts to impinge the movement of Qi and Blood, the conflict of Cold with the Normal Qi generates combative activity. The pulse feels as if it is moving from left to right and can be compared to the tautness of a stretched rope. Clinically, this pulse often accompanies a pattern of External Cold Wind with body aches, or Deficient Cold of the Middle Burner with pain, or Cold Stagnant Food with pain.

Common Pulse Combinations: Tight Pulse

Pulse	Associated Symptoms and/or Patterns
Tight and rapid	simultaneous Heat and Cold pattern
Tight and wiry	Cold obstruction
Tight and full	distention and pain
Tight and choppy	Cold obstruction

TABLE 27 *The Various Positions and a Tight Pulse*

First position	
Bilateral (Li Shi-zhen)	(omitted)
Left Side	feverish head; stiff neck; Heart pain
Right Side	External Cold; asthma; cough; tight diaphragm
Second position	
Bilateral (Li Shi-zhen)	Cold Dampness Obstructing Middle Burner; pain
Left Side	abdominal distention and pain; flank pain; cramps
Right Side	distended epigastrium and abdomen
Third position	
Bilateral (Li Shi-zhen)	external genitals are Cold; running piglet illness;* hernia
Left Side	pain underneath navel; sore legs; constipation
Right Side	running piglet illness; hernia

* Running piglet (ben-tun) illness is mentioned in the *Ling Shu* (sec. 1, chap. 4, p. 45) and is discussed at length in other early texts. Its symptoms are very unpleasant sensations of pain that come and go and run from the navel to the throat. The pattern most associated with these symptoms is Deficient Kidney Yang with Excess Cold, although Liver Fire is also cited.

⊣ Knotted Pulse

A knotted pulse signifies Yin in ascendancy. If the pulse is also weak, the lack of smooth movement signifies extreme and chronic insufficient Kidney Fire or insufficient Qi and Blood to fill and move within the Blood pathways. If the pulse is also strong, the obstruction probably involves extreme Mucus, Cold, or Stagnant Qi/Congealed Blood.

Common Pulse Combinations: Knotted Pulse

PULSE	ASSOCIATED SYMPTOMS AND/OR PATTERNS
Knotted and floating	Cold Obstructing Meridians
Knotted, sinking, and strong	Stagnant Qi with lumps
Knotted sinking, and frail	Life Gate Fire exhausted
Knotted and slippery	chronic Mucus
Knotted and choppy	Congealed Blood with lumps

⊣ HURRIED PULSE

This pulse signifies Excess Heat, often accompanied by aspects of obstruction from Stagnant Qi, Congealed Blood, or Mucus or Food blocking movement. A hurried pulse, especially when it is also weak, is sometimes a sign of "Organ Qi in Perverse Violation" and signifies extreme Deficiency and Cold. This is similar to the rapid pulse in a Cold pattern. Clinically, a hurried pulse is often seen in patterns of Excess Yang that include such symptoms as red eruptions, extreme anger, coarse breathing, violent insanity. The pulse is also seen in Hot asthmatic conditions where Mucus obstructs. Finally, this pulse may accompany patterns of Heart Qi and Heart Yang both exhausted.

Common Pulse Combinations: Hurried Pulse

PULSE	ASSOCIATED SYMPTOMS AND/OR PATTERNS
Hurried, flooding, and full	Pernicious Influence Obstructing Meridian
Hurried and weak	Deficiency approaching separation of Yin and Yang
Hurried and floating	Yang-ming Heat

⊣ INTERMITTENT PULSE

This pulse is generally a sign that all the Yin Organs are exhausted. Sometimes this pulse specifically accompanies a Deficient Heart Qi pattern with palpitation and pain, or a Middle Burner Deficient Cold pattern with vomiting. If, however, this pulse suddenly arises and is strong, it may be part of a momentary obstruction of Qi associated with a Wind pattern, pain condition, an emotional situation of great stress, or an injury.

Common Pulse Combinations: Intermittent Pulse

PULSE	ASSOCIATED SYMPTOMS AND/OR PATTERNS
Intermittent, thin, and sinking	Deficiency with diarrhea
Intermittent, minute, and thin	Fluids dry
Intermittent and moderate	Spleen Qi exhausted

⊣ SHORT PULSE

This pulse is usually a label for a pulse that cannot be felt in either the first or third positions or in both positions. Sometimes a pulse is called short even when it is felt in all three positions but the beats touching the fingers feel too small in length. Signifying Deficient Qi (especially when the pulse is also weak), it is most commonly seen in Lung, Heart, or Kidney Deficiencies. A short pulse can also accompany a condition of Mucus, Stagnant Food, or alcoholic intoxication (which generates Damp Heat), but in these cases the pulse will also have strength and be slippery and rapid.

Common Pulse Combinations—Short Pulse

PULSE	ASSOCIATED SYMPTOMS AND/OR PATTERNS
Short and floating	Deficient Lung Qi or Congealed Blood
Short and sinking	Deficient Kidney Qi
Short and rapid	Heart pain and irritability
Short and slow	Deficient Cold
Short, slippery, and rapid	alcohol injuring Spirit

⊣ Long Pulse

If a long pulse is also moderate, it can be a sign of a strong constitution. If it has a hard, urgent, tight, or wiry feeling, it suggests Excess. Clinically, this pulse combined with a wiry pulse is often seen with Constrained Liver Qi and with such symptoms as flank pain, headaches, red eyes, and tinnitus. A long pulse together with a flooding pulse can be seen in Yang-Ming (Stomach and Large Intestine) Heat disharmonies, especially when accompanied by Mucus and such signs as epilepsy or Yang insanity. Cold/Excess with pain and asthma can have a long and wiry pulse. Lung Heat with coughing of blood often displays this pulse together with a rapid pulse. A long pulse is often felt in Heat patterns in general, characterized by such symptoms as irritability, thirst, and constipation.

Common Pulse Combinations—Long Pulse

Pulse	Associated Symptoms and/or Patterns
Long and floating	External Pernicious Influence or Deficient Yin
Long and flooding	Yang insanity or epilepsy
Long, sinking, and thin	Lumps or tumors
Long and slippery	Mucus Heat
Long and soggy	alcohol intoxication or Cold
Long and wiry	Liver disharmony

⊣ Moderate Pulse

A moderate pulse is the stereotypical normal pulse. Clinically, it is quite rare, for most people have constitutional tendencies to particular disharmony patterns, and even when they are healthy, those tendencies can be detected in their pulses. A pure moderate pulse accompanied by signs of disharmony is, according to some sources, a sign of Dampness. Most sources, however, seem to think that within a disharmony, a moderate pulse will take on the shading of other pulse types so that its interpretation would depend on the complete configuration.

Common Pulse Combinations—Moderate Pulse

Pulse	Associated Symptoms and/or Patterns
Moderate and floating	External Dampness or Wind
Moderate and sinking	Dampness Obstructing
Moderate and choppy	Deficient Blood
Moderate, slow, and thin	Deficient Yang

⊣ Flooding Pulse

A flooding pulse is a sign of Excess/Heat with aspects of Deficient Yin. Treatment therefore consists of both cooling Heat and nourishing the Yin. This pulse is usually felt during febrile illnesses with thirst, irritability, and vomiting of blood, or in diseases with red, swollen skin ulceration. Occasionally, there is a flooding pulse whose surging forward movement is big but lacks strength and which recedes like a regular flooding pulse. If this pulse is accompanied by such signs as diarrhea, the interpretation is that the bigness signifies Deficiency (as does an empty pulse), and the pulse is then considered a sign of Deficiency. Heart disharmonies are also associated with this pulse. Another possible interpretation of a flooding pulse is that it implies a situation in which Heat on the Interior is being restrained or bottled up by Cold on the Exterior.

Common Pulse Combinations—Flooding Pulse

Pulse	Associated Symptoms and/or Patterns
Flooding and big	Heat Ascending
Flooding and floating	External Heat or Deficient Yin
Flooding and sinking	Internal Heat or Cold Restraining Heat
Flooding and tight	chest distention or constipation with bleeding
Flooding and slippery	Heat/Mucus

⊣ Minute Pulse

A minute pulse signifies Deficient Yang and often accompanies patterns of
extreme weakness with such signs as loose stools, bright face, little Spirit, fear
of cold, Cold diarrhea, or Cold uterine bleeding. This pulse frequently arises
in the clinically urgent situations of "Vanquished Yang" (*wang-yang*) and "Vanquished Yin" (*wang-yin*). Vanquished Yang can arise when the Yang is so
extremely weak (signified by such signs as much oily perspiration, cold body,
no thirst, very faint respiration, cold limbs, coma) that it cannot nourish the
Yin. This causes the Yin and Yang to separate, leading to possible "collapse"
(fainting or shock) or even death. Vanquished Yin can occur because of great
loss of fluids evidenced by severe sweating, vomiting, diarrhea, and bleeding,
and is accompanied by weakness, fear of heat, warm skin, thirst, coarse respiration, warm limbs, red, dry tongue, and a flooding but weak pulse. In this
case the Yin can no longer nourish the Yang, and the result may be similar to
that of Vanquished Yang—separation, collapse, or death. Vanquished Yin or
Yang can turn into one another, so even a Vanquished Yin situation can finally
develop a minute pulse.

Common Pulse Combinations—Minute Pulse

Pulse	Associated Symptoms and/or Patterns
Minute and soggy	spasms
Minute and soft	spontaneous sweating
Minute and choppy	great loss of Blood

TABLE 28 *The Various Positions and a Minute Pulse*

First position	
Bilateral (Li Shi-zhen)	asthma; Heart palpitations
Left Side	Qi and Blood both Deficient
Right Side	Mucus obstructed; asthma

Second position	
Bilateral (Li Shi-zhen)	Deficient Spleen Qi; distended abdomen
Left Side	sensation of pressure in chest; spasms in four limbs
Right Side	Stomach Cold; food not transformed

continued

TABLE 28 *The Various Positions and a Minute Pulse (continued)*

THIRD POSITION	
Bilateral (Li Shi-zhen)	Deficient Essence; fear of cold; diabetes
Left Side	injured sperm; uterine bleeding
Right Side	Kidney diarrhea; pain in navel region; extremely Deficient Yang

⊣ FRAIL PULSE

This pulse shows that the Yang cannot raise the pulse, and so it is a sign of Deficient Yang and/or Deficient Essence. It is primarily seen in Deficient Kidney patterns along with such symptoms as sore bones, weak back and legs, asthma, tinnitus, or dizziness. A frail pulse is sometimes also seen in Deficient Cold Spleen patterns. Li Shi-zhen mentions that it is understandable and even normal to see this pulse in an elderly person, but if it is seen in a young person, the physician must be on the alert for a problem.

Common Pulse Combinations—Frail Pulse

PULSE	ASSOCIATED SYMPTOMS AND/OR PATTERNS
Frail and choppy	Deficient Blood
Frail and rapid	excessive loss of sperm, or uterine bleeding
Frail, wiry, and thin	Deficient Blood and flaccid tendons
Frail and soft	spontaneous sweating

TABLE 29 *The Various Positions and a Frail Pulse*

FIRST POSITION	
Bilateral (Li Shi-zhen)	Deficient Yang
Left Side	Heart palpitations; forgetfulness
Right Side	shortness of breath; spontaneous sweating
SECOND POSITION	
Bilateral (Li Shi-zhen)	Deficient Spleen Qi and Deficient Stomach Qi
Left Side	spasms
Right Side	diarrhea

continued

TABLE 29 *The Various Positions and a Frail Pulse (continued)*

Third position	
Bilateral (Li Shi-zhen)	Yang collapses; Deficient Yin
Left Side	Deficient Yin
Right Side	Yang collapses

⊣ Soggy Pulse

This pulse is a sign of either Deficient Yin or Deficient Yin and Yang both. It is most often seen after loss of blood, as well as in many serious Deficiency patterns that are slightly more Deficient of Yin than of Yang. Li Shi-zhen says that if this pulse appears after a severe illness or postpartum, it is normal and recovery will be easy. (The tradition speaks of Deficiency that can easily receive tonification and Deficiency that cannot. This situation is Deficiency that can receive tonification.) If a person has this pulse but has no accompanying symptoms of Deficiency, it is said that the pulse is "without root," but the person should be treated in order to prevent disease.

A soggy pulse can also appear along with a Damp pattern, because the Dampness "spreads everywhere" and obstructs Qi and Blood movement. In this case, the soggy pulse is likely to have a tight, hindered quality. Sometimes a soggy, weak pulse appears with simultaneous Dampness Distress and Deficient Spleen patterns.

Common Pulse Combinations—Soggy Pulse

Pulse	**Associated Symptoms and/or Patterns**
Soggy and wiry	dizziness or numb fingers
Soggy and choppy	loss of Blood
Soggy and rapid	Damp Heat

⊣ Leather Pulse

This pulse is a sign of Deficient Essence, Yin, or Blood. It is more serious than an ordinary empty pulse since in this case the Yang Qi is less controlled by the Yin, so that along with an empty feeling in the middle, the very surface of the pulse is hard and wiry. A leather pulse often appears with miscarriages, uterine bleeding, or spermatorrhea.

Common Pulse Combinations—Leather Pulse

Pulse	Associated Symptoms and/or Patterns
Leather, slippery, and big	excess of perspiration, or diarrhea
Leather and moderate, without Spirit	"dead" Yin, not treatable

⊣ Hidden Pulse

This pulse is usually a sign of serious obstruction. If a hidden pulse is strong, the obstruction is usually Excess/Cold or Stagnant Food, and is often accompanied by violent pain. When an extreme Heat situation displays a hidden rapid pulse, it is a situation in which the pattern and pulse do not match and is therefore serious and difficult to treat.

If the hidden pulse is without strength, it is usually a sign that Yang Qi is insufficient to raise the pulse. This is often seen in chronic illnesses accompanied by vomiting, diarrhea, cold limbs, or fainting. Occasionally, a person with a chronic pattern combining Arrogant Liver Yang and Deficient Kidney Yin will suddenly collapse (apoplexy or "succumbing" to Wind) and develop hemiplegia, and this pulse will appear. Some sources say that this can be a normal pulse during pregnancy.

Common Pulse Combinations—Hidden Pulse

Pulse	Associated Symptoms and/or Patterns
Hidden and slow	Extreme Cold: Extreme Yin Ascending
Hidden and rapid	Extreme Heat: Extreme Yang Ascending

⊣ Confined or Prison Pulse

This pulse is basically a subcategory of the hidden pulse with strength. It again signifies Cold obstruction with pain and the presence of lumps, tumors, or hernia. Li Shi-zhen cautions that if this pulse arises in a Deficiency pattern, the situation is dangerous. Other sources mention it as appearing with "running piglet" illness.

⊣ Spinning Bean or Moving Pulse

This pulse is said to result from the chaotic movement of Yin and Yang. When severe pain interrupts the Blood flow, or fright causes the Qi to "sneak" away, the Qi and Blood lose their mutual nourishing function and generate this unharmonious pulse. Although a spinning bean pulse is generally rapid, it does not necessarily imply a Heat condition; it just implies great imbalance.

Common Pulse Combinations—Spinning Bean Pulse

Pulse	Associated Symptoms and/or Patterns
Spinning bean and frail	palpitations
Spinning bean and full	pain; obstruction
Spinning bean and hollow	loss of Essence
Spinning bean and floating	External Pernicious Influence

⊣ Hollow Pulse

This pulse generally appears after great loss of blood, but not in chronic patterns of Deficient Blood. It can also appear after depletion of fluids due to vomiting, diarrhea, excessive perspiration, and loss of sperm.

Common Pulse Combinations—Hollow Pulse

Pulse	Associated Symptoms and/or Patterns
Hollow and rapid	Deficient Yin
Hollow, empty, and soft	Deficient Essence; loss of Blood
Hollow and knotted	Congealed Blood

⊣ Scattered Pulse

A scattered pulse is a sign of extreme Deficiency, especially of Yang or of Original Qi. When seen in a chronic Deficiency illness with Deficiency signs, however, this pulse is unlike the weak pulse mentioned earlier, in which matching pulse and pattern meant the condition would be relatively easy to treat. In this case, because a scattered pulse is superficial, it shows that the Normal Qi or Yang is "floating" away. This is extreme weakness, and the pattern is difficult to reharmonize. Some sources say that this pulse can have the uneven quality sometimes associated with a choppy pulse. This pulse is usually seen in chronic patterns or in patterns of exhaustion.

The signification of the scattered pulse tends to remain the same no matter what other pulses it is found in combination with. The chart of combinations has therefore been omitted.

NOTES

1. The *Nei Jing* opinion is found in *Su Wen*, sec. 5, chap. 17, pp. 106–107. The *Nan Jing* opinion is in "Difficulty 18," pp. 45–46. Its schema is about Meridians, makes no distinction between left and right hands, and is very unclear. The data in this table are only one interpretation. Following these correspondences, the *Nan Jing* goes on to say that the first, second, and third positions represent the Upper, Middle, and Lower Burner, respectively. Wang Shu-he's opinion is found in the Classic of Pulse [22], p. 6. Wang also says that the first, second, and third positions correspond to the sections of the Triple Burner. Li Shi-zhen also emphasizes this Triple Burner relation and his opinion is found in Pulse Studies [16], p. 4. The Zhang Jie-bing opinion is from his landmark *Complete Works of Jing-yue* (*Jing-yue Quan-shu*), 1624 C.E. [Taipei: Guofeng, 1980], sec. 5, p. 86.

   Alternative styles of pulse correspondence at the radial artery also exist in early texts. The *Nan Jing* describes the horizontal layers of the pulse as matching the various Organs: "With three beans of pressure the skin is reached, which is the Lung position. Six beans of pressure reaches the Blood Vessels and is the Heart position. Nine beans of pressure reaches the flesh and muscles and is the Spleen position. Twelve beans of pressure is level with tendons and is the Liver position. Pressing to the bone . . . reaches the Kidneys" (*Nan Jing*, "Difficulty 5," p. 12). Related to this *Nan Jing* method is the method whereby the qualities of pulses are fitted into a correspondence schema. For instance, the *Nei Jing* states that the "Liver is wiry; the Heart pulse is 'hooked' [interpreted to mean flooding]; the Spleen is 'substitutelike' [interpreted to mean soft]; the Lung is 'featherlike' [interpreted to mean superficial]; the Kidneys are 'stonelike' [interpreted to mean deep]" (*Su Wen*, sec. 7, chap. 23, p. 154).

   An elaborate comparative pulse correspondence system also exists in the earliest texts. The schema depends mainly on the relative sizes of the entire radial artery as compared with the pulse at the acupuncture point *ren-ying* (Stomach 9) at the common carotid artery of the neck. For example, if the radial pulse is twice as big as the carotid pulse, the illness is in the Gall Bladder Meridian. This method continues for the other Meridians (*Ling Shu*, sec. 2, chap. 9, pp. 89–92; *Su Wen*, sec. 3, chap. 10, p. 69).

2. Li Shi-zhen's opinion is from his Pulse Studies. If an opinion concerning both sides is omitted, it is usually because Li did not mention the case. The summary of opinions of individual positions on each hand is taken from Selections from Pulse Examination [17]. This comprehensive study excerpts pulse discussions from many early texts and catalogs them under the twenty-eight types in historical order.

3. See Zhang Zhong-jing, Discussion on Cold-Induced Disorders [27], secs. 208, 225, and 234, for some examples of this situation. Liu Guan-jin (Pulse Examination

[61], p. 82) mentions that if the Western disease entity meningitis is accompanied by increased cerebral pressure and high fever, a slow pulse can occasionally be felt. This is a dangerous sign in both medical systems.

4. An example of this situation is discussed in Liaoning Institute, *Lecture Notes on Traditional Chinese Medicine* [48], p. 34.

5. Yang Ji-zhou, Great Compendium of Acupuncture and Moxibustion [26], (1601 C.E.), sec. 5, p. 164. Originally based on *Su Wen*, sec. 7, chap. 24, p. 54.

6. *Su Wen* [1], sec. 40, chap. 53, p. 280.

7. Pulse Studies [16], p. 58.

8. Wang Shu-he, Classic of Pulse [22], p. 30.

9. Many classical physicians such as Zhang Zhong-jing and Zhang Jie-bing discuss this possibility.

APPENDIX D

THE CURIOUS ORGANS

The *Nei Jing* mentions six miscellaneous or Curious Organs and occasionally refers to one or another of them in passing. These Organs—the Brain, Marrow, Bones, Uterus, Blood Vessels, and Gall Bladder—are said to resemble the Yang Organs in form but the Yin Organs in function. They "store the Yin and imitate Earth; therefore, they store and do not disperse,"[1] whereas the Yang Organs "disperse and do not Store."[2] These Curious Organs are actually of little importance, in both theory and practice; any distinct function they may have is subsumed under, and accessory to, the functions of the primary Organs. Treatment, therefore, is almost always aimed at one of the primary Organs or Meridians.

The Gall Bladder has been discussed earlier, with the Yang Organs (see Chapter 3).

The Brain, Marrow, and Bones are often indistinguishable from each other in the *Nei Jing* and are always inseparable from the Kidney, in both conception and function. Like the Kidneys, they are dependent on the combination of prenatal and postnatal Essence (Jing). "When an individual is created, first the Essence (Jing) is formed; from the Essence (Jing) comes the Brain and Marrow."[3] "The five-grain Essence (Jing) [postnatal Jing] forms a cream, seeping into the empty spaces of the Bones to nourish the Brain and Marrow."[4]

The main function of the Marrow is to nourish the bones. It should be noted that the Chinese word here translated as "Marrow" refers not only to bone marrow but also to the spinal cord. If the Marrow is sufficient, the Bones are strong.[5] If the Marrow is insufficient, the Bones will be weak. Children with insufficient Marrow have problems with Bone growth.

The Brain is the "sea of Marrow."[6] It is responsible for the fluidity of movement in the body and for the sensitivity of the eyes and ears. The Brain, like the Bones, is nourished by the Marrow. When the Brain is not nourished, because the "Marrow is insufficient, the Brain lacks coordination and there is ringing in the ears, tremors, dizziness, poor vision, and languid idleness."[7]

The Bones are "ruled by the Kidneys" and give the body structural support.

Later in the medical tradition, there developed greater understanding of these Organs. Li Shi-zhen, for example, believed the Brain to be the sea of consciousness.[8] But however the Brain, Marrow, and Bones have been understood, their disorders have been treated with herbs or needles directed to the Kidneys or the Kidney Meridian.[9]

The Uterus is important to two major processes, menstruation and gestation. The Chinese believe, however, that both of these processes are governed, *functionally* if not anatomically, by other Organs and by the Meridians.

Menstrual periods cannot occur without a "communicating" Conception Meridian and a "full" Penetrating Meridian.[10] (The Penetrating Meridian is one of the extra Meridians and is known as the "sea of the Twelve Meridians.")[11] Both of these Meridians are said to "arise in the Uterus."[12] Menstruation also depends on the Kidney Essence (Jing) and on the Blood functions of the Spleen and Liver. Therefore, although the Uterus is involved in the proper function of menstruation, treatment for menstrual disorders is generally directed toward the Liver, Spleen, or Kidneys and toward related Meridians.

Since the Uterus is also the place where the fetus resides during pregnancy, the word for Uterus in Chinese literally means "palace of the child." Most of the functions of pregnancy, however, are thought to be the province of the Conception and Penetrating Meridians and of the Spleen, Liver, and Kidneys. This is an example of Chinese medicine's emphasis on function and its relative indifference to structure.

The Blood Vessels are the "Yang Organ of the Blood"[13] and the means by which most Blood is transported through the body. The tradition states that Qi is associated with Blood in the Vessels[14] and that Qi and Blood are both in the Meridians, but the distinction between Blood Vessels and Meridians is not clearly stated. The implication is that Blood Vessels carry relatively more Blood and the Meridians relatively more Qi. Disorders of the Blood Vessels are treated through the other Organs; for instance, the Heart rules regularity of flow, the Liver rules evenness of distribution, and the Spleen rules the ability to keep the Blood within its pathways.[15]

NOTES

1. *Su Wen* [1], sec. 3, chap. 11, p. 77.
2. Ibid.
3. *Ling Shu* [2], sec. 3, chap. 10, p. 104.
4. Ibid., sec. 6, chap. 36, p. 289.
5. *Su Wen*, sec. 24, chap. 81, p. 573.
6. *Ling Shu*, sec. 6, chap. 33, p. 275.
7. Ibid., p. 277.
8. Shanghai Institute, *Foundations* [53], p. 97.
9. One exception is found in the *Nan Jing*, in which the Bones and Marrow are thought to have their own "meeting point" that allows them to be treated not through the other Organs, but as distinct entities. The Bone point is Bladder 11 (*Da-zhu*) and the Marrow point is Gall Bladder 39 (*Jue-gu*, also called *Xuan-zhong*). *Nan Jing*, "Difficulty 45," p. 104.
10. *Su Wen*, sec. 1, chap. 1, p. 4.
11. *Ling Shu*, sec. 6, chap. 33, p. 275.
12. Ibid. sec. 10, chap. 65, p. 447.
13. *Su Wen*, sec. 5, chap. 17, p. 98.
14. *Ling Shu*, sec. 6, chap. 30, p. 267.
15. One exception, in which the Blood Vessels are treated as an entity independent of the other Organs, is in the discussion of "meeting points" in the *Nan Jing*. Acupuncture point Lung 9 (*tai-yuan*), the Blood Vessels' "meeting point," is said to treat the Blood Vessels directly. *Nan Jing* [3], "Difficulty 45," p. 104.

THE SCIENTIFIC ENCOUNTER WITH EAST ASIAN MEDICINE: EFFICACY AND ADVERSE EVENTS

Until about 1955, both East Asian medicine and biomedicine shared similar explicit standards for determining the acceptability of a medical intervention: legitimacy was defined by beneficial outcome. While physicians in both traditions also spoke of medicine based on "proven" or "recognized" principles, and inevitably were influenced by cultural assumptions, acceptable therapy was ultimately expected to deliver relief if not cure.[1]

In the years after World War II, biomedicine underwent a dramatic shift. Major reforms were undertaken in medical research that sought to free therapeutic evaluations from human judgment based on clinical experience and impressions. Comparative experiments were rare before World War II. The first controlled clinical trial that allocated treatment arms by random assignment was performed in 1948; inferential statistics was gradually accepted as a surrogate for determinism in the 1950s; placebo controls were slowly incorporated in the 1950s and 1960s.[2] American and European regulatory agencies only mandated these methodological safeguards in the 1960s and 1970s.[3] The apparatus of the double-blind randomized controlled trial (RCT) gradually established itself as the "gold standard" for determining legitimate therapy.

A major shift had occurred. A medical intervention was now scientifically justifiable only if it was superior to a placebo: method became more important than outcome.[4] Superiority to placebo replaced ability to confirm health benefits as judgment criteria in medicine. Ideally, an acceptable treatment was now a *relative* outcome that could be isolated, disguised, and compared to the entire matrix of effects embodied in an identical healing ritual lacking this single ingredient.* Healing was no longer an *absolute* outcome that comprised multiple interactive dimensions. Biomedicine reconceptualized legitimate healing as "a cause and effect relationship between a specific agent or treatment and a specific biological result."[5] Therapeutics that imitated the laboratory and depended on an isolatable, precise, and single mechanism were privileged. For biomedicine, the masked RCT significantly realigned the power relationships between "art" and "science" in medicine, as it was itself a product of this transformation.[6]

Employing this new research agenda and methodology has been a challenge for conventional medicine. The commitment, resources, and skills needed for its implementation have been immense.[7] Unquestionably, valuable achievements have been made.[8]

In the West, East Asian medicine has recognized that acceptance (and possibly survival) may depend on how successfully it addresses these recently introduced biomedical standards of legitimacy. Whether as a defensive measure or because of genuine scientific commitment, a serious scientific inquiry has begun. The following discussion is an attempt to summarize these ongoing efforts. It also addresses the issue of adverse events, because, from a scientific perspective, the value of a therapy must include a comparison of its benefits with its risks.[9]

In general, this appendix looks at East Asian medicine from the critical conceptual apparatus one would usually expect from academic biomedicine. While the rest of *The Web That Has No Weaver* attempts to allow the inner world of Oriental medicine to become visible to the outside world, this appendix examines how science has begun to penetrate and quantify the inner Asian world. The appendix offers a Yang balance to the Yin unfolding portrayed elsewhere in the book.

---

*Theoretically, it was now possible for a "proven" drug to have a smaller effect size on a particular ailment than a "debunked" therapy (i.e., an intervention that equals its dummy control).

⊣ CLINICAL RESEARCH IN EAST ASIA

The modernization of East Asia has meant the universal adoption of bio-medicine as the foundation of health care systems. While traditional medicine has always played an important role, it has often had to defend its continued existence and compete for the allocation of limited resources.[10] Undoubtedly, the Western-style research mentioned in Chapter 1 has been a major factor in the scientific, cultural, political, and rhetorical struggles in Asian countries.[11]

Some of the methodological problems with research performed in China have also already been discussed in Chapter 1. The early research in East Asia lacked control groups. Later efforts adopted controls but still had serious flaws (see description below). In the West, a general skepticism has developed that the evidence produced in Asia lacks rigor and may be questionable. This suspicion has been partially confirmed by systematic reviews of controlled trials on acupuncture and other interventions performed in China, Japan, Hong Kong, and Taiwan, which show that trial results are uniformly favorable.[12] Such unlikely outcomes have reinforced already existing serious doubt on the reliability of scientific evidence performed in East Asia. Other studies demonstrate that even research performed in biomedicine in China does not meet Western standards.[13] (Recent indications point to an improvement in the situation.[14]) Because of such problems, this appendix will mostly be limited to reviewing the scientific evidence concerning East Asian medicine produced in the West.

⊣ CLINICAL RESEARCH ON ACUPUNCTURE IN THE WEST

Since the early 1970s, more than 500 randomized controlled trials (RCTs) have been performed on acupuncture in North America, Europe, Australia, and New Zealand.[15] While these trials cover a wide range of clinical concerns, the bulk address various pain conditions. Other especially well studied areas include emesis (nausea and vomiting), ophthalmology and otolaryngology, substance abuse, cerebrovascular illnesses, neurological problems, gynecological complaints, asthma, and gastrointestinal problems. (Most of these trials are listed at the end of this appendix.)

A National Institutes of Health's Consensus Development Panel on Acupuncture (November 1997) sifted through this mountain of evidence and reached the following conclusions:

> *There is clear evidence that needle acupuncture is efficacious for adult post-operative and chemotherapy nausea and vomiting and probably for the nausea of pregnancy. Much of the research is on various pain problems. There is evidence for efficacy for postoperative dental pain. There are reasonable studies (although sometimes only single studies) showing relief of pain with acupuncture on diverse pain conditions such as menstrual cramps, tennis elbow and fibromyalgia. This suggests that acupuncture may have a more general effect on pain. However, there are also studies that do not find efficacy for acupuncture in pain. . . . Although many other conditions have received some attention in the literature, and, in fact, the research suggests some potential areas for the use of acupuncture, the quality and quantity of the research evidence is not sufficient to provide firm evidence of efficacy at this time.*[16]

For such a prestigious panel to give a positive endorsement for the validity of acupuncture in at least some indications has meant a significant advance for acupuncture's acceptance in the scientific community. This nod also demonstrated that, in some situations, acupuncture can successfully negotiate the methodological hurdles of rigorous RCTs.

It is, however, possible to look at the evidence that the NIH Consensus Conference evaluated from another perspective. It could also be argued, as two leading acupuncture researchers have, that "disappointingly little has been achieved by literally hundreds of attempts to [scientifically] evaluate acupuncture."[17] It would seem that, with so much research, more clarity and conclusions should have been possible. What has been the problem?

Designing, implementing, and interpreting RCTs is never simple. As a group, acupuncture researchers in the West have not had the resources and/or skills to perform trials that the scientific community would consider relatively conclusive and convincing. The simple fact is that, while research in the West is much better than in Asia, it is still methodologically weak. Researchers may have underestimated the challenges necessary to overcome systematic error (bias) and random error (chance) with an intervention as complex as acupuncture. Some of the problems in acupuncture RCTs are the common short-comings that plague other RCTs in any research domain.[18] One of the most important of these shared problems has been that many (if not most) acupuncture trials have had too few participants enrolled; this creates the situation of insufficient statistical power to show a significant differential between the acupuncture and the controls when in fact a difference really exists.[19] (This is technically called a *beta*, or type II, error.) Also, the comparability of groups in trials with small numbers is not easily guaranteed, which again increases the likelihood of confounding results. Other common problems include difficulties with assumptions underlying statistics and statistical analyses such as choice of appropriate statistical procedure and hypothesis testing; choice of measurable endpoints versus clinically meaningful endpoints or patient-relevant endpoints; testing of poorly defined illnesses or vague enrollment criteria leading to heterogeneous study groups; high dropout rates; and inadequate follow-up. Any one of these problems could make the results of an RCT questionable and subject to inaccuracy.

Besides typical problems, many of the limitations with existing acupuncture RCTs have to do with unique acupuncture constraints that do not arise in drug trials.[20] For example, it is unclear whether the acupuncturist(s) in many RCTs have adequate training. (The training and qualifications of the acupuncturist are often not mentioned in reports of clinical trials.) For many trials, it is unclear what type of acupuncture was performed.[21] Frequently, there is an insufficient "dose" of acupuncture (not enough treatment given to the patient) for there to be reasonable expectation of success. There may have been occasions when what was considered the active intervention in RCTs was actually placebo control points.[22] Few trials attempt to take into consideration the conceptual models of East Asian medicine or stratify for distinct Oriental diagnoses that may not easily correspond to Western diagnosis.[23] Almost no trials attempted to measure for the relative suitability for acupuncture treatments from the Oriental perspective. The difficulty or impossibility of blinding the acupuncturist(s) and preventing their enthusiasm from being communicated is a serious handicap and may also contribute to inaccurate evidence.[24]

Finding a suitable placebo or sham control in an acupuncture RCT remains a serious obstacle in acupuncture research. Many researchers worry that needling at "non-acupuncture" is not analogous to a dummy inert pill as a placebo control. The concern is that needling anywhere in the body (at both real acupuncture sites or non-acupuncture sites) may have physiological effects. Aside from normal nonspecific placebo outcomes, random needling may have counter-irritation properties that initiate neurological processes or stimulate other physiological mechanisms (such as the release of neurotransmitters).[25] These responses can modulate pain and might produce effects beyond what are expected from an inert sham control. Especially in pain trials, using non-acupuncture needling sites as a control design may make the possibility of detecting a difference between treatment arms unusually difficult and lead to a type II error. This problem of finding a suitable and credible inert sham control in an acupuncture trial has actually generated an enormous debate in the research literature that is still not resolved.[26]

Review of Systematic Reviews of Acupuncture RCTs

The methodological problems of acupuncture RCTs outlined above made the deliberations of the NIH Consensus Panel difficult. Much of the potential evidence may have been confounded.[27] Caution was necessary and continues to be warranted in interpreting acupuncture RCTs. (In fact, one of the primary conclusions of the panel was that research needed to be performed on how best to conduct an acupuncture RCT.)

With this serious caveat, this section will summarize the seventeen peer-reviewed systematic reviews and meta-analyses of acupuncture RCTs currently available.[28] (A systematic review is an approach where each RCT is methodologically analyzed, evaluated, and often scored. A meta-analysis is a statistical approach which treats all subjects of comparable studies as members of a larger pool of subjects and then aggregates the results of these multiple trials into a single outcome.) It is hoped that this review of reviews will provide interested readers with a better sense of the state of the scientific evidence for the efficacy of acupuncture.

As mentioned earlier, pain is the most explored domain for the clinical efficacy of acupuncture. At least eight reviews concerning pain have been published. The earliest such acupuncture meta-analysis was performed by a team from the Institut Universitaire de Médecine Sociale et Préventive in Lausanne, Switzerland. They meta-analytically pooled fourteen randomized clinical trials of acupuncture for chronic pain and analyzed them in a variety of sub-groups (e.g., acupuncture for all pain, for low-back pain, for head/neck pain, larger clinical trials versus smaller trials, partially blind trials versus no blinding).[29] The researchers believed that methodological shortcomings pre-cluded conclusive results, but found that, overall, most results "apparently favored acupuncture." The subgroup of those six acupuncture trials that com-pared acupuncture with sham did not produce significant positive results for acupuncture.[30]

Subsequent to this meta-analysis, a team from the University of Limberg in the Netherlands published a more extensive review of fifty-one controlled clinical trials on the efficacy of acupuncture in chronic pain.[31] Their review was a "voting" meta-analysis (which simply counts positive and negative trials and does not aggregate outcomes across trials). They found twenty-four stud-ies had significant positive results and twenty-seven studies had negative out-comes. Because the results were "highly contradictory," their opinion was that acupuncture's efficacy remained "doubtful." Also, they found the quality of the studies deficient and urged that future studies have a larger number of patients, more homogeneous entry criteria, fewer dropouts, longer follow-up, and bet-ter outcome assessments.[32]

A systematic review from the University of Exeter of sixteen trials of acu-puncture for dental pain reached the same conclusion as the NIH Consensus Panel. Most of these trials used acupuncture in a clinical situation, e.g., as pain relief during dental operations, while five studies (predominantly the early ones) related to experimental setups where dental pain was induced to volunteers in a laboratory situation. While the authors could not aggregate across trials, they still concluded that "the vast majority of these investigations suggest that acupuncture is more effective than control treatments and only four trials imply the contrary."[33] Again the authors underscore that these findings are "cautious" and that many of the trials have significant method-ological flaws.

Another meta-analysis performed by a group also from Exeter focused on acupuncture for back pain. Twelve randomized trials were included in their study, of which nine presented data suitable for meta-analysis. By aggregating across studies, it was found that the overall evidence pointed to acupuncture as being effective for this condition. The authors noted that the trials included in their analysis "are heterogeneous in terms of study population, type of acupuncture used, outcome measure employed and length of follow-up. Thus it is problematic to form a firm judgment.[34] The difficulty in interpreting RCTs in acupuncture research is underscored by a later systematic review of basically the same trials for low-back pain performed by a team lead from the Free University of Amsterdam. Reviewing identical evidence, this team found that due to the poor quality of research, "there is no convincing scientific evidence to show that acupuncture is effective in the management of acute and chronic low-back pain."[35]

Neck pain was the subject of another systematic review of acupuncture from Exeter. Overall, the outcomes of fourteen RCTs were equally balanced between positive and negative.[36] Acupuncture was superior to waiting-list in one study, and either equal or superior to physiotherapy in three studies. Acupuncture was not superior to indistinguishable sham controls in four out of five studies. The study concluded that the hypothesis that acupuncture is efficacious in the treatment of neck pain is not based on evidence from RCTs.

Researchers from the University of Maryland examined acupuncture's efficacy in the treatment of fibromyaliga.[37] The study found only three RCTs. The single high-quality RCT suggested that real acupuncture is more effective than sham acupuncture. The authors called for further high-quality studies to provide more robust data on effectiveness.

Recurrent headaches was the subject of a systematic review by investigators from the Technische Universität in Munich, Germany. A total of twenty-two trials including a total of 1042 patients met the inclusion criteria. Fifteen trials were in migraine patients, six in tension headache patients, and in one trial, patients with various headaches were included. The majority of the fourteen trials comparing true and sham acupuncture showed at least a trend in favor of true acupuncture. The eight trials comparing acupuncture and other treatment forms had contradictory results. The team concluded that the existing evidence "suggests that acupuncture has a role in the treatment of recurrent headaches. However, the quality and amount of evidence is not fully convincing. There is urgent need for well-planned, large-scale studies to assess efffectiveness and efficacy of acupuncture under real life conditions."[38]

At least nine systematic reviews of acupuncture exist for non-pain conditions. As already mentioned, those for acupuncture in the treatment of nausea and vomiting have established the most positive scientific evidence to date on acupuncture's value. A researcher from the Research Council for Complementary Medicine in London found thirty-three controlled trials; of the twenty-nine trials performed on people awake and not under anesthesia, twenty-seven demonstrated acupuncture to be statistically superior to the control. A second analysis was restricted to twelve high-quality randomized placebo-controlled trials. Eleven of these trials, involving nearly 2,000 patients, showed acupuncture to be effective. The reviewed papers showed consistent results across different investigators, different groups of patients (e.g., adult postoperative and chemotherapy nausea and vomiting), and different forms of acupuncture-point stimulation (e.g., needles, electro-acupuncture, acupressure.) The author concluded that, except when administered under anesthesia, acupuncture "seems to be an effective antiemetic technique."[39] Peculiarly, the acupuncture performed in all these trials was a single point (Pericardium 6, *Nei Guan*), not the elaborate acupuncture discussed in this book. This may suggest that the methodology of the RCT can most easily detect efficacy when an acupuncture intervention is well-defined and discrete which may create a simple "drug-like" replicable model.

The three systematic reviews of acupuncture for asthma reached two different conclusions and again underscores the difficulty in interpreting acupuncture RCTs. The first review was performed by the same team from the University of Limberg mentioned earlier. They found thirteen trials, which were reviewed on the basis of eighteen predefined methodological criteria. They found "the results from the better studies [to be] highly contradictory" and that "claims that acupuncture is effective in the treatment of asthma are not based on the results of well-performed clinical trials."[40] A later review, from Oxford University, of sixteen trials for bronchial asthma, chronic bronchitis, and chronic disabling breathlessness reached a different conclusion. This review felt that the earlier review was confounded because in some trials what were considered to be inactive sham points were actually, according to traditional Chinese principles, active and real points. By retrospectively changing the definitions of "real" acupuncture to what was felt to be a more traditional criteria, the reviewer found that "the literature to date provides evidence that acupuncture treatment can be effective and safe."[41] However, an even later review from Ludwig-Maximilians-Universität, Munich, Germany, of fifteen trials agreed with the Limberg team and stated that "there is insufficient data to draw conclusions about the effectiveness of acupuncture treatment for asthma."[42]

The University of Limberg team also performed a meta-analysis on addiction. They found twenty-two studies and concluded that acupuncture was not helpful in relation to smoking and had an inconclusive profile in relation to heroin or alcohol.[43] A systematic review from the University of Exeter of four studies on acupuncture for weight reduction found a similar absence of convincing evidence.[44]

Two preliminary reviews have been performed on acupuncture in stroke recovery. A team from the University of Exeter reviewed six RCTs and found that "without exception, these trials suggest positive effects of acupuncture on functional recovery. . . . The evidence that acupuncture is a useful adjunct for stroke rehabilitation is encouraging but not compelling."[45] All trials compared acupuncture with other treatment or no additional treatment and the researchers felt that acupuncture's placebo effect was taken into account by any of the RCTs reviewed. Another more narrative review from Hythe Hospital in Southampton, United Kingdom, reviewed seven trials and concluded that "the studies done so far have opened up the field but have not been conclusive."[46]

Temporomandibular joint dysfunction (TMJD) was also the subject of a systematic review by Exeter researchers. Three trials met the inclusion criteria and "overall, their results suggested that acupuncture might be an effective therapy for TMJD. However, none of the studies was designed to control for a placebo effect."[47] The study called for more rigorous investigation.

Besides systematic reviews, as mentioned earlier, there exist a large number of clinical trials on other conditions treated by acupuncture. Unfortunately, because of their small study size, lack of replication, or because of other methodological shortcomings, none of these particular single trials is able to offer reasonable definitive evidence for acupuncture's efficacy. Some of the trials are nonetheless promising and provocative. Perhaps the most important conclusion one can draw from this entire body of evidence is to repeat the refrain from the NIH Consensus Panel and most of the reviews: More research of a higher caliber needs to be performed.

— BASIC SCIENCE SUPPORTIVE EVIDENCE

Despite the inconclusiveness of the bulk of the RCT evidence, at least the work in emesis and dental pain has created a general consensus that "something is going on" with acupuncture therapy in a scientific sense. This has allowed acupuncture to enjoy enormous credibility within the biomedical community.[48] But this positive consensus would not be possible without the parallel basic research investigations into acupuncture's possible mechanism. In fact, the RCTs may have been interpreted differently if this mechanistic work had not already been ongoing.[49] This work has significantly created the underlying plausibility that exists within the medical community towards acupuncture therapy (if not its philosophical theories). Chapter 4 note 11 has already reviewed this basic science evaluation. These investigations have demonstrated that acupuncture analgesia may be initiated by stimulation of high-threshold, small-diameter nerves in the muscles that send messages to the spinal cord and then activate three centers—spinal cord, brainstem (periaqueductal gray), and hypothalamic (arcuate) neurons—to stimulate endogenous opioid mechanisms. These responses include changes in plasma or corticospinal fluid levels of endogenous opioids such as endorphins and enkephalins or stress-related hormones such as ACTH.[50] Evidence also supports the notion that one of the mechanisms of acupuncture may involve stimulation for the gene expression of neuropeptides.[51] Functional Magnetic Resonance Imaging (fMRI) has also begun to show that stimulation of specific acupuncture points may have regionally specific, quantifiable effects on relevant structures of the human brain.[52] For a fuller discussion of this aspect of acupuncture's encounter with science, the reader should see Chapter 4, note 11.

ADVERSE EVENTS ASSOCIATED WITH ACUPUNCTURE

Classical East Asian sources including the *Nei Jing* were concerned with potential iatrogenic effects that could result from the improper use of acupuncture needles.[53] For the scientific evaluation of the value of acupuncture, benefits must be weighted against risks.

Numerous clinical reports have appeared in biomedical journals concerned with harmful outcomes associated with acupuncture needling. The reports of injuries are essentially what would be expected with the use of any needles. Most of the side effects reported have been transient and have included bleeding, hematoma, bruising, erythema, drowsiness, dermatitis, nausea, and fainting. A few large prospective systematic surveillance studies of acupuncture's adverse effects also exist. The chart below summarizes all eleven events and the incident rates from a large study of an acupuncture training facility in Japan.[54]

Reported Adverse Events Related to Acupuncture Treatment

REPORTED ADVERSE EVENTS	# OF CASES
forgotten needles	16
dizziness, discomfort or perspiration (transient hypotension)	13
burn injury (caused by thermotherapy, including moxibustion)	7
ecchymosis accompanied by pain	6
ecchymosis without pain	5
malaise	5
minor hemorrhage	3
aggravation of complaint	3
itching and/or redness (suspected contact dermatitis)	3
pain in the puncture region	2
fall from bed	1

November 1992 through October 1997. Total number of acupuncture treatments was 55,291. Reprinted with permission from H. Yamashita et. al. "Adverse Events Related to Acupuncture." *Journal of the American Medical Association*, 1998; 280: 1563–1564.

Besides minor problems, major complications have also been reported from acupuncture treatment. These have included transmission of infectious diseases, most commonly hepatitis B but also subacute bacterial endocarditis; tissue damage, including pneumothorax and other organ punctures, including cardiac tamponade; and broken needles with remnants migrating to other locations, including the spine. Some reviews believe as many as five incidents may have resulted in fatalities while others contest these allegations.[55]

Six major systematic reviews summarizing the totality of adverse events associated with acupuncture have been published in peer review journals. While every review has recognized that serious injuries have resulted from acupuncture, all agree that "considering the frequency with which the technique is applied, complications and adverse effects of acupuncture seem to be anecdotal and rare"[56] and "acupuncture can generally be considered a safe treatment."[57]

It is also important to note that the bulk of adverse events seem to result from acupuncturists with inadequate training. A large study of Australian acupuncturists demonstrated that an acupuncturist's adverse event rate was inversely proportional to the quality and length of training of the practitioner.[58] Another major review concluded that "knowledge of normal anatomy and anatomical variation [is] considered essential for safe practice and should be reviewed by regulatory bodies and those responsible for training courses."[59] Also, all the systematic reviews of acupuncture's adverse effects support the idea that "a system of self regulation across the [acupuncture] profession, firmly based on ethical principles," is sorely needed to prevent adverse effects,[60] as is the "maintenance of national standards of training and standard licensure."[61] None of the other five systematic summaries or the NIH panel found any evidence to disagree with the first review of acupuncture's safety, which stated that "the majority of [complications] can be avoided with cautious and prudent use. . . . [and] we conclude that acupuncture is a safe technique when administered in the correct way."[62] All the reviews also seemed to agree with the NIH Consensus Panel that "one of the advantages of acupuncture is that the incidence of adverse effects is substantially lower than that of many drugs or other accepted medical procedures used for the same conditions."[63]

⊣ SCIENTIFIC RESEARCH ON EAST ASIAN HERBAL MEDICINE

Oriental herbal medicine has also received much scientific attention. By far the largest investigation concerning East Asian herbal medicine has been a laboratory-centered effort related to drug discovery, isolation, and development. Besides scientific and medical interest, this effort has been propelled by commercial concerns and the inertia inherent in "standard" methods in the pharmaceutical industry. Academic institutions, pharmaceutical companies, and government organizations continue to subject the Oriental pharmacopia to the standard gamut of pharmacological studies. The chemical composition of most herbs has been determined; cell lines (such as various cancers) and isolated animal organs have been subjected to different extracts in multiple concentrations; the lethal dose upon which half of a cohort of animals die (LD-50) has been studied extensively; countless mice, guinea pigs, rats, pigs, cats, rabbits, and dogs, in pieces or whole, healthy and intentionally made sick, awake or under anesthesia, have had physiological functions and organ activities challenged by oral, intravenous, intra-arterial, or intraventricular injections of herbal concentrates; and a wide assortment of bacteria, viruses, fungi, and parasites have been bombarded with countless herbal preparations.[64] Serious pharmacokinetic studies (which deal with the effects of the body on the herbs) have begun to supplement these more traditional pharmacodynamic studies.[65] This effort has been mentioned in Chapter 1 and seeks to translate Chinese experience into the standard scientific and commercial methods of biomedicine. This effort has clearly documented that the *materia medica* has potent pharmacological activity; unfortunately, and not unusual for the effort, only a few potential drugs have made it through the drug development process.[66]

For a pharmacologist, the presence of such physiological activity in herbal material is not surprising. But, whatever the outcome of such studies, laboratory investigations ultimately tell us little about the effectiveness (or lack of effectiveness) of Chinese medicinals on human beings. First, pharmacological activity on cell lines or animals does not necessarily translate into clinical effectiveness in humans. Second, these approaches tend to be based on a reductionist drug development models of assessment that overlooks the actual practice of East Asian herbal medicine. For any ultimate judgment on Oriental herbalism's efficacy, RCTs on human participants using traditional methods of delivery must provide the decisive scientific evidence.

— RANDOMIZED CONTROLLED TRIALS ON EAST ASIAN HERBAL MEDICINE

Clinical research on Chinese herbs in the West is in its infancy.[67] There have been only a handful of rigorously performed double-blind RCTs of Chinese herbal therapy. The first important such trial was for recalcitrant adult atopic dermatitis. Performed in London, it used a crossover design whereby patients are alternatively switched to either true herbs or dummy treatment.[68] The herbs were a standardized formula and not individually tailored for each patient. Of the thirty-one patients who completed the study, there was a highly significant objective improvement in erythema and surface damage scars as well as itching and sleep during the Chinese herbal treatment phase. The placebo was a decoction of equally bad-tasting and -smelling herbs that were thought to have no effect on the skin. This trial was preceded by an earlier RCT on forty-seven children with non-exudative atopic eczema, which had equally impressive results.[69]

The most sophisticated study, so far, that managed to fully adhere to traditional Chinese diagnostic and treatment processes while using a strict and accepted double-blind Western methodological protocol took place in Sydney.[70] A total of 116 patients with irritable bowel syndrome were randomly allocated to one of three arms: a placebo treatment, a standardized Chinese herbal formulation, and an individualized herbal prescription that was regularly adjusted by a traditional Chinese herbalist. The standard formula contained twenty ingredients; the tailored prescriptions consisted of herbs chosen from a total of eighty-one herbs to match the unique pattern of disharmony of each patient. To enforce concealment, besides having a placebo designed to taste, smell, and look similar to the herbal formulas, all patients, after consulting a Chinese herbalist who was ignorant as to whether they were to receive real or dummy treatment, were required to complete a series of questionnaires and wait thirty minutes for the preparation of their herbs. The wait time was used to avoid patients identifying whether they were receiving standard, placebo, or customized formulations that take time to prepare. Compared with the placebo group, patients in the active treatment groups had significant improvement on all outcome measures. Standardized and individualized formulations were equally effective at the end of the sixteen-week treatment phase. At the fourteen-week followup, only those patients treated with individualized herbs maintained improvement.

A large double-blind RCT to test Chinese herbs was performed on a standardized Chinese herbal extract for males with alopecia androgenetica in Holland. Three hundred ninety-six males were randomly assigned to one of two groups for six months; the active preparation group had a modest but statistically significant improvement based on hair counts and blind reviews of photo-report.[71]

Several other trials have been published by Western researchers, another Australian pilot study randomly allocated forty-four patients with chronic hepatitis C to either placebo or a standardized Chinese herbal formula of nineteen ingredients.[72] Active Chinese herbal medication was associated with a significant reduction in alanine aminotransferase (ALT) levels over the six-month study period. No patient cleared the virus, but four normalized their ALT on treatment. No patients in this pilot study were cured and one experienced a lasting normalization of LFT on cessation of the herbs.

A Danish team gave 100 elderly volunteers a fixed Chinese herbal formula that was designed to help deteriorating memory. No desirable effect on memory functions was achieved by the active treatment group.[73] A San Francisco group performed a pilot twelve-week study on thirty adults with symptomatic HIV infection to see whether using a standardized Chinese herbal formula for twelve weeks could improve general life satisfaction, perceived health, and severity of symptoms.[74] No differences between the herbal group or placebo were detected.

The effects of Chinese herbal medicines in acute respiratory infections and the health promoting effects of ginseng have been investigated in multiple RCTs. At least two systematic reviews have been performed. A team from the Australian National University found twenty-seven studies of Chinese herbs in the management of acute respiratory infections. (The study included mostly trials performed in Asia.) The authors concluded that the "trial methodology of these studies was often inadequate or insufficiently documented. . . . More rigourous evaluation is needed."[75]

Ginseng used as single herb (one of the very few Chinese herbs to sometimes be used alone) has probably received the most attention in clinical trials. A systematic analysis performed at the University of Limberg found twenty-one double-blind RCTs (mostly performed in Germany, Italy, and Switzerland) and reported that "among elderly people who suffer from fatigue, about 75 percent appear to benefit from ginseng, of which 50 percent is a ginseng effect and 25 percent a placebo effect. Moreover, certain psychological tests give better results."[76] These trials are very small, tend to use self-report psychometric measures, and seem to decide the main outcomes retrospectively. Illustrative of these ginseng trials is one performed in Italy where sixteen healthy volunteers were given ginseng and another group of sixteen subjects given identical placebo capsules under randomized double-blind conditions.[77] Ginseng subjects performed better on certain psychomotor function tests (e.g., mental arithmetic). This study was similar in design to a study of twelve duty nurses in London in a double-blind crossover study comparing the effects of ginseng or placebo on competence, mood, and performance.[78] More recent trials have been larger. An Oslo team assigned sixty geriatric patients to either a ginseng vitamin capsule or placebo. After eight weeks, there was no difference between either group in various functional outcomes measures.[79] In Mexico City, a large double-blind clinical trial compared a multivitamin complex supplemented with ginseng versus a multivitamin complex without ginseng in 625 patients complaining of stress or fatigue.[80] The ginseng group had significant improvement in some measures, including quality of life index after 4 months.[81]

⊣ EAST ASIAN HERBS AND ADVERSE EVENTS

Safety has been the main focus of the biomedical literature's discussion of Chinese herbs. A serious perception has developed in the biomedical literature that herbs, especially those from East Asia, pose significant risks to patients.[82]

This recognition of the potential harm involved with herbal medicine is not new or confined to the West. In fact, the classic texts of East Asia have always understood the potential toxic effects of herbs. China's earliest *materia medica*, the *Shen-nong Ben Cao Jing* (Pharmacopoeia Classic of the Divine Husbandman, c. 150 B.C.E.) says that 125 of its herbs "have poison" (*you du*) and should not be taken over a long period of time; and another 120 of its herbs also have poison and must be used "carefully." Out of the 365 herbs it describes, only 120 are said to be "without poison" (*wu du*) and can be taken safely for a long period of time.[83] Tao Hong-jing (456–636 B.C.E.), the earliest commentator on the Divine Husbandman (in his *Shen-nong Ben Cao Jing Ji-Zhu*, Annotations to the Phamacopoeia Classic of the Divine Husbandman), describes the fact that herbs can "cause suffering."[84] All major historical and modern Chinese *materia medica* have extensively discussed toxicity and methods to avoid it.

The East Asian tradition has always understood that any pharmacodynamic substance implies possible toxicity. Unfortunately, this Oriental concern for potential danger has, until very recently, had a tendency to be buried or overlooked in the public/popular discussion of Chinese herbal medicine. This avoidance is undoubtedly partly related to the polemical tug-of-war that has dominated the conflict between Oriental and biomedicine in Asia and unconventional and conventional medicine in the West. In the rhetoric between the two camps, East Asian and unconventional medicine practitioners have tended to emphasize the potential and genuine dangers of biomedicine and emphasize their own purported safety. Modern Asian and Western alternative medicine have often come to defensively believe, at least in their popular utterances, that nature is uniformly innocent, wholesome, and benevolent.[85] It seems that the traditional notion of nature and such forces as Wind, Damp, and Cold as embodying multivalent and complex potential dynamics has been lost. A false expectation has arisen that no injury is possible from "natural" herbs, which has until recently allowed the Oriental medical profession to neglect its historic responsibility to critically evaluate its work.[86] In the absence of clear self-regulation mechanisms and surveillance systems, it has been biomedical and scientific vigilance that has alerted the East Asian medical community of its professional responsibility to monitor and protect the public from potential iatrogenic damage.[87] The discussion below summarizes the main categories of adverse events that have been discussed in the scientific literature.

Direct Toxic Effects

A very few Chinese herbs are dangerously toxic; their toxicity is an extension of the therapeutic effects. These adverse effects are pharmacologically predictable. Professionally trained herbalists are aware of this toxicity and understand that the use of these herbs is only possible in a *very* narrow therapeutic window. Most such herbs are very rarely used; in fact, most practitioners would understand that such herbs have become a historical curiosity for situations not applicable in societies where surgery and precise pharmacological methods are available and safer. Herbs such as *Datura metel* (*yan jin hua*) and *Rhodendenri mollis* (*nao yang hua*) contain scopolamine, hypscamine, and atropine and have understandably been mentioned as causing adverse effects in Hong Kong.[88] So has cinnabar (*Cinnabaris*), which contains mercuric sulfide.[89] This author has never used such herbs and never includes them in his herbal teaching except as historical artifacts, no longer relevant to actual clinical practice. Such herbs are also not generally available in the West.

A more important problem has been *Aconitum kusenzoffi* (*cao wu*) and *Aconitum carmichael* (*chuan wu*). These herbs contain highly toxic alkaloids, including aconitine, which have created serious side effects.[90] The accessory root of aconite (*Radix Laterals Aconiti Carmichaeli Praeparate*) is more commonly used in Chinese medicine, is less toxic than the main root, and is always further processed to reduce toxicity.[91] And while it is often unclear which form of aconite is being referred to, there seems to have been reports of adverse events from the milder form of aconite also.[92] Most (if not all) of the reports of toxicity have resulted from East Asian patients self-medicating without proper professional guidance.

Toxicity Due to Dosage Extension

Some herbs in the East Asian *materia medica* have toxicity that is a consequence of an extension of their therapeutic dosage. For example, *Pruni Armeniacae* (bitter almond, *xing ren*) has amygdalin and amygdalase, which combine in the digestive tract to produce prusnasis and mandelonitrile, which are further broken down to benzaldehyde and hyrocyanic acid, the latter of which is highly toxic. In low therapeutic dosage, the herb is a cough suppressant, but in very excessive dosages the effect can be very dangerous. *Perillaei Frutescen-*

tis (*su ye*), a common ingredient of Japanese cooking, is another example of this problem. The perilla ketone, derived from its essential oil, in one dosage is valuable for cough but in another can have serious adverse effects.[93] When dosages are kept within therapeutic range, such dangers are not expected.

Licorice root (*Glycyrrhiza glabra*) is routinely used in Chinese herbal medicine in small doses. It contains glycyrrhizic acid and glycyrrhitic acid, which have mineralocorticoid-like actions. Reports of inappropriate usage of this herb (especially when taken in large quantities) with subsequent adverse effects have been reported in the biomedical literature in both the context of Chinese herbalism and Western herbalism.[94] Many other herbs can become toxic if they are used in incorrect quantities.

Idiosyncratic Toxicity Besides predictable adverse effects, Chinese herbal medicines have been associated with rare reactions that could be considered idiosyncratic allergy or hypersensitivity reactions.[95] Even in safe doses with very benign herbs, it s possible to see unexpected developments. A totally safe medicine, just like perfectly safe food, can become dangerous for unusually responsive individuals.[96]

There have been associational reports of adverse effects from ginseng (*Panax ginseng*), which suggest an estrogen-like effect and a danger with hypertension.[97] There is also one very poorly performed uncontrolled observational study that reported a "ginseng abuse syndrome" with a myriad of positive and negative effects that has affected the biomedical discussion.[98] In rare cases, ginseng seems to be able to cause estrogenic effects, even though it does not actually contain phytoestrogens.[99]

Several other problems have been noted in the literature. A number of cases of allergic contact dermatitis have been reported from topically applied Chinese herbs.[100] Also there are reports of Chinese herbs being taken with the intention of producing adverse side effects (such as deliberate self-poisoning)[101] or to produce peculiar forms of excitement and recreation such as the incidents of *Ephedra sinica* (*ma huang*) poisoning in teenagers.[102]

Hepatotoxic Effects Pharmacological active drugs are first metabolized in the liver. Thus, liver damage is not an altogether unexpected consequence of the use of some medications. Predictably, this problem has been a major finding.

Perhaps, the most well-known incident of liver toxicity is related to the very impressive clinical trial on skin disease described above. In the follow-up study, two children whose eczema was so well controlled that the therapy was stopped, developed elevated liver enzymes (serum asparatate aminotransferase to 7–10 times normal values).[103] The damage was reversible and liver function tests returned to normal after 8 weeks of cessation of therapy. Subsequently, several patients who received Chinese herbs for skin disease in nonexperimental clinical situations have reported hepatatis (though the effects of prior use of such drugs as cyclosporin and azathiprine could not be ruled out).[104] Upwards of two dozen other cases have been reported.[105] Most Oriental practitioners have been alerted to the potential danger and concrete steps have been taken to avoid a reoccurrence.[106]

Another troubling report has come from the Hospital for Traditional Chinese Medicine in southeast Germany near Munich, in which 1507 consecutive patients treated with traditional Chinese herbs had liver enzymes measured at admission and during the last 3 days before discharge. A more than two-fold elevation of alanine aminotransferase (ALT) was observed in fourteen (0.9 percent) of the patients. Two of the fourteen patients had temporary clinical symptoms (nausea or itching). A causal relationship between the herbs and enzyme elevation seemed possible although all patients were also on previously prescribed drugs (e.g. minocycline, mesalazine, and diclofenac) before their admission and all during their hospital stay. Such medications can also cause liver damage. ALT returned to normal within eight weeks of discharge. The authors of this study suggested that liver functions should be monitored in patients using Chinese herbs.[107] Again such reports have alerted the Oriental medical profession that herbs have the ability to both benefit and harm and that extreme vigilance is necessary to reduce adverse effects.[108]

Herbs Adulterated with Western Drugs and Camouflaged Drugs

Chinese herbal manufacturers in Hong Kong, until recently, were not regulated and it is unclear whether the regulations in the People's Republic of China and other parts of East Asia are adequately enforced.[109] This has allowed fraudulent and unscrupulous manufacturers to adulterate their products with Western drugs, causing great concern in the biomedical literature (as well as the East Asian practitioner community). A survey of 260 Asia-manufactured patent medicines collected from California retail herbal stores found seventeen (7 percent) that contained undeclared pharmaceuticals including ephedrine, chlorpheniramine, methyltestosterone, and phenacetin.[110] This survey confirmed numerous earlier studies that found such drugs as diazepam, phenylbutazone, prednisolone, and hydrocortisone hidden in other Chinese pills.[111] Occasionally, a plant-derived pharmaceutical has been identified as an "herbal product" to take advantage of popular beliefs that *herbal* means harmless.[112] No incidents of adulteration or camouflaged drugs have been reported by Chinese herbal products manufactured in the West.

Contamination with Heavy Metals and Poor Manufacturing Practices

Again, the problem arises with herbal products manufactured in Asia. Products manufactured in developing countries lack the standards and quality control expected for medical substances in the West. Even for Western pharmaceutical drugs, only 20 percent of Chinese-manufactured medicines meet the Food and Drug Administration (FDA) standards for quality control.[113] Reports in the biomedical literature concerning the quality of Chinese herbal products reflect this predicament. Various types of heavy-metal contamination including lead, arsenic, mercury, cadmium, and thallium have caused serious problems.[114] Only one published report, printed in the Oriental medical literature, has found contamination due to microorganisms, or pesticides.[115]

Interaction with Western Drugs

Little reliable information is available concerning Chinese herbs and biomedicine interactions. Clearly it is possible for herbs to affect the pharmacodynamic and pharmokinetic effects of Western drugs. Even common foods have this potential.[116]

The most serious incident of a Chinese herbal iatrogenic effect reported in the biomedical literature first seemed to be due to an interaction between herbs and drugs in a combined drug/herbal product once used in a weight reduction clinic in Belgium. This mixture was prescribed by Western physicians with no training in Chinese medicine. At least 100 women developed interstitial renal fibrosis with terminal or preterminal renal failure.[117] The epidemiology of this tragic incident is still unclear and confusing. One possibility is that a Western drug in the slimming pill cocktail may have made the urine alkaline and increased the half-life of aristocholoic acid (found in *Aristolochiae Fangchi, guang fang ji*), and increased the slight toxicity that already existed in the herb and drug individually. Another analysis notes the different outcomes between the two practitioners at the single clinic and points a finger at what was called a "homemade" solution of a serotonin derivative or a serotonin enhancer.[118] This report believed that only the interaction between these serotonin-type drugs and the oral dexfenfluramine prescribed can explain the nature of the lesions and their very high incidence in such a limited population. Further complicating the picture, a subsequent report of serious nephropathy associated with Chinese herbs containing aristolochic acids (identification of the exact herb is confusing) raises the distinct possibility that this tragic event should be classified as a toxicity incident and not a herb-drug interaction.[119]

Other incidents of Chinese herbs interacting with drugs and enhancing or reducing the pharmacological effects of either component have also been reported. Several cases of *Salvia miltiorrhize* (danshen) interacting with warfarin and causing profound anticoagulation has been observed.[120] While the exact mechanism of the salvia-warfarin interaction has not yet been elucidated, it is not totally surprising given the herb's properties of improving microcirculation, causing coronary vasodilation and inhibiting platelet adhesion and aggregation.[121] The important Chinese herb *Angelica sinensis* (dong gui), which contains natural coumarin derivatives, has also been reported to interact with warfarin.[122] Ginseng has also been reported to interact with various drugs but these reports are especially difficult to interpret.[123] Given that future incidents of herb-drug interaction are inevitable, a system of herbal vigilance with the active cooperation of East Asian practitioners, other complementary practitioners, biomedical physicians, toxicologists, and government regulatory bodies is clearly needed. Practitioners of East Asian medicine are increasingly aware that only an understanding of the traditional use of herbs is not enough. Practitioners need to anticipate that herbs can interact with potent pharmaceuticals and that Chinese herbalism can never be viewed in isolation.

Cross-Cultural Differences

One potential danger for Chinese herbal medicine's transmission to the West is the fact that, although the herbs have been used for thousands of years in Asia, there may exist cross-cultural differences (due to genetic makeup, dietary habits, or environmental conditions) that could modify their effects in Western patients. This has been shown to be possible with some important Western pharmaceuticals when used in Asian patients.[124] No publication has appeared reporting such a problem with herbs, but systematic observations of herbal Chinese practices in the West have raised this possibility.[125]

Are East Asian Herbs Safe?

It is clear that Chinese herbs, especially when improperly or poorly manufactured, can be harmful. How dangerous are they? Are they relatively safe? Obviously an answer to such a question is complex. First, it should be said that safety is a judgment; one-hundred percent safety never exists. Safety is always relative because the chances are that absolutely no foreign substance in some dosage can be introduced into the human body without producing some harm in at least some individuals. For scientific medicine, safety is a judgment given after weighing benefits against risks. From this scientific perspective, the balance is not favorable for Chinese herbal medicine. Chinese herbs have not demonstrated sufficient reproducible efficacy in RCTs, and herbs (however incorrectly used) have definitely been shown in the biomedical literature to be associated with adverse effects. Therefore, the biomedical literature has serious concerns with the safety of Chinese herbs. There is a perception of risk that tends to accept the hazards of routine care (drugs, surgery, diagnostic devices) but becomes extremely fearful and concerned with the dangers of Chinese herbs.

Within scientific circles, the index of suspicion towards Chinese herbs is high. This perception of risk can be as influential as any complex mathematical algorithm for determining benefit/risk. For example, people tend to be more concerned with their safety in airplanes than in automobiles, although the risk of being killed in a motor vehicle accident is twice that of an air crash.[126]

From the East Asian perspective, the counter argument is that, when used by properly trained practitioners who use herbs and products from reputable distributors who guarantee quality, the herbs are relatively safe and the benefits have been reasonably documented in a long historical tradition. Additionally, they argue that the Chinese herbs produce less harm than conventional medicine. (See note 108.)

There seem to be only pieces of direct evidence on the relative risks of Chinese herb treatment as compared to biomedical treatment in the scientific literature. In 1992, a team of scientists prospectively studied all 1,701 patients admitted to two general medical wards at the Prince of Wales Hospital in Hong Kong over an eight-month period. Three patients (0.2 percent) were admitted for reactions to Chinese herbs (allergy to dates [*Ziziphus jujuba, da zao*] and licorice and a third case of undetermined origin) while seventy-four patients (4.4 percent) were admitted because of adverse reactions to Western drugs.[127] This data looks favorable for Chinese herbs, but the study lacked information on the comparative usage of herbs to drugs, which makes the comparison difficult to interpret. Probably the debate concerning safety will not be settled for some time.[128]

—| CONCLUSION

A serious effort to investigate the efficacy of acupuncture has begun in the West. Some of the results have been positive. Adverse events due to acupuncture have been described, but the consensus is that acupuncture is relatively safe. High professional standards can ensure safety.

The laboratory investigation of Oriental herbal medicine has been extensive. The clinical investigation of herbal medicine is beginning. The medical literature has produced evidence of significant adverse events associated with Chinese herbal medicine. It is likely that Western consumers will not tolerate such iatrogenic possibilities. East Asian herbalists need to rely on reputable suppliers and inquire about their quality-control measures to prevent fraudulent substitution, adulteration, and contamination. Herbal training needs to be cognizant of potential dangers, including possible herb-drug interactions. Cooperation between Western and Eastern practitioners must be established to ensure that drug surveillance systems attentively monitor herbal medicine safety.

In the most general terms, it seems that the Western quantitative, "no-nonsense," "Yang" assessment of East Asian medicine has contributed to East Asian medicine's acceptance in the West. Besides this legitimacy, the contrasting style of scientific inquiry has contributed to Chinese medicine's own self-awareness, self-identity, and internal reflections. Both sides of East-West dialectic undoubtedly have more to learn from one another. This cooperation needs to expand. Rhetorical debates and conflict over "market shares" and medical resources need to be avoided. Mutual respect, careful attention to the concerns of the other side, and deep patience needs to underscore all collaboration. Undoubtedly, finding joint agendas will provide both the Eastern and Western approaches opportunities to grow and, most importantly, better serve the needs of patients.

NOTES

1. The explicit notion that medicine was acceptable because of positive outcomes was significantly supplemented by the often-unacknowledged process whereby legitimate therapy was determined by prestige, cultural associations, and sociopolitical power relationships. For example, biomedicine was adopted by Asian and African countries most often not because of medical outcomes but because of the prestige associated with the other developments of science. James Nelson Riley provides many examples where "the efficacious therapeutic techniques that Western medicine has gathered from modern science have come much more recently than the zeal for promoting science within medicine and for exporting somewhat scientific medicine to other cultures. . . . An ideological commitment to science antedates pragmatic benefits from science." "Western Medicine's Attempt to Become More Scientific: Examples from the United States and Thailand," *Social Science and Medicine* 1977; 11: 549–560, pp. 551, 557. For a discussion on how "efficacy" can be seen as a linguistic tool to control medical knowledge, see Elizabeth Hsu, "The Polyglot Practitioner: Towards Acceptance of Different Approaches in Treatment Evaluation." In Erling Hog and Sorew Olesew (eds.), *Studies in Alternative Therapy*, 3, Odense: Odense University Press, 1996. For a discussion on how prestige and authority influence acceptance of therapeutics within

biomedicine, see Samuel Hellman, "Dogma and Inquisition in Medicine," *Cancer* 1993; 71: 2430–2433. For a discussion on how such issues pertain to the Chinese encounter with Western medicine, see Theron Kue-Hing Young, "A Conflict of Professions: The Medical Missionary in China, 1835–1890," *Bulletin of the History of Medicine*, 1973: 47: 250–272; AnElissa Lucas, *Chinese Medical Modernization: Comparative Policy Continuities, 1930s–1980s*, (New York: Praeger, 1982); Bridie Andrews, *The Making of Modern Chinese Medicine, 1895–1937.* The importance of public health (as opposed to therapeutics) in influencing the wholesale adoption of biomedicine in China should also be noted. For example, see Carol Benedict, *Bubonic Plague in Nineteenth-Century China* (Stanford: Stanford University Press, 1996).

2. For a discussion on the history of the double-blind randomized controlled trial, see Ted J. Kaptchuk, "Intentional Ignorance: A History of Blind Assessment and Placebo Controls in Medicine," *Bulletin of the History of Medicine* 1998, 72: 389–433; Abraham M. Lilienfeld, "*Ceteris Paribus:* The Evolution of the Clinical Trial," *Bulletin of the History of Medicine* 1982; 56: 1–18; Harry M. Marks, *The Progress of Experiment* (Cambridge: Cambridge University Press, 1997).

3. For a history of regulatory requirements concerning therapeutics, see Richard A. Merrill, "Regulation of Drugs and Devices: An Evolution," *Health Affairs* 1994; 47–69; Peter Temin, *Taking Your Medicine: Drug Regulation in the United States* (Cambridge: Harvard University Press, 1980); James Harvey Young, "Federal Drug and Narcotic Legislation," *Pharmacy in History* 1995; 37: 59–67.

4. For a discussion of the philosophic implications of making method more important than outcome, see Mark D. Sullivan, "Placebo Controls and Epistemic Control in Orthodox Medicine," *Journal of Medicine and Philosophy* 1993; 18: 213–231. This shift from emphasizing oucomes to the purity of the means, directly parallels developments in modern bioethics and the movement away from "beneficience" centered ethics to an "informed consent" ethics focused on the method of performing medicine. For a discussion of the scientific, historical, ethical, and rhetorical implications created by post–World War II methodological innovations, see Ted J. Kaptchuk, "Powerful Placebo: The Dark Side of the Randomised Controlled Trial," *Lancet* 1998; 351: 1722–1725.

5. M. M. Lyon, "Order and Healing: the Concept of Order and Its Importance in the Conceptualization of Healing," *Medical Anthropology* 1990; 12: 249–268, p. 257. For a more complex discussion on the competition within biomedicine between ontological concepts of disease versus a concept of physiological aberration (which see disease as a continuum of quantifiable functions between the normal and pathological), see Alfred I. Tauber, "Darwinian Aftershocks: Repercussions in Late Twentieth Century Medicine," *Journal of the Royal Society of Medicine* 1994; 87: 27–31, and Georges Canguilhem, *Ideology and Rationality in the History of the Life Sciences* (Cambridge: MIT Press, 1988).

6. For a discussion of the relationship of tension between art and science in modern clinical biomedicine, see David Armstrong, "Clinical Sense and Clinical Science," *Social Science and Medicine* 1977; 11: 599–601.

7. For a discussion of the expansion of resources required for the implementation of more rigorous research in medicine, see Donald C. Swain, "The Rise of a Research Empire: NIH, 1930 to 1950," *Science* 1962: 1233–1237; George Rosen, "Patterns of Health Research in the United States, 1900–1960," *Bulletin of the History of Medicine* 1965; 39: 201–221; Peter Temin, *Taking Your Medicine: Drug Regulation in the United States* (Cambridge: Harvard University Press, 1980); Russell F. Doolittle, "Biotechnology—The Enormous Cost of Success," *New England Journal of Medicine* 1991; 324: 1360–1361.

8. For a discussion on the medical significance of the introduction of the RCT into biomedicine, see Alejandro R. Jadad and Drummond Rennie, "The Randomized Controlled Trial Gets a Middle-Aged Checkup," *Journal of the American Medical Association* 1998; 279: 319–320; David P. Byar et al., "Randomized Clinical Trials," *New England Journal of Medicine* 1976; 295: 74–80; David A. Grimes, "Techology Follies: The Uncritical Acceptance of Medical Innovation," *Journal of the American Medical Association* 1993; 269: 3030–3033.

9. Evaluating a benefit/risk ratio is a complex and often imprecise process. See, for example, S. Eriksen and L. R. Keller, "A Multiattribute-Utility-Function Approach to Weighing the Risks and Benefits of Pharmaceutical Agents," *Medical Decision Making* 1993; 13: 118–125.

10. The question of competition between biomedicine and traditional medicine in China is discussed in Paul U. Unschuld, "Medico-Cultural Conflicts in Asian Settings: An Explanatory Theory," *Social Science and Medicine* 1975; 9: 303–312; and Paul U. Unschuld, "Western Medicine and Traditional Healing Systems: Competition, Cooperation or Integration?" *Ethics in Science and Medicine* 1976; 3: 1–20. For a discussion of this issue in Korea, see Soon Young Yoon, "A Legacy Without Heirs: Korean Indigenous Medicine and Primary Health Care," *Social Science and Medicine* 1993; 17: 1467–1576; for a discussion on Japan, see Margaret Lock, "Rationalization of Japanese Herbal Medication: The Hegemony of Orchestrated Pluralism," *Human Organization* 1990; 49: 41–47.

11. For a discussion on how the RCT era fits into the long-term history of East Asian medicine, see Ted J. Kaptchuk, "Acupuncture: History, Context and Long-Term Perspectives," NIH *Consensus Development Conference on Acupuncture* (Bethesda, MD: NIH, 1997), pp. 25–30.

12. See Andrew Vickers, Niraj Goyal, Robert Harland, and Rebecca Rees, "Do Certain Countries Produce Only Positive Results? A Systematic Review of Controlled Trials," *Controlled Clinical Trials* 1998; 19: 159–166. This systematic review sought to determine whether clinical trials originating in certain countries always produce positive results. Two separate studies were conducted. The first included trials

(with English-language reports) in which the clinical outcomes of a group of subjects given acupuncture were compared to those of a group receiving placebo, no treatment, or a non-acupuncture treatment. All acupuncture trials originating in China, Japan, Hong Kong, and Taiwan were positive. The second study looked at interventions other than acupuncture. Positive results were reported in 99 percent, 89 percent, and 95 percent of the studies performed in China, Japan, and Taiwan, respectively. No trial published in China found a test treatment to be ineffective. Vickers and colleagues blamed "publication bias," which has to do with the fact that it is more likely that positive trials are published or even submitted. This is undoubtedly true, but additional cultural reasons (e.g., the Asian emphasis on "face" versus "guilt") and historical reasons (e.g., the RCT is an Anglo-American invention and has more cultural acceptance in the West) may also contribute to the predicament. It is also possible that some of these results reflect the interaction of modern science with the persistance of Confucian expectations about the nature and use of knowledge. See Peter Buck, "Order and Control: The Scientific Method in China and the United States," *Social Studies of Science* 1975; 5: 237–267.

Other reviews of randomized controlled trials from China concerning traditional Chinese medicine have pointed to a host of methodological shortcomings which may have also caused some of the puculiar results noted in the Vicker's study. One review summarizing RCTs performed in China before 1997 found such problems as lack of description of randomization, use of blinding in only 15 percent of trials, small sample sizes, short term follow-up, and the absense of intention-to-treat analysis in the statistical analysis. J. L. Tang, S. Y. Zhang and E. Ernst, "Review of Randomised Controlled Trials of Traditional Chinese Medicine," *British Medical Journal* 1999; 319: 160–161. Other imortant reviews of Chinese clinical research include Z. Xie and N. Li, "Methodological Analysis of Clinical Articles on Therapy Evaluation Published in *Chinese Journal of Integrated Traditional and Western Medicine* (in Chinese) 1982–1994," *Chinese Journal of Integrated Traditional and Western Medicine* [English] 1995; 1: 301–206 and G. P. Yu and S. W. Gao, "Quality of Clinical Trials of Chinese Herbal Drugs: A Review of 314 Published Papers," *Chinese Journal of Integrated Traditional and Western Medicine* [*Zhong-guo Zhong-xi-yi Jie-he Za-zhi*] 1994; 14: 50–52.

13. A recent review of Chinese biomedical research found significant shortcomings in methodology. See Qian Wang and Boheng Zhang, "Research Design and Statistical Methods in Chinese Medical Journals," *Journal of the American Medical Association* 1998; 280: 283–285.

14. Ibid. This article notes that, since 1985, there has been significant improvement in the quality of biomedical research in China.

15. The Cochrane Collaboration has 554 RCTs on acupuncture in its registry. A. J. Vickers, "Bibliometric Analysis of Randomized Trials in Complementary Medi-

cine," *Complementary Therapies in Medicine* 1998; 6: 185–189. Also, see National Library of Medicine, *Current Bibliographies in Medicine: Acupuncture* (Bethesda, MD: US DHHS PHS NIH, NCM, 1997). The bulk of acupuncture RCTs are cited at the end of this appendix.

16. National Institutes of Health Consensus Development Panel on Acupuncture. "Acupuncture," *Journal of the American Medical Association* 1998; 280: 1518–1524; p. 1519. The panel also stated that "there are other situations, such as addiction, stroke rehabilitation, headache, menstrual cramps, tennis elbow, fibromyalgia, myofascial pain, osteoarthritis, low-back pain, carpal tunnel syndrome, and asthma, in which acupuncture may be useful as an adjunct treatment or an acceptable alternative or be included in a comprehensive management program." Ibid. p. 1518. For a discussion of NIH consensus statements, see Robert M. Veatch, "Consensus of Expertise: The Role of Consensus of Experts in Formulating Public Policy and Estimating Fact," *Journal of Medicine and Philosophy* 1991; 16: 427–445.

17. G. Lewith and C. Vincent, "The Clinical Evaluation of Acupuncture," In: J. Filshie (ed.) *Medical Acupuncture: A Western Scientific Approach*, 1998.

18. Methodological difficulties and imperfections exist in most RCTs. For example, one review of the conventional medical literature concluded that "serious widespread problems exist in the published clinical literature." J. W. Williamson, P. G. Goldschmidt, and T. Colton, "The Quality of Medical Literature: An Analysis of Validation Assessments," *Medical Uses of Statistics*, J. C. Bailer and F. Mosteller (eds.), Waltham, MA: NEJM Books, 1986), p. 381.

19. The problem of insufficient sample size in all RCTs is examined in J. A. Freiman et al., "The Importance of Beta, the Type II error, and Sample Size in the Design and Interpretation of the Randomized Controlled Trial: A Survey of 71 'Negative' trials," *New England Journal of Medicine* 1978; 299: 690–694. M. S. Mulward and P. C. Gøtzsche, "Sample Size of Randomized Double Blind Trials 1976–1991," *Danish Medical Bulletin* 1996; 43: 96–98 and J. F. Reed and W. Slaichert, "Statistical Proof in Inconclusive 'Negative' Trials," *Archives of Internal Medicine* 1981; 141: 1302–1310. Scientists have noted that trials of inadequate size "may have the potential to actually do scientific harm, if, for example, their results are misinterpreted as evidence of no effect or an intervention when the trial simply had inadequate power to detect an effect even if it truly existed." J. E. Buring and C. H. Hennekens, "The Contribution of Large, Simple Trials to Prevention Research," *Preventive Medicine* 1994; 23: 595–598, p. 595.

20. For a general discussion of methodological difficulties in acupuncture research, see Ted J. Kaptchuk, Roger A. Edwards, and David M. Eisenberg, "Complementary Medicine: Efficacy Beyond the Placebo Effect," In: *Complementary Medicine: An Objective Appraisal* Edzard Ernst (ed.), (Oxford: Butterworth Heinemann, 1996). For other analyses, see George L. Lewith, "Can We Assess the

Effects of Acupuncture," *British Medical Journal* 1984; 288: 1475–1476; Richard Hammerschlag, "Methodological and Ethical Issues in Clinical Trials of Acupuncture," *Journal of Alternative and Complementary Medicine* 1998; 4: 159–171; E. Ernst and A. R. White, "A Review of Problems in Clinical Acupuncture Research," *American Journal of Chinese Medicine* 1997; 25: 3–11; George Lewith and Charles Vincent, "Evaluation of the Clinical Effects of Acupuncture: A Problem Reassessed and a Framework for Future Research," *Pain Forum* 1995; 4: 29–39.

21. This book has emphasized traditional Chinese acupuncture. In fact, multiple variants of acupuncture exist that can produce distinct intervention methods. Some of these forms of acupuncture have been developed in the various countries of East Asia and depend on different interpretations of classical texts. For a discussion of Japanese acupuncture, see Kiiko Matsumoto and Stephen Birsch, *Hara Diagnosis: Reflections on the Sea* (Brookline, MA: Paradigm, 1988); for a discussion of Korean acupuncture, see Johng Kyu Lee and Sang Kook Bae, *Korean Acupuncture* (Seoul: Ko Mun Sa, 1978); for Vietnamese acupuncture, see J. M. Levinson, "Traditional Medicine in the Democratic Republic of North Vietnam," *American Journal of Chinese Medicine* 1974; 2: 159–162). Also, distinct approaches to clinical acupuncture have developed in the West (most often by Western physicians) that combine aspects of traditional methods and modern physiological understandings of the body. (For a discussion of these approaches, see various chapter in *Medical Acupuncture*, J. Filshie and A. White [eds.]). Also see Joseph M. Helms, *Acupuncture Energetics: A Clinical Approach for Physicians* (Berkeley, CA: Medical Acupuncture Publishers, 1995). Each of these approaches can produce a different treatment protocol, which can confuse the issue of exactly what acupuncture is being tested in an RCT and the generalizability of the results. For example, in the fifteen RCTs of acupuncture for asthma (discussed below) only two trials by the same author used the same points. See K. Linde and W. B. Jonas, "Evaluating Complementary and Alternative Medicine: The Balance of Rigor and Relevance," In: W. B. Jonas and J. S. Levin (eds.) *Essentials of Complementary and Alternative Medicine* (Philadelphia: Lippincott Williams & Wilkins, 1999).

22. Ted J. Kaptchuk, "Acupuncture and Amitriptyline for HIV-Related Peripheral Neuropathic Pain," *Journal of the American Medical Association*, 1999; 281: 1270.

23. It could also be argued that integrating an Oriental diagnosis into the structure of the RCT can increase variability in the acupuncture intervention and make the detection of a treatment effect more difficult. Certainly, the dramatically positive outcome of the emesis RCTs (see below) is related to the simplicity and replicability of the model, not the sophistication of the acupuncture intervention. Such research questions probably need to be concretely investigated and as Kenneth Ottenbacher has noted "the influence of design quality factors should not be an *a priori* assumption but an empirical question." "Impact of Random Assignment

on Study Outcome: An Empirical Examination," *Controlled Clinical Trials* 1992; 13: 50–61.

24. All single-blind RCTs have the problem that provider expectations can easily be communicated. (e.g., see R. P. Reilly and T. W. Findley, "Research in Physical Medicine and Rehabilitation," *American Journal of Physical Medicine & Rehabilitation* 1989: 196–201; S. J. Haines, "Randomized Clinical Trials in the Evaluation of Surgical Innovation," *Journal of Neurosurgery* 1979; 51: 5–11.) For a quantitative verification of how provider expectations can be communicated in a single-blind RCT, see Richard H. Gracely et al., "Clinicians' Expectations Influence Placebo Analgesia," *Lancet* 1985; 1: 43. Most of the acupuncture RCTs have been single-blind. (A very few trials have managed to devise clever ways in particular situations to actually blind the therapist; e.g., C. M. Godfrey and P. Morgan, "A Controlled Trial of the Theory of Acupuncture in Musculoskeletal Pain," *Journal of Rheumatology* 1978; 5: 121–124. In this trial, patient populations with different conditions were mixed, and the acupuncturist was kept blind. Several trials for nausea and vomiting have also managed to blind the therapist. See, e.g., J. Bayreuther et al., "Acupressure for Early Morning Sickness: A Double Blind, Randomized Controlled Crossover Study," *Complementary Therapies in Medicine* 1994; 2: 70–76.; L. A. Warwick-Evans et al., "A Double-Blind Placebo Controlled Evaluation of Acupressure in the Treatment of Motion Sickness," *Aviation, Space, and Environmental Medicine* 1991; 62: 776–778 and S. Hu et al., "Electrical Acustimulation Relieves Vection-Induced Motion Sickness," *Gastroenterology* 1992; 102: 1854–1858. These trials were able to blind the therapist because the acupressure/acupuncture was kept very primitive so a "naive" therapist could perform it or because the acupressure was self-administered by "naive" patients.

25. The phenomenon of nonspecific physiological effects induced by random needling, called "diffuse noxious inhibitory control (DNIC)," has been reasonably well established in research in experimental models. See, e.g., J. C. Willer et al., "Psychophysical and Electrophysiological Approaches to the Pain-Relieving Effects of Heterotopic Nonreceptive Stimuli," *Brain* 1984; 107: 105–112; D. le Barsi et al., "Diffuse Noxious Inhibitory Controls (DNIC) in Animals and in Man," *Acupuncture in Medicine* 1991; 9: 47–56. For a discussion of acupuncture and neurotransmitters see Chapter 4, note 11.

26. See for example, Ted J. Kaptchuk, "Placebo Needle for Acupuncture," *Lancet* 1998; 352; 992; K. Streitberger and J. Kleinhenz, "Introducing a Placebo Needle into Acupuncture Research," *Lancet* 1998; 352: 364–365; Charles Vincent and George Lewith, "Placebo Controls for Acupuncture Studies," *Journal of the Royal Society of Medicine* 1995; 88: 199–202. Also acupuncture may have a "megaplacebo" effect which could make detection of an acupuncture-placebo difference inordinately difficult. See: Ted J. Kaptchuk et al., "Do Medical Devices Have Enhanced Placebo Effects?" *J. Clinical Epidemiology* 2000; 53: 314–321. The pre-

cise location of the sham needling can also confound trials. See: M. Araujo, "Does the Choice of Placebo Determine the Results of Clinical Studies on Acupuncture? A Meta-Analysis of 100 Clinical Trials." *Forschende Komplementänmedizin* 1998; 5: 8–11.

27. For a systematic discussion of thirty-five types of bias, see David L. Sackett, "Bias in Analytic Research," *Journal of Chronic Diseases* 1979; 32: 51–63; and "Bias and Confounding Factors," Bert Spilker, *Guide to Clinical Trials* (Philadelphia: Lippincott-Raven, 1996).

28. It would be noted that, besides acupuncture, other East Asian nonpharmacological interventions exist. Acupressure is included in the discussion below (especially in emesis). East Asian traditional bone-setting is another important modality. There is at least one RCT in this domain. On some measures, bone-setting was significantly better than regular Western physical therapy. See H. M. Hemmilä et al., "Does Folk Medicine Work? A Randomized Clinical Trial on Patients with Prolonged Back Pain," *Archives of Physical Medicine and Rehabilitation* 1997; 78: 571–577. Moxibustion (the use of burning herbs to stimulate acupuncture points) has rarely been the subject of an RCT. An important exception is the dramatic trial performed to determine whether moxibustion at acupuncture point Bladder 67 (*Zhi yin*) could promote versions of fetuses in breech presentation. Two hundred sixty patients were randomized either to the moxibustion or a no-treatment control. The moxa increased fetal activity during the treatment phase and cephalic presentation after the treatment period and at delivery. Francesco Cardini and Huang Weixin, "Moxibustion for Correction of Breech Presentation: A Randomized Controlled Trial," *Journal of the American Medical Association* 1998; 280: 1580–1584. This trial was performed in Jiangxi, China under the direction of Italian researchers.

29. M. Patel, F. Gutzwiller, F. Paccaud, and A. Marazzi, "A Meta-Analysis of Acupuncture for Chronic Pain," *International Journal of Epidemiology* 1989; 18: 900–906. Most of the acupuncture meta-analyses do not actually aggregate data. Because of the heterogeneity of acupuncture RCTs, most reviews mainly tabulate and systematically evaluate all trials and look at the preponderance of positive and negative trials. For a general discussion on the dangers of meta-analysis see Alvan R. Feinstein, "Meta-Analysis: Statistical Alchemy for the 21st Century," *Journal of Clinical Epidemiology* 1995; 48: 71–79. For a general discussion on how biomedicine interprets multiple RCTs with contradictory results see R. I. Horwitz, "Complexity and Contradiction in Clinical Trials Research," *American Journal of Medicine* 1987; 82: 498–510.

30. It should be mentioned that this appendix emphasizes acupuncture versus placebo as the "gold standard" for providing evidence for efficacy. In fact, many of the acupuncture RCTs have been equivalence trials where acupuncture was compared to a conventional medical treatment. For a discussion of this approach, see Richard

Hammerschlag and M. M. Morris, "Clinical Trials Comparing Acupuncture with Biomedical Standard Care: A Criteria-Based Evaluation of Research Design and Reporting," *Complementary Therapies in Medicine* 1997; 5: 133–140. For a discussion on the limitations of inferring causality in equivalence trials see R. J. Temple, "When Are Clinical Trials of a Given Agent vs. Placebo No Longer Appropriate or Feasible?" *Controlled Clinical Trials*, 1997; 18: 613–620, and B. Jones et al., "Trials to Assess Equivalence: The Importance of Rigorous Methods," *British Medical Journal* 1996; 313: 36–39. This appendix's reviews of acupuncture RCTs includes both placebo controlled and comparative trials.

31. G. ter Riet et al., "Acupuncture and Chronic Pain: A Criteria-Based Meta-Analysis," *Journal of Clinical Epidemiology* 1990; 43: 1191–1199.

32. The ter Riet group, like the Patel team, also performed a separate subgroup analysis of acupuncture versus sham for chronic pain. Again the evidence was inconclusive; of the thirty-two studies, fifteen were positive and seventeen were negative. Many other reviews of acupuncture for pain conditions exist. These reviews are not systematic and do not quantitatively score each trial. Rather, they present the evidence in a more discussive format. One important study is Stephen Birch, Richard Hammerschlag, and Brian M. Berman, "Acupuncture in the Treatment of Pain," *Journal of Alternative and Complementary Medicine* 1996; 2: 101–124. This study included animal and human basic science studies and experimental induced pain conditions. It concluded "the evidence [is] building as to how acupuncture treats pain conditions and for which conditions and to what extent it is effective" (p. 101). This team also worried that it is "critical to determine the extent to which the outcome [of an acupuncture RCT] was due to poor study design rather than to an actual failure of acupuncture to ameliorate the condition" (ibid.). Several other earlier studies exist that review acupuncture's effectiveness in pain. These studies do not describe their search, appraisal, and synthesis methods in a manner which would, in theory, permit replication of the review. Nonetheless, they are still informative and include G. T. Lewith, "How Effective Is Acupuncture in the Management of Pain?" *Journal of the Royal College of General Practitioners* 1984; 34: 275–278; J. Filshie and P. J. Morrison, "Acupuncture for Chronic Pain: A Review," *Palliative Medicine* 1988; 2: 1–14; P. H. Richardson and C. A. Vincent, "Acupuncture for the Treatment of Pain: A Review of Evaluative Research," *Pain* 1986; 24: 15–40.

One additional narrative review that is at least partially related to chronic pain conditions deserves mention. This review examined seventeen studies of inflammatory rheumatoid diseases (including rheumatoid arthritis, spondarthropathy, lupus erthematosus, and local and progressive systematic scleroderma). The author concluded that "acupuncture cannot be recommended for treatment of these diseases" because the evidence is of insufficient quality. J. Lautenschläger, "Akupunktur bei der Behandlung Entzündlich-Rheumatischer Erkrankugen," *Zeitschrift für Rheumatologie* 1997; 56: 8–20.

33. E. Ernst and M. H. Pittler, "The Effectiveness of Acupuncture in Treating Acute Dental Pain: A Systematic Review," *British Dental Journal* 1998; 184: 443–447.

34. E. Ernst and A. R. White, "Acupuncture for Back Pain: A Meta-Analysis of Randomised Controlled Trials," *Archives of Internal Medicine* 1998; 158: 2235–2241. The authors noted that in the subgroup analysis of the four sham-controlled studies there is a positive trend toward acupuncture's effectiveness but that this trend lacks statistical significance. They suggest that further trials are needed to determine whether acupuncture works through specific or nonspecific means. Another narrative review (but not a systematic one) of acupuncture for specific types of back pain reached a similar conclusion to Ernst and White. See Wendy Longworth and Peter W. McCarthy, "A Review of Research on Acupuncture for the Treatment of Lumbar Disc Protrusions and Associated Neurological Symptomatology," *Journal of Alternative and Complementary Medicine* 1997; 3: 55–76.

35. M. W. van Tulde, D. C. Cherkin, B. Berman, L. Lao, and B. Koes, "The Effectiveness of Acupuncture in the Treatment of Low Back Pain," *Spine* 1999; 24: 1113–1123. This study accepted only eleven out of twelve trials reviewed by Ernst and White. But this difference does not explain the conflicting conclusions.

36. A. R. White and E. Ernst, "A Systematic Review of Randomized Controlled Trials of Acupuncture for Neck Pain," *Rheumatology* 1999; 38: 143–147.

37. B. M. Berman, J. Ezzo, V. Hadhazy, and J. B. Swyers, "Is Acupuncture Effective in the Treatment of Fibromyalgia?" *Journal of Family Practice* 1999; 48: 213–218.

38. D. Melchard, K. Linde, P. Fischer, A. White, G. Allais, A. Vickers, and B. Berman, "Acupuncture for Recurrent Headaches: A Systematic Review of Randomized Controlled Trials," *Cephalalgia* 1999; 19: 779–786.

39. A. J. Vickers, "Can Acupuncture Have Specific Effects on Health? A Systematic Review of Acupuncture Antiemesis Trials," *Journal of the Royal Society of Medicine* 1996; 89: 303–311, p. 303. A similarly positive evaluation of acupressure for nausea was found by E. Ernst, "Acupressure for Nausea: A Best Evidence Analysis," *European Journal for Physical Medicine and Rehabilitation* 1996; 6: 29–30. This evidence is especially impressive because several of the RCTs actually were able to keep the therapist blind. See note 24.

40. J. Kleijnen, G. ter Riet, and P. Knipschild, "Acupuncture and Asthma: A Review of Controlled Trials," *Thorax* 1991; 46: 799–802, p. 802.

41. K. A. Jobst, "A Critical Analysis of Acupuncture in Pulmonary Disease: Efficacy and Safety of the Acupuncture Needle," *Journal of Alternative and Complementary Medicine* 1995; 1: 57–85; p. 82.

42. K. Linde et al., "Randomized Clinical Trials of Acupuncture for Asthma—a Systematic Review," *Forschende Komplementärmededizin* 1996; 3: 148–155; p. 148.

43. G. ter Riet, J. Kleijnen, and P. Knipschild, "A Meta-Analysis of Studies into the Effect of Acupuncture on Addiction," *British Journal of General Practice* 1990; 40: 379–382. A similar conclusion is reached by A. R. White and H. Rampes, "Acupuncture in Smoking Cessation," T. Lancaster and C. Silagy (eds.), "Tobacco

Addiction Module of the *Cochrane Database of Systematic Reviews*," Issue 1, Oxford: Update Software, 1997; and in A. R. White, K. L. Resch and E. Ernst, "Smoking Cessation with Acupuncture? A 'Best Evidence Synthesis,'" *Forschende Komplementärmededizin* 1997; 4: 102–105. A more optimistic assessment of the substance abuse research is presented in the narrative review by P. D. Culliton and T. J. Kiresuk, "Overview of Substance Abuse Acupuncture Treatment Research," *Journal of Alternative and Complementary Medicine* 1996; 2: 149–159. These authors felt that while acupuncture research shares the methodological weaknesses found in most substance abuse research and the early findings "suggests positive treatment effects."

The addictional literature also points to an interesting conundrum. For example, while it seems that acupuncture's effect on smoking cessation in RCTs is no different from the placebo treatment, there is also no difference between acupuncture and the conventional treatments for smoking cessation. See: K. Linde and W. B. Jonas, "Evaluating Complementary and Alternative Medicine: The Balance of Rigor and Relevance," In: W. B. Jonas and J. S. Levin (eds.) *Essentials of Complementary and Alternative Medicine* (Philadelphia: Lippincott Williams & Wilkins, 1999).

44. E. Ernst, "Acupuncture/Acupressure for Weight Reduction? A Systematic Review," *Wiener Klinische Wochenschrift* 1997; 109: 60–62.

45. E. Ernst and A. White, "Acupuncture as an Adjuvant Therapy in Stroke Rehabilitation?" *Wiener Medizinische Wochenschrift* 1996; 146: 556–558. Ernst and White felt that none of the trials tried to account for the placebo effect.

46. H. Hopwood, "Acupuncture in Stroke Recovery: A Literature Review," *Complementary Therapies in Medicine* 1996; 4: 258–263. This study felt that while the studies have been carefully controlled and blinded, the numbers have been too small and the inherent variability of stroke was not accounted for. The stroke RCTs include one of the most important cost benefit analysis of acupuncture treatment ever performed. In one stroke study, B. Jahansson et al. showed that the acupuncture group had, overall, fewer days in nursing homes and rehabilitation facilities with a subsequent savings over the control group of $26,000 per patient. "Can Sensory Stimulation Improve the Functional Outcome in Stroke Patients?" *Neurology* 1993; 43: 2189–2195.

47. E. Ernst and A. R. White, "Acupuncture as a Treatment for Temporomandibular Joint Dysfunction: A Systematic Review of Randomized Trials," *Archives of Otolaryngology, Head, and Neck Surgery* 1999; 125: 269–272.

48. J. A. Astin et. al., "A Review of the Incorporation of Complementary and Alternative Medicine by Mainstream Physicians," *Archives of Internal Medicine* 1998; 158: 2303–2310. This study points out that acupuncture is the most accepted of the complementary therapies within the biomedical community.

49. For the classic epidemiological discussion on biological plausibility as one of the criteria for evidence of causality see Austin Bradford Hill, "The Environment and Disease: Association or Causation?" *Proceedings of the Royal Society of Medicine* 1965; 58: 295–300. For an example of more recent discussion see M. C. Sutter, "Assigning Causation in Disease: Beyond Koch's Postulates," *Perspectives in Biology and Medicine* 1996; 39: 581–591. For discussion on how plausability and theoretical constructs effects the interpretation of RCT evidence see Jan P. Vandenbroucke, "Medical Journals and the Shaping of Medical Knowledge," *Lancet* 1998; 352: 2001–2006. This essay specifically discusses the rejection of the positive RCT evidence in homeopathy because of lack of biological plausability.

50. B. Pomeranz and G. Stux (eds.) *Scientific Bases of Acupuncture* (New York: Springer-Verlag, 1989).

51. See: H. F. Guo et al., "Brain Substrates Activated by Electroacupuncture (EA) of Different Frequencies (II): /Role of Fos/Jun Proteins in EA-Induced Transcription of Preproenkephalin and Preprodynorophin Genes," *Molecular Brain Research* 1996; 43: 167–173 and M. Gao M et al., "Changes of Mu Opioid Receptor Binding Sites in Rat Brain Following Electroacupuncture," *Acupuncture and Electro-Therapeutic Research* 1997; 22: 161–166.

52. Z. N. H. Cho et al., "New Findings of the Correlation Between Acupoints and Corresponding Brain Cortices Using Functional MRI," *Proceedings of the National Academy of Science* 1998; 95: 2670–2673; M. T. Wu et al., "Central Nervous Pathway for Acupuncture Stimulation: Localization of Processing with Functional MR Imaging of the Brain," *Radiology* 1999; 212: 133–141; K. K. S. Hui et al., "Acupuncture Modulates the Limbic System and Subcortical Gray Structures of the Human Brain," Human Brain Mapping 2000; 9: 12–25.

53. Lixing Lao, "Safety Issues in Acupuncture," *Journal of Alternative and Complementary Medicine* 1996; 2: 27–31.

54. H. Yamashita, H. Tsukayama, Y. Tanno, and K. Nishijo, "Adverse Events Related to Acupuncture," *Journal of the American Medical Association* 1998; 280: 1563–1564

55. E. Ernst and A. R. White, "Life-Threatening Adverse Reactions After Acupuncture? A Systematic Review," *Pain* 1997; 71: 123–126. Hugh MacPherson contends that an examination of the original reports allows for the attribution of acupuncture in only one of the five cases. The rest of the evidence is seriously flawed. "Fatal and Adverse Events from Acupuncture: Allegations, Evidence, and the Implications," *Journal of Alternative and Complementary Medicine* 1999; 5: 47–56.

56. E. Ernst, "The Risks of Acupuncture," *International Journal of Risk and Safety in Medicine* 1995; 6: 179–186, p. 184.

57. A. J. Norheim, "Adverse Effects of Acupuncture: A Study of the Literature for the Years 1981–1994," *Journal of Alternative and Complementary Medicine* 1996; 2: 291–297, p. 291. The use of indwelling needles seems to carry greater risk than

the use of conventional acupuncture techniques. E. Ernst and A. R. White, "Indwelling Needles Carry Greater Risks than Acupuncture Techniques," *British Medical Journal*, 1999; 318: 536.

58. A. Bensoussan and S. P. Myers, *Toward a Safer Choice: The Practice of Traditional Chinese Medicine in Australia* (Campbelltown, NSW, Australia: University of Western Sydney, Macarthur, 1996.) This study was commissioned by the Victorian Department of Human Services.

59. E. T. Peuker, et al., "Traumatic Complications of Acupuncture: Therapists Need to Know Human Anatomy," *Archives of Family Medicine* 1999; 8: 553–558.

60. E. Ernst and A. R. White, "Acupuncture: Safety First: Training Programmes Should Include Basic Medical Knowledge and Experience," *British Medical Journal* 1997; 314: 1362.

61. Lixing Lao, op. cit. p. 29.

62. H. Rampes and R. James, "Complications of Acupuncture," *Acupuncture in Medicine* 1995; 13: 26–33, pp. 26, 31. Rampes is also co-author of an extensive monograph on adverse events associated with acupuncture. This review is more extensive and detailed than those published in the peer-reviewed journal literature. See Hagen Rampes and Elmar Peuker, "Adverse Effects of Acupuncture," In: *Acupuncture: A Scientific Appraisal*, E. Ernst and A. White (eds.) (Oxford: Butterworth Heinemann, 1999). This review concludes that "there is a need for practitioners and patients to be aware of possible adverse effects of acupuncture, the majority of which can be avoided with cautious and prudent use of this ancient therapy. . . . The serious adverse effects reported in the literature may easily be prevented by straightforward precautions." p. 145.

63. National Institutes of Health Development Panel on Acupuncture, p. 1520. The panel noted "as an example, musculoskeletal conditions, such as fibromyalgia, myofascial pain, and epicondylitis (tennis elbow) are conditions for which acupuncture may be beneficial. These painful conditions are often treated with, among other things, anti-inflammatory medications (aspirin, ibuprofen) or with steroid injections. Both medical interventions have a potential for deleterious side effects but are still widely used and are considered acceptable treatments. The evidence supporting these therapies is no better than that for acupuncture." Ibid.

64. The best summary of this extensive research can be found in Hson-Mou Chang and Paul Pui-Hay But (eds.), *Pharmacology and Application of Chinese Materia Medica* Vol.1–2, (Singapore: World Scientific, 1986); W. Tang and G. Eisenbrand, *Chinese Drugs of Plant Origin* (Berlin: Springer-Verlag, 1992); Kee Chang Huang, *The Pharmacology of Chinese Herbs* (Boca Raton, FL: CRC Press, 1993). Relatively little of this work has concerned how the various herbs in combinations may interact and influence one another beneficially or adversely. See E. L. Way and C. F. Chen, "Modern Clinical Applications Related to Chinese Traditional Theories of Drug Interactions," *Perspectives in Biology and Medicine*, 1999; 42: 512–525.

65. Peter A. G. M. DeSmet and Jacobus R. B. J. Brouwers, "Pharmacokinetic Evaluation of Herbal Remedies," *Clinical Pharmacokinetics* 1997; 32: 427–436. Pharmacokinetics studies the metabolic process of absorption, distribution, biotransformation, and elimination of the drug once it is introduced into the body. This study can be critical for the scientific understanding of herbal medicine. A recent example is the work performed on a classical variant of Minor Bupleurum Soup *(xiao chai hu tang)*, which adds *Magnoliae cortex* and *Perillae herba* and is extensively used in Japan for severe asthma. Some of the presumed active compounds are recoverable from the urine after ingestion (including magnolol from the magnolia); but, surprisingly, none of the expected major trierpenoids in the source plants can be recovered from either the urine or blood. See M. Homma et al., "Liquid Chromatographic Determination of Magnolol in Urine Collected from Volunteers After a Single Dose of Saiboku-To, an Oriental Herbal Medicine for Bronchial Asthma," *Journal of Pharmacy and Pharmacology* 1993; 45: 839–841; M. Homma et al., "A Pharmacokinetic Evaluation of Traditional Chinese Herbal Remedies," *Lancet* 1993; 341: 1595.

66. The classic example of herb to drug is ephedrine from the Chinese herb *ma huang (Ephedra sinica)*. (See "Back to Folk Medicine: The Pros and Cons," *Medical World News* 1977; 65–68.) A more recent potential example is artemisinin. (See Daniel L. Klayman, "Qinghausu (Artemisinin): An Antimalarial Drug from China," *Science* 1985; 220: 1049–1055.

67. This review of clinical evidence is confined to experiments performed in the West. But it should be mentioned that rigorous RCTs have begun to take place in East Asia, and they deserve mention. Several of these RCTs performed in China or Japan seem relatively well performed and have even been published in European-language peer review journals. For example, a RCT of Chinese herbs for nasopharyngeal carcinoma randomized 188 patients to either radiotherapy with Chinese herbs versus just radiotherapy. It found significantly reduced rates of local recurrence at the primary site in the Chinese herbal group versus the controls. (G. Z. Xu et al., "Chinese herb 'Destagnation' Series I: Combination of Radiation with Destagnation in the Treatment of Nasopharyngeal Carcinoma: A Prospective Randomized Trial on 188 Cases," *International Journal of Radiation and Oncology* 1989; 196: 297–300. Another study concerned the important herbal formula Minor Bupleurum Soup, which randomized in a double-blind manner 222 patients with chronic active hepatitis to either herbs or placebo. The difference of the mean value in such liver tests as serum AST and ALT between the herbal treatment group and the placebo group was significant after twelve weeks. (C. Hirayama et al., "A Multicenter Randomized Controlled Clinical Trial of Shosaiko-To in Chronic Active Hepatitis," *Gastroenterologia Japonica* 1989; 24: 715–719. Another study from Harbin, China, showed in a randomized single-blind trial that Chinese herbs for bronchiolitis were effective compared to placebo in terms of cough,

fever, wheezing, chest signs, and duration of stay in the hospital. (X. T. Kong et al., "Treatment of Acute Bronchiolitis with Chinese Herbs," *Archives of Diseases in Childhood* 1993; 68: 468–471.) A joint Chinese-Japanese study compared a classic Chinese herbal formula (Ziziphus Soup) versus diazepam for controlling anxiety. This double-blind RCT showed that both had almost the same anxiolytic effect but that the Chinese herbs (and not the diazepam) improved psychomotor performance during the daytime. (C. H. Chen et al., "Suanzaorentang Versus Diazepam: A Controlled Double-Blind Study in Anxiety," *International Journal of Clinical Pharmacology, Therapy and Toxicology* 1986; 24: 646–650). A double-blind randomized crossover study performed in Beijing showed that Chinese herbs were effective for rheumatoid arthritis in most measures. (S. L. Tao et al., "A Prospective, Controlled, Double-Blind, Cross-Over Study of Triptergygium Wilfoddii Hook in Treatment of Rheumatoid Arthritis," *Chinese Medical Journal* 1989; 102: 327–332). Forty-two patients with chronic idiopathic dyspepsia in Osaka were randomized to either the Six Gentleman Soup or a placebo. After seven days of treatment, gastric emptying was significantly accelerated and gastrointestinal symptoms were significantly reduced in patients taking herbs. M. Tatsuta and H. Hshi, "Effect of Treatment with Liu-Jun-Zi-Tang (TJ-43) on Gastric Emptying and Gastrointestinal Symptoms with Dyspeptic Patients," *Alimentary Pharmacology and Therapy* 1993; 7: 459–462.

68. M. P. Sheehan et al., "Efficacy of Traditional Chinese Herbal Therapy in Adult Atopic Dermatitis," *Lancet* 1992; 340: 13–17. Each patient received a decoction of ten herbs; the herbs were not individualized for each patient but were a standardized mixture. Part of the reason that this trial was so well received may be that the potential chemical component may have been identified. See J. H. Galloway, "Chinese Herbs for Eczema, the Active Compound?" *Lancet* 1991; 337: 566. For additional basic science research on this herbal approach to eczema, see X. J. Xu et al., "Modulation by Chinese Herbal Therapy of Immune Mechanisms in the Skin of Patients with Atopic Eczema," *British Journal of Dermatology* 1997; 136: 54–59; Y. Latchman et al., "Association of Immunological Changes with Clinical Efficacy in Atopic Eczema Patients Treated with Traditional Chinese Herbal Therapy (Zemaphyte)," *International Archives of Allergy and Immunology* 1996; 109: 243–249 and Y. Latchman et al., "Efficacy of Traditional Chinese Herbal Therapy *In Vitro*. A Model System for Atopic Eczema: Inhibition of CD23 Expression on Blood Monocytes," *British Journal of Dermatology* 1995; 132: 592–598. For a general clinical summary of Chinese herbs and skin disease see J. Koo and S. Arain, "Traditional Chinese Medicine for the Treatment of Dermatologic Disorders," *Archives of Dermatology* 1998; 134: 1388–1393.

69. P. Sheehan and D. J. Atherton, "A Controlled Trial of Traditional Chinese Medicinal Plants in Widespread Non-Exudative Atopic Eczema," *British Journal of*

Dermatology 1992; 126: 179–184. Also see: M. P. Sheehand and D. J. Atherton, "One-Year Follow Up of Children Treated with Chinese Medicinal Herbs for Atopic Eczema," *British Journal of Dermatology* 1994; 130: 488–493. Parents of thirty-seven children in the original study were offered the opportunity to continue treatment. In every case, parents agreed. After one year of treatment, eighteen children had at least 90 percent reductions in eczema activity scores and five showed lesser degrees of improvement. A recent RCT using a slightly different treatment regimen failed to replicate the positive findings of the two earlier eczema trials. A. Y. P. Fung et al., "A Controlled Trial of Traditional Chinese Herbal Medicine in Chinese Patients with Recalcitrant Atopic Dermatitis," *International Journal of Dermatology* 1999; 38: 387–392.

70. Alan Bensoussan, Nick J. Talley, Michael Hing, Robert Menzies, Anna Guo, and Meng Ngu, "Treatment of Irritable Bowel Syndrome with Chinese Herbal Medicine: A Randomized Controlled Trial," *Journal of the American Medical Association* 1998; 280: 1585–1589. For a discussion on the possible pharmacological actions of the herbs involved in this study see Weindong Lu, "Chinese Herbal Medicine for Irritable Bowel Syndrome," [Letter] *Journal of the American Medical Association* 1999; 282: 1035. For further discussion concerning the design of the study see Ted J. Kaptchuk, "Chinese Herbal Medicine for Irritable Bowel Syndrome," [Letter] *Journal of the American Medical Association* 1999; 282: 1035–1036.

71. A. G. H. Kessels et al., "The Effectiveness of the Hair-Restorer 'Dabao' in Males with Alopecia Androgenetica: A Clinical Experiment," *Journal of Clinical Epidemiology* 1991; 44: 439–447.

72. R. G. Batey, A. Bensoussan, Yang Yi Fan, S. Bollipo, M. A. Hossain, "Preliminary Report of a Randomized, Double-Blind Placebo-Controlled Trial of a Chinese Herbal Medicine Preparation CH-100 in the Treatment of Chronic Hepatitis C," *Journal of Gastroenterology and Hepatology* 1998; 13: 244–247.

73. T. Iversen, K. M. Fiirgaard, P. Schriver, O. Rasmussen, F. Andreasen, "The Effect of NaO Li Su on Memory Functions and Blood Chemistry in Elderly People," *Journal of Ethnopharmacology* 1997; 56: 109–116.

74. J. H. Burack, M. R. Cohen, J. A. Hahn, D. I. Abrams, "Pilot Randomized Controlled Trial of Chinese Herbal Treatment for HIV-Associated Symptoms," *Journal of Acquired Immune Deficiency Syndromes and Human Retrovirology* 1996: 12: 386–393.

75. C. Liu and R. M. Douglas, "Chinese Herbal Medicines in the Treatment of Acute Respiratory Infections: A Review of Randomised and Controlled Clinical Trials," *Medical Journal of Australia* 1998; 579–582.

76. P. Knipschild, "Ginseng: Pep of Nep? "Een Overzicht van Experimenten bij Oudern met Stoornissen van de Vitaliteit," *Phrameceutisch Weekbland* 1988; 123: 4–11, p. 4.

77. L. D'Angelo et al., "A Double-Blind, Placebo-Controlled Clinical Study on the Effect of a Standardized Ginseng Extract on Psychomotor Performance in Healthy Volunteers," *Journal of Ethnopharmacology* 1986; 16: 15–22.

78. Cosmo Hallstrom et al., "Effects of Ginseng on the Performance of Nurses on Night Duty," *Comparative Medicine East and West* 1982; 6: 227–282.

79. B. Thommessen and K. Laake, "No Identifiable Effect of Ginseng (Gericomplex) as an Adjunct in the Treatment of Geriatric Patients," *Aging and Clinical and Experimental Research* 1996; 8: 417–420.

80. C. Maracos et al., "Double-Blind Study of a Multivitamin Complex Supplemented with Ginseng Extract," *Drugs and Experimental and Clinical Research* 1996; 22: 323–329.

81. A more recent systematic review of ginseng has also been performed. Sixteen trials met the inclusion criteria. The trials related to such conditions as physical and psychomotor performance, immunomodulation, and diabetes. The review concluded that the evidence is contradictory and the "efficacy of ginseng root is not established beyond reasonable doubt." B. K. Vogler et al., "The Efficacy of Ginseng. A Systematic Review of Randomised Clinical Trials," *European Journal of Clinical Pharmacology* 1999; 55: 567–575.

82. The concern for the danger of herbal medicine extends to all herbal preparations, not just Eastern ones. For examples of this general concern see such articles as Anne Savage and Anne Hutchings, "Poisoned by Herbs," *British Medical Journal* 1987; 295: 1650–1651; Edzard Ernst, "Harmless Herbs? A Review of the Recent Literature," *American Journal of Medicine* 1998; 104: 170–178; Thomas L. Delbanco, "Bitter Herbs: Mainstream, Magic, and Menace," *Annals of Internal Medicine* 1994; 121: 803–804; Ryan J. Huxtable, "The Harmful Potential of Herbal and Other Plant Products," *Drug Safety* 1990; 5: 126–136; Raymond Koff, "Herbal Hepatotoxicity: Revisiting a Dangerous Alternative," *Journal of the American Medical Association* 1995; 273: 502. The most exhaustive discussion of herbal toxicity is P. A. G. M. DeSmet et al. (eds.), *Adverse Effects of Herbal Drugs* vols. 1, 2, 3 (Berlin: Springer-Verlag, 1990, 1993, 1997).

It should also be mentioned that the methodology for attribution in adverse effects and toxicity events resembles the pre-RCT standards where judgment was decisive. Objective or statistical proof of a causal relationship between a drug or herb and a specific adverse event is quite exceptional. The rate of disparity in the clinical identification of adverse drug reactions is extremely high, and the evaluation often relies on subjective and imprecise information. The method of prospectively randomizing people to comparative groups to primarily look for adverse or unintended effects is considered unethical. For adverse effects, the methods used to make inferences of causality resemble the pre-RCT standards of evidence. See, for example, M. Auriche and E. Loupi, "Does Proof of Causality Ever Exist in Pharmacobigilance?" *Drug Safety* 1993; 9: 230–235; J. Koch-

Weser et al., "The Ambiguity of Adverse Drug Reactions," *European Journal of Clinical Pharmacology* 1977; 11: 75–78; F. E. Karch et al., "Adverse Drug Reactions: A Matter of Opinion," *Clinical Pharmacology and Therapeutics* 1976; 19: 489–492.

83. *Pharmacopoeia Classic of the Divine Husbandman with Investigations (Shen-nong Ben-Cao Jiao-Zhng)*. Wang Zhu-mo (ed.) (Jilin: Science and Technology Press, 1988), p. 33. For a discussion of poisons and toxic herbs in early Chinese medical history see Frédéric Obringer, *L'Aconit et L'Orpimement: Drogues et Poisons en Chine Ancienne et Médiévale* (Paris: Fayard, 1997). Obringer notes that the Chinese character *du* (poison) means both "toxic" and "pharmacologically active."

84. P. U. Unschuld, *Medicine in China: A History of Pharmaceutics* (Berkeley: University of California Press, 1986), p. 33. For a historical discussion in English on toxicity from the perspective of Chinese herbal tradition see P. P. H. But, "Attitudes and Approaches of Traditional Chinese Medicine to Herbal Toxicity," *Journal of Natural Toxins* 1995; 4: 207–217.

85. The rhetorical dimensions of the "nature" discussion have been noted by various scholars. For example, Bray notes that the Chinese medical discussion of "natural" "is to some extent a conscious or unconscious exercise in marketing, the dramatic differentiation of a product which today has to survive the competition with . . . biomedicine." Francesca Bray, "Chinese Medicine," in W. F. Bynum and R. Porter (eds.), *Companion Encyclopedia of the History of Medicine*. London: Routledge, 1993, p. 728. Sivin has noted that there is no term equivalent to "nature" (*zi-ran*) in China before the late nineteenth century when the early term *zi-ran* ("what is so of itself," which carried the meaning of "spontaneous process") was redefined as nature for use in translating Western scientific writings. Nathan Sivin, "State, Cosmos, and Body in the Last Three Centuries B.C.," *Harvard Journal of Asiatic Studies*, 1995; 55: 5–37. For a discussion of how unconventional medicine in general has turned "nature" into an iconographic symbol of virtue, see Ted J. Kaptchuk and David M. Eisenberg, "The Persuasive Appeal of Alternative Medicine," *Annals of Internal Medicine* 1998; 129: 1061–1065. For further discussions on this theme, see Ted J. Kaptchuk and David M. Eisenberg, "The Health Food Movement," *Nutrition* 1998; 14: 471–473. Ted J. Kaptchuk, "Uptake of Alternative Medicine," *Lancet* 1996; 347: 972; Catherine L. Albanese, *Nature Religion In America* (Chicago: University of Chicago Press, 1990).

86. For an example of the recent Oriental medicine profession's discussion on its responsibility to prevent herbal adverse effects, see Richard Blackwell, "Adverse Events Involving Certain Chinese Herbal Medicines and the Response of the Profession," *Journal of Chinese Medicine* 1996; 50: 12–22.

87. For a discussion on how the failure to detect adverse effects, incompetence and professional errors, mistakes, and inappropriate interventions can automatically become a societal issue if health providers neglect their responsibility, see

R. S. Broadhead and N. J. Facchinetti, "Drug Iatrogenesis and Clinical Pharmacy: The Mutual Fate of a Social Problem and a Professional Movement," *Social Problems* 1985; 32: 425–436.

88. T. Y. K. Chan et al., "Chinese Herbal Medicines Revisited: A Hong Kong Perspective," *Lancet* 1993; 1532–1534. Also see, for example, T. Y. K. Chan and J. A. J. H. Critchley, "Usage and Adverse Effects of Chinese Herbal Medicines," *Human & Experimental Toxicology* 1996; 15: 5–12; J. C. Chan et al., "Anticholinergic Poisoning from Chinese Herbal Medicines," *Australian & New Zealand Journal of Medicine* 1994; 24: 317–318. For a list of toxic herbs controlled by goverment regulations in China and Taiwan see P. P. H. But, "Attitudes and Approaches of Traditional Chinese Medicine to Herbal Toxicity." *Journal of Natural Toxins* 1995; 4: 207–217.

89. E. Kang-Yum and S. H. Oransky, "Chinese Patent Medicine as a Potential Source of Mercury Poisoning," *Veterinary and Human Toxicology* 1992; 34: 235–238.

90. For examples of aconite poisoning reports, see T. Y. Chan et al., "Aconitine Poisoning Due to Chinese Herbal Medicines: A Review," *Veterinary & Human Toxicology* 1994; 36: 452–455; T. Y. Chan et al., "Aconite Poisoning Following the Ingestion of Chinese Herbal Medicines: A Report of Eight Cases," *Australian & New Zealand Journal of Medicine* 1993; 23: 368–371.

91. The traditional processing of the crude aconite botanical changes the aconitine alkaloid into the much less poisonous benzoylaconines. See H. Hikino et al., "Change of Alkaloid Composition and Acute Toxicity of Aconitum Roots During Processing," *Yakugaku Zasshi* 1977; 97: 359–366.

92. T. Y. K. Chan et al., 1993 op. cit.; Y. T. Tai et al., "Cardiotoxicity After Accidental Herb-Induced Aconite Poisoning," *Lancet* 1992; 340: 1254–1255. The Chinese-language literature has also had serious concern with aconite. See, for example, Yun Wu, "Aconite Poisoning: Review of Experience in China Over the Past 30 Years," *Jiangsu Zhong Yi* [Jiangsu Traditional Chinese Medicine] 1988; 12: 39–42.

93. B. J. Will et al., "Perilla Ketone: A Potent Lung Toxin from the Mint Plant, *Perilla Frustescens Britton*," *Science* 1977; 573–574.

94. T. Y. K. Chang and J. A. J. H. Critchley, "Usage and Adverse Effects of Chinese Herbal Medicines," *Human & Experimental Toxicology* 1996; 15: 5–12. The biomedical literature has many reports of negative incidents due to licorice in the context of Western herbalism or candy consumption. See, for example, J. W. Conn et al., "Licorice-Induced Pseudoaldosteronism," *Journal of the American Medical Association* 1968; 205: 80–84. A. van der Zwan, "Hypertension Encephalopathy After Liquorice Ingestion," *Clinical Neurology and Neurosurgery* 1993; 95: 35–37; M. Schambelan, "Licorice Ingestion and Blood Pressure Regulating Hormones," *Steroids* 1994; 59: 127–130. (Incidentally, most licorice candy is flavored with anise seed oil [*Pimpinella anisum*], not licorice.)

95. The most exhaustive list of idiosyncratic reactions to Chinese herbs is actually found in the Chinese-language literature. Important review articles include Hiu-nan Yuan and De-jiang Tan, "Review of the Adverse Reactions of Chinese Herbs from the Major Medical Journals in the Nation in 1990," *Zhong-guo Zhong-yao Za-zhi* [China Medical Journal] 1991; 16: 628–634. Other important sources are the Yearbooks of Traditional Chinese Medicine published in China, which usually have a section on allergic reactions and adverse effects. For example, see Shanghai Institute of Chinese Medicine (ed.), *Yearbook of Traditional Chinese Medicine (Zhong-guo Nian-jian)*. Beijing: People's Health Press, 1985, pp. 148–153. It should be mentioned that royal jelly (which could also be considered either a food or a Chinese herb) has been noticed to produce significant allergic reactions (mostly asthma, anaphylaxis, and rash). See, for example, J. R. Loporte et al., "Bronchospasm Induced by Royal Jelly," *Allergy* 1996; 51: 440–445; R. Leung et al., "Royal Jelly Consumption and Hypersensitivity in the Community," *Allergy* 1997; 27: 333–336. The royal jelly effect is likely an IgE mediated hypersensitivity to a number of various proteins in royal jelly, and not a reaction to preservatives or impurities.

96. An example of a safe Western herb becoming dangerous might be a helpful illustration of this problem. See, for example, M. H. Benner and H. J. Lee, "Anaphylactic Reaction to Chamomile Tea," *Journal of Allergy and Clinical Immunology* 1973; 52: 307–308; C. Casterline, "Allergy to Camomile Tea," *Journal of the American Medical Association* 1980; 4: 330–331; and G. W. Smith et al., "Vasculitis Associated with Herbal Preparation Containing Passiflora Extract," *British Journal of Rheumatology* 1993; 32: 87–88. A good example of potentially serious but rare food allergy is peanut allergy.

97. See, for example, T. G. Hammond and J. A. Whitworth, "Adverse Reactions to Ginseng," *Medical Journal of Australia* 1981; 492.

98. R. K. Siegel, "Ginseng Abuse Syndrome: Problems with the Panacea," *Journal of the American Medical Association* 1979; 241: 1614–1615.

99. E. M. Greenspan, "Ginseng and Vaginal Bleeding," *Journal of the American Medical Association* 1983; 249: 2018; M. O. Hopkins et al., "Ginseng Face Cream and Unexplained Vaginal Bleeding," *American Journal of Obstetrics and Gynecology* 1988; 159: 1121–1122; O. M. Koriech, "Ginseng and Mastalgia," *British Medical Journal* 1978; 1: 1556; B. V. Palmer et al., "Ginseng and Mastalgia," *British Medical Journal* 1978; 1: 1284 and G. Koren et al., "Maternal Ginseng Use Associated with Neonatal Androgenization," *Journal of the American Medical Association* 1979; 241: 1614–1615.

100. For example, see T. Y. Lee and T. H. Lam, "Allergic Contact Dermatitis to Yunnan Paiyao," *Contact Dermatitis* 1987; 17: 59–60; A. Barbaud et al., "Contact Allergy to Colophony in Chinese Musk and Tiger-Bone Plaster," *Contact Der-*

matitis 1991; 25: 324–325; T. Y. Lee and T. H. Lam, "Irritant Contact Dermatitis Due to a Chinese Herbal Medicine Lu-Shen-Wan," *Contact Dermatitis* 1988; 12: 213–218.

101. Cases of deliberate poisoning can be found in T. Y. Chan et al., "Drug Overdosage and Other Poisoning in Hong Kong—the Prince of Wales Hospital (Shatin) Experience," *Human & Experimental Toxicology* 1994; 13: 512–515.

102. See, for example, T. C. Theoharides, "Sudden Death of a Healthy College Student Related to Ephedrine Toxicity from a Ma-Huang-Containing Drink," *Journal of Clinical Psychopharmacology* 1997; 17: 437–439; T. Powell et al., "Ma-Huang Strikes Again: Ephedrine Nephrolithiasis," *American Journal of Kidney Disease* 1998; 32: 153–159, H. Doyle et al., "Herbal Stimulant Containing Ephedrine Has Also Caused Phychosis," *British Medical Journal* 1995; 152: 647. Cf. L. M. White et al., "Pharmacokinetics and Cardiovascular Effects of Ma-Huang (*Ephedra sinica*) in Normotensive Adults," *Journal of Clinical Pharmacology* 1997; 37: 116–122.

103. M. P. Sheehan and D. J. Atherton, "One-Year Follow Up of Children Treated with Chinese Medicinal Herbs for Atopic Eczema," *British Journal of Dermatology* 1994; 130: 488–492.

104. Examples of the discussion of the relationship of the Chinese herbs for skin disease and liver disease appear in R. Graham-Brown, "Toxicity of Chinese Herbal Remedies, *Lancet* 1992; 340: 673–674; and J. A. Kane et al., "Hepatitis Induced by Traditional Chinese Herbs; Possible Toxic Components," *Gut* 1995; 36: 146–147; L. Perharic et al., "Possible Association of Liver Damage with the Use of Chinese Herbal Medicine for Skin Disease," *Veterinary & Human Toxicology* 1995; 37: 562–566. In the skin case, the dangerous herb seems to be *Dictamnus dasycarpus* (*bai xian pi*); some suspicion also has been directed at *Paeonia suffructicosa* (*chi shao*). Chinese herbal treatment of skin disease has also been implicated in one case of cardiomyopathy. See J. E. Ferguson et al., "Reversible Dilated Cardiomyopathy Following Treatment of Atopic Eczema with Chinese Herbal Medicine," *British Journal of Dermatology* 1997; 136: 592–593.

105. For a tabulation of liver damage associated with Chinese herbs and the treatment of skin disease, see D. Shaw et al., "Traditional Remedies and Food Supplements: A 5-Year Toxicological Study (1991–1995)" *Drug Safety* 1997; 17: 342–355, p. 350. Shaw et al. report a total of twenty-one cases, with fourteen cases having good evidence. In two patients reexposure provoked a severe response. The effects seem to be dose-independent and the reactions may be idiosyncratic. Despite such reports of serious side effects, the potentional value of East Asian herbs to positively influence liver disease should not be dismissed. Besides the RCT mentioned earlier on hepatitis C, much basic research has produced provocative evidence for the potential value of Chinese herbs in liver disease. See, for example, G. T. Liu, "Effects of Some Compounds Isolated from Chinese Medicinal Herbs on

Hepatic Microsomal Cytochrome P-450 and Their Potential Biological Consequences," *Drug Metabolism Reviews* 1991; 23: 439–465; I. Schimizu et al., "Effects of Sho-Saiko-To, A Japanese Herbal Medicine, on Hepatic Fibrosis in Rats," *Hepatology* 1999: 29: 149–160.

106. J. Young and R. Blackwell, "Liver Toxicity and Herbal Medicine," *Journal of Chinese Medicine* 1993; 41: 28–29. For a parallel discussion in the biomedical literature, see, for example, G. Vautier and R. C. Spiller, "Safety of Complementary Medicines Should Be Monitored," *British Medical Journal* 1995; 311: 633.

107. D. Melchart et al., "Liver Enzyme Elevations in Patients Treated With Traditional Chinese Medicine," *Journal of the American Medical Association* 1999; 282: 28–29. Other reports of liver damage can be found in the biomedical literature. For example, S. Itoh et al., "Liver Injuries Induced by Herbal Medicine, Syo-Saiko-To (Xiao-Chai-Hu-Tang)," *Digestive Diseases and Science* 1995; 40: 1845–1848; Cf. D. Melchart et al., "Monitoring of Liver Enzymes in Patients Treated with Chinese Drug," *Complementary Therapies in Medicine* 1999; 7: 208–216. "Hepatitis Related to the Chinese Medicine Shou-Wu-Pian Manufactured from *Polygonum Multiflorum*," *Veterinarian and Human Toxicology* 1996; 38: 280–282. For a discussion on the overall medical outcomes on the patients in the German hospital see D. Melchert et al., "Systematic Clinical Activity In Complementary Medicine: Rationale, Concept, and a Pilot Study," *Alternative Therapies* 1997; 3: 33–39.

    One additional aspect of the herbal toxicity debate needs mention. It is easy to demonstrate acute toxic reactions. Chronic toxicity and cumulative toxicity are much harder to detect. Morbidity and mortality patterns can disguise such toxicity. The most important example of this is the recent discovery of plants that contain pyrrolizidine alkaloids, which can produce hepatic veno-occlusive disease and cancer after long-term usage. *Flos Tussilago Farfarae* (*dong hua*, Chinese coltfoot) is an example of a Chinese herbal that may have such a problem, although this author is unaware of any published report on the flower of this species with such findings. The literature on pyrrolizidine alkaloids in plants and toxicity is large. See, for example, P. M. Ridker et al., "Hepatic Veno-occlusive Disease Associated with the Consumption of Pyrrolizidine-Containing Dietary Supplements," *Gastroenterology* 1985; 88: 1050–1054; P. J. Abbott, "Comfrey: Assessing the Low-Dose Health Risk," *Medical Journal of Australia* 1998; 149: 678–682. Only a few important studies of subacute toxicity have been published on Chinese herbs in English. The most impressive one is Hsing-Yi Yang and Chieh-Fu Chen, "Subacute Toxicity of 15 Commonly Used Chinese Drugs(1)," *Journal of Chinese Medicine* 1995; 6: 127–128. They uncovered no problems.

108. The iatrogenic effects of biomedicine have been extensively described. For example, it has been estimated that in 1994, 106,000 fatal events occurred in U.S. hospitals from adverse drug reactions, making these reactions between the fourth and

sixth leading cause of death. This report studied only events that occurred from correctly administered drugs. (It excluded errors in drug administration, non-compliance, overdose, drug abuse, therapeutic failures, and possible adverse events.) It also found the overall incidence of serious effects was 6.7 percent of hospitalized patients. J. Lazarou, B. H. Pomeranz, P. N. Corey, "Incidence of Adverse Drug Reactions in Hospitalized Patients: A Meta-Analysis of Prospective Studies," *Journal of the American Medical Association* 1998; 279: 1200–1205. Also see David W. Bates, David J. Cullen, Nan Laird et al., "Incidence of Adverse Drug Events and Potential Adverse Drug Events," *Journal of the American Medical Association* 1995; 274: 29–34. Besides adverse events from correctly prescribed medications, biomedicine also has a serious problem with complications caused by mistakes. A report by the Institute of Medicine claimed that research suggests medical errors in United States hospitals alone kill 44,000 to 98,000 people a year. This compares unfavorably with the toll from highway accidents, about 43,450, breast cancer 42,300, or AIDS, 16,500. Medication error alone (as oppposed to surgical and diagnostic mistakes) results in 7,000 deaths compared with about 6,000 deaths from workplace injuries. *New York Times*, November 30, 1999, pp. A1, A18.

109. K. Tsutani, "The Evaluation of Herbal Medicines: An East Asian Perspective," in *Clinical Research for Complementary Medicine*, G. T. Lewith and D. Aldridge (eds.), London: Hodder & Stoughton, 1993.

110. R. J. Ko. "Adulterants in Asian Patient Medicines," *New England Journal of Medicine* 1998; 339: 847. The original survey was published as Richard Ko and Alice Au, *1997–1998 Compendium of Asian Patent Medicines* (Sacramento, CA: California Department of Health Services, 1998).

111. For examples of reports of adulteration of Chinese herbs, see W. F. Huang et al., "Adulteration by Synthetic Therapeutic Substances of Traditional Chinese Medicines in Taiwan," *Journal of Clinical Pharmacology* 1997; 37: 344–350; E. Gertner et al., "Complications Resulting from the Use of Chinese Herbal Medications Containing Undeclared Prescription Drugs," *Arthritis and Rheumatism* 1995; 38: 614–617; R. Karunanithy and K. P. Sumita, "Undeclared Drugs in Traditional Chinese Antirheumatoid Medicine," *International Journal of Pharmacy Practice* 1991; 1: 117–119. For a relatively complete list of adulterant pharmaceuticals found in Chinese patent remedies, see Alan Bensoussan and Stephen P. Myers, *Toward a Safer Choice: The Practice of Traditional Chinese Medicine in Australia* (Campbelltown, Australia: University of Western Sydney Macarthur, 1996), p. 72.

Chinese herbal creams seem especially prone to adulteration. In one study, an analysis of eleven herbal creams obtained from patients attending general and pediatric dermatology clinics found eight which contained potent steroids (dexamethasone). F. M. Keane et al., "Analysis of Chinese Herbal Creams Prescribed for Dermatological Conditions," *British Medical Journal* 1999; 318: 563–564.

112. An example of a plant-derived pharmaceutical labeled as an herbal product was the case of Jin Bu Wan, which contained tetrahydropalmatine, a concentrated alkaloid fraction derived from plant material. See Ted J. Kaptchuk, "Acute Hepatitis Associated with Jin Bu Wan," *Annals of Internal Medicine* 1995; 122: 636. For a detailed discussion, see Subhuti Dharmananda, *The Story of Jin Bu Huan* (Portland, OR: START Group Manuscripts, ITM, 1994).

113. C. Drew, "Medicines from Afar Raise Safety Concerns," *New York Times*, October 29, 1995, pp. 1, 32.

114. Many reports exist. See, for example, S. Brown and R. Ede, "Occult Lead Poisoning," *British Journal of Hospital Medicine* 1996; 53: 469–476; H. H. Schaumburg and A. Berger, "Alopecia and Sensory Polyneuropathy from Thallium," *Journal of the American Medical Association* 1992; 268: 3430–3431; S. B. Markowitz et al., "Lead Poisoning Due to Hai Ge Fen," *Journal of the American Medical Association* 1994; 271: 932–934; C. A. W. Mitchell-Heggs et al., "Herbal Medicine as a Cause of Combined Lead and Arsenic Poisoning," *Human & Experimental Toxicology* 1990; 195–196; E. O. Espinoza and M. I. Mann, "Arsenic and Mercury in Traditional Chinese Herbal Balls," *New England Journal of Medicine* 1995; 333: 803–804.

115. The most systematic analysis published on the quality of Chinese herbs was performed at the Hospital for Traditional Chinese Medicine in Bavaria, Germany. This is an inpatient hospital facility for Chinese medicine, and from December 1990 to June 1994 it analyzed 967 herbal samples from 15 consignments from the People's Republic of China. One hundred sixty herb samples were analyzed in designated laboratories for heavy metal, pesticides, afatoxin, and microbial contamination. Because of the small size of the consignments and the very labor-intensive and expensive analyses, only random samples of "suspect" herbs were performed. Twenty-five (15.6 percent of the 160 analyzed herbs exceeded the upper limits of normal values and resulted in discarding. In eight samples, the upper limit of microbial contamination (especially fungus) was registered; ten herb samples were found to have elevated heavy metal content and there were high levels of pesticides in several samples (mostly HCH isomers). Further reasons for rejecting the herbs included lack of identification, poor pharmaceutical quality, and evidence of destruction by beetles. A total of 6.1 percent of the herbs were rejected and the hospital has taken measures to perform sample checks on all batches of herbs in the future. See Stephan Hager, "Chinese Herbal Formulas: Problems with Toxic Contamination and Discussion of Relevant Side Effects," *The Magazine of the Anglo-Dutch Institute of Oriental Medicine* 1996; 1: 8–9. Most Western manufacturers of Chinese herbs have taken suitable precautions.

116. That even ordinary food can significantly change bioavailability of some drugs has been established. See, for example, D. G. Bailey et al., "Grapefruit Juice and

Drugs: How Significant Is the Interaction?" *Clinical Pharmacokinetics* 1994; 26: 91–98. Also, many cases of interactions between Western herbal remedies and pharmaceuticals have been reported. See D. Shaw et al., "Traditional Remedies and Food Supplements: A 5-Year Toxicological Study (1991–1995)," *Drug Safety* 1997; 17: 342–356, pp. 349–350. Also see E. Ernst, "Second Thoughts on St John's Wort," *Lancet* 1999; 354: 2014–2015. Of course drug-drug interaction is a major issue in biomedicine. For an overview of herb-drug interactions that includes both Western and Asian herbs, see Adrianne Fugh-Berman, "Herb-Drug Interactions," *Lancet* 2000; 355: 134–138.

117. J. L. Vanherweghern et al., "Rapidly Progressive Interstitial Renal Fibrosis in Young Women: Association with Slimming Regimen Including Chinese Herbs," *Lancet* 1993; 341: 387–391. These women are also at great risk of urothelial malignancy. See J. P. Cosyns, "Urothelial Lesions in Chinese-Herb Nephropathy," *American Journal of Kidney Diseases* 1999; 33: 1011–1017. The episode also included a misidentification of the Chinese herb. See M. Vanhaelen et al., "Identification of Aristolochic Acid in Chinese Herbs," *Lancet* 1994; 343: 174. Besides two Chinese herbs, the clinic used a bizarre mixture of such Western herbs as artichoke extract, kelp, and cascara and a mixture of drugs such as fenfluramine, diethylpropion, meprobamate, and acetazolamide. Cf. C. van Ypersele de Strihou, "Chinese Herbs Nephropathy or the Evils of Nature," *American Journal of Kidney Diseases* 1998; 32: i–iii.

118. J. Malak, "Chinese Herb Nephropathy Is Not a (Dex)Fenfluramine Nephropathy but a Serotonin Nephropathy," *Journal of Alternative and Complementary Medicine* 1998; 4: 131–135. A third theory, based on the fact that only women in one particular clinic had reactions (and not the other clinics that used the same concoction) was that there was contamination of the herbs with a nephotoxic mildew such as ochratoxin. A. Delcour, "Can Chinese Herbal Remedies Be Trusted?" *Magazine of the Anglo-Dutch Institute of Oriental Medicine* 1996; 116–117.

119. G. M. Lord et al., "Nephropathy Caused by Chinese Herbs in the UK," *Lancet* 1999; 354: 481–482. The report concerns two cases which resulted in renal failure. The investigators isolated a known nephrotoxin and carcinogen from Chinese herbal preparations taken by these patients that were unconnected to the isolated outbreak in Belgium and were prescribed for a different reason. The herb that is responsible for the two case reports is probably *Aristolochia manshuriensis* or various species of akebia or clematis. Again, a case of herbal misidentification probably occurred. For an extensive discussion on the question of the confusion in the identification of the entire class of Chinese herbs called *fangi* see Subhuti Dharmananda, *The Strange Story of Stephania: Lessons About Herb Substitution, Toxicity, and Modern Research* (Portland, OR: START Group Manuscripts, ITM, 1997). Supporting the thesis that the Belgium nephropathy is a case of toxicity is a report on aristolochic acid DNA adducts in renal tissue samples of some victims. The existence of the deoxyadenosine adduct of aristolochic acid 1 showed that

sufficient aristolochic acid had been consumed to alter cellular DNA. H. H. Schmeiser et al., "Detection of DNA Adducts Formed by Aristolochic Acid in Renal Tissue from Patients with Chinese Herbs Nephropathy," *Cancer Research* 1996; 56: 2025–2058. That Chinese herbs are implicated in the increased risk of urothelial malignancy in this case is supported by the fact that the aristolochic acids in *Aristolochia* plants are carcinogenic in rats. See: P. A. G. M. DeSmet, "*Arisolochia* species," In: P. A. G. M. DeSmet et al., (eds.) *Adverse Effects of Herbal Drugs*, vol. 1 (Heidelberg: Springer-Verlag, 1992) pp. 79–89.

120. For example, C. M. Yu, "Chinese Herbs and Warfarin Potentiation By 'Danshen,'" *Journal of Internal Medicine* 1997; 241: 337–339; M. B. Izzat et al., "A Taste of Chinese Medicine," *Annals of Thoracic Surgery* 1998; 66: 941–941; L. S. Tam, "Warfarin Interactions with Chinese Traditional Medicines: Danshen and Methyl Salicylate Medicated Oil," *Australia and New Zealand Journal of Medicine* 1995; 25: 258.

121. T. O. Cheng, "Warfarin Danshen Interaction," *Annals of Thoracic Surgery* 1999; 67: 894.

122. J. D. Lawrence, "Potentiation of Warfarin by Dong Quai," *Pharmacotherapy* 1999; 19: 870–876; G. R. Ellis et al., "Minerva," *British Medical Journal* 1999; 319: 650.

123. There have been at least two reported cases of ginseng interacting with phenelzine (Nardil) to cause symptoms of headache and tremulousness. See R. I. Shader et al., "Bees, Ginseng and MAOIs Revisited," *Journal of Clinical Psychopharmacology* 1988; 8: 255; B. D. Jones et al., "Interaction of Ginseng with Phenelzine," *Journal of Psychopharmacology* 1987; 7: 202. Like all herb-drug interaction reports the lack of a control group, absence of dosage, simultaneous use of other drugs, and lack of botanical authentication makes inferences of causality difficult.

124. See, for example, H. H. Zhou et al., "Differing Effects of Atropine on Heart Rate in Chinese and White Subjects," *Clinical Pharmacology and Therapy* 1992; 52: 120–124. K. Ming and W. W. Shen, "Pharmacology for Southeast Asian Psychiatric Patients," *Journal of Nervous and Mental Diseases* 1991; 179: 346–350, which summarizes the differences found in pharmacokinetic and pharmacody-namic profiles of various psychotropic medications between Asian and non-Asian patients. Cf. C. Wu, "Drug Sensitivity Varies with Ethnicity," *Science News* 1997; 152: 165. Curiously, issues of cross-cultural differences of drug effects has already been raised by both Chinese and Western physicians during the early penetration of Western medicine into China. See, Bridie J. Andrews, "Tuberculosis and the Assimilation of Germ Theory in China, 1895–1937," *Journal of the History of Medicine* 1997; 52: 114–157. This debate also occurred in sixteenth- and seventeenth-century Europe. See A. Wear, "The Early Modern Debate About Foreign Drugs: Localism Versus Universalism in Medicine," *Lancet* 1999; 354: 149–151.

125. The director of the Chinese Medical Hospital mentioned in note 115, Stephan Hager, described in a personal communication with the author that his staff of senior Chinese physicians from Beijing caused an unacceptably high incidence of

unpleasant gastrointestinal reactions with Chinese herbs. This required that the hospital insist on a significant reduction in usual dosage of the herbs. Curiously, the Chinese physicians noticed no reduction in effectiveness of treatments. Dr. Hager attributed the problem to a German sensitivity to the herbs. A prospective outcome study of 1597 in-patients at this hospital reported 2 percent of patients with such side effects as flatulence, nausea, vomiting, diarrhea, and allergic erythema. D. Melchart, K. Linde, W. Weidenhammer, S. Hager, J. Z. Liao, R. Bauer, H. Wagner, "Use of Traditional Drugs in a Hospital of Chinese Medicine in Germany," *Pharmacoepidemiology and Drug Safety* 1999; 8: 84–89. The reported medical outcomes on these patients can be found in D. Melchart, K. Linde, J. Z. Liao, S. Hager, and W. Weiderhanmer, "Systematic Clinical Auditing in Complementary Medicine: Rationale, Concept, and a Pilot Study," *Alternative Therapies* 1997; 3: 33–39.

126. See discussion in P. A. G. M. DeSmet, "Is There Any Danger in Using Traditional Remedies?" *Journal of Ethnopharmacology* 1991; 21: 43–50. Another example of this problem would be the acceptance of the dangers of the most common Western medicaments. For example, the use of nonsteroidal anti-inflammatory drugs (NSAIDs) has been conservatively estimated to lead to 16,500 deaths among people with rheumatoid arthritis or osteoarthritis every year in the United States. This figure is similar to the number of deaths from HIV and considerably greater than the number of deaths from multiple myeloma, asthma, or cervical cancer. If deaths from gastrointestinal toxic effects of NSAIDs were tabulated separately, these effects would consitute the fifteenth most common cause of death in the United States. The annual number of hospitalizations in the United States for serious gastrointestinal complications due to NSAIDs is conservatively estimated to be at least 103,000 at a cost of $15,000 to $20,000 per hospitalization. For details see M. M. Wolfe et al., "Gastrointestinal Toxicity of Nonsteroidal Anti-Inflammatory Drugs," *New England Journal of Medicine* 1999; 340: 1888–1999.

127 T. Y. K. Chan et al., "Hospital Admissions Due to Adverse Reactions to Chinese Herbal Medicine," *Journal of Tropical Medicine and Hygiene* 1992; 95: 296–298; T. Y. K. Chan et al., "Adverse Reactions to Drugs as a Cause of Admissions to a General Teaching Hospital in Hong Kong," *Drug Safety* 1992; 7: 235–240. The authors felt that the rate of 4.4 percent that they found for the Western drugs was comparable to earlier studies on rates of admission in hospitals for adverse drug events. The most important drugs responsible for problems included sulphoylurea, NSAIDs, insulin, diuretics, and aspirin.

128. For a discussion on precautions Oriental practitioners need to undertake to avoid adverse herbal events, see J. Young and R. Blackwell, "Liver Toxicity and Herbal Medicine," *Journal of Chinese Medicine* 1993; 41: 28–29 and G. Maciocia, *Safety of Chinese Herbs*. (Chesham Bois, UK: Su Wen Press, 2000.)

—| ADDENDUM: SELECTED CLINICAL TRIALS INVOLVING
ACUPUNCTURE

Abel SM, Barber HO, Briant TD. A study of acupuncture in adult sensorineural hearing loss. *Journal of Otolaryngology* 1976; 6: 166–172.

Ader L, Hansson B, Wallin, G. "Parturition pain treated by intracutaneous injections of sterilae water," *Pain* 1990; 41: 133–38

Aglieeti L, Roila F, Tonato, M et al. "A pilot study of metoclopramide, dexamethasone, diphenhydramine and acupuncture in women treated with cisplatin." *Cancer Chemother Pharmacol* 26: 239–240.

Ahonen E, Hakumaki M, Mahlamaki S. Acupuncture and physiotherapy in the treatment of tension neck patients: pain relief and EMG activity. *Pain* 1981; Suppl 1: S278.

Ahonen E, Hakumaki M, Mahlamaki S. Effectiveness of acupuncture and physiotherapy on myogenic headache: a comparative study. *Acupunct Electrother Res* 1984; 9: 141–150.

al-Sadi M, Newman B, Julious SA. Acupuncture in the prevention of postoperative nausea and vomiting. *Anaesthesia* 1997; 52: 658–661.

Allen DL, Kitching AJ, Nagle C. P6 acupressure and nausea and vomiting after gynecological surgery. *Anaesthesia and Intensive Care* 1994; 22: 691–693.

Ammer K, Petschnig R. Comparison of the effectiveness of acupuncture and physical therapy in ambulatory patients with gonarthrosis. *Wiener Medizinische Wochenschrift* 1988; 138: 566–569.

Anderson DG, Jamieson JL, Man SC. Analgesic effects of acupuncture on the pain of ice water: a double-blind study. *Can J Psychol* 1974; 28: 239–244.

Andrzejowski J, Woodward D. Semi-permanent acupuncture needles in the prevention of postoperative nausea and vomiting. *Acupuncture in Medicine* 1996; 14: 68–70.

Appiah R, Hiller S, Caspary L et al. Treatment of primary Raynaud's syndrome with traditional Chinese acupuncture. *J Inter Med* 1997; 241: 119–124.

Arseni A, Zbaganu G. Electroacupuncture in the treatment of headache. *Neurolog Psychiat* 1988; 26: 265–270.

Arseni A, Zbaganu G, Rosca T. Acupuncture in the treatment of craniofacial pain. *Neurolog Psychiat* 1988; 26: 85–92.

Ashton H, Ebenezer I, Golding JF, Thompson JW. Effects of acupuncture and transcutaneous electrical nerve stimulation on cold-induced pain in normal subjects. *Journal of Psychosomatic Research* 1984; 28: 301–308.

Aune A, Alraek T, Lihua H et al. Acupuncture in the prophylaxis of recurrent lower urinary tract infection in adult women. *Scand J Prim Health Care* 1998; 16: 37–39.

Avants SK, Margolin A, Chang P, Kosten TR, Birch S. Acupuncture for the treatment of cocaine addiction. Investigation of a needle puncture control. *Journal of Substance Abuse Treatment* 1995; 12: 195–205.

Axelsson A, Andersson S, Gu LD. Acupuncture in the management of tinnitus: a placebo-controlled study. *Audiology* 1994; 33: 351–360.

Aydin S, Crcan M, Caskurlu T et al. Acupuncture and hypnotic suggestions in the treatment of non-organic male sexual dysfunction. *Scand J Urol Nephrol* 1997; 31: 271–274.

Bakke M. Effect of acupuncture on the pain perception thresholds of human teeth. *Scand J Dent Res* 1976; 84: 404–408.

Ballegaard S, Christophersen SJ, Dawids SG, Hesse J, Olsen NV. Acupuncture and transcutaneous electric nerve stimulation in the treatment of pain associated with chronic pancreatitis. A randomized study. *Scand J Gastroenterol* 1985; 20: 1249–1254.

Ballegaard S, Jensen G, Pedersen F, Nissen VH. Acupuncture in severe, stable angina pectoris: a randomized trial. *Acta Med Scand* 1986; 220: 307–313.

Ballegaard S, Meyer CN, Trojaborg W. Acupuncture in angina pectoris: does acupuncture have a specific effect? *Journal of Internal Medicine* 1991; 229: 357–362.

Ballegaard S, Pedersen F, Pietersen A, Nissen VH, Olsen NV. Effects of acupuncture in moderate, stable angina pectoris: a controlled study. *J Intern Med* 1990; 227: 25–30.

Barber J, Mayer D. Evaluation of the efficacy and neural mechanism of a hypnotic analgesia procedure in experimental and clinical dental pain. *Pain* 1977; 4: 41–48.

Barsoum G, Perry EP, Fraser IA. Postoperative nausea is relieved by acupressure. *Journal of the Royal Society of Medicine* 1990; 83: 86–89.

Batra YK, Chari P, Negi ON. Comparison of acupuncture and placebo in treatment of chronic shoulder pain. *American Journal of Acupuncture* 1985; 13: 69–71.

Baust W, Sturtzbecher KH. Management of migraine using acupuncture in a double-blind study. *Medizinische Welt* 1978; 29: 669–673.

Beer AM, Munstermann M. Comparative studies on the treatment of post partum hemoglobin decrease with acupuncture. *Akupunktur* 1994; 22: 182–187.

Belgrade MJ, Solomon LM, Lichter EA. Effect of acupuncture on experimentally induced itch. *Acta Derm Venereol* 1984; 64: 129–133.

Berger D, Nolte D. Hat akupunktur einen nachweisbaren bronchospasmolytischen effekt beim asthma bronchiale? *Med Klin* 1975; 70: 1827–1830.

Berlin FS, Bartlett R, Black JD. Acupuncture and placebo: effects on delaying the terminating response to a painful stimulus. *Anesthesiology* 1975; 42: 527–531.

Berlin J, Erdman W, David E. Psychosomatic correlations in chronic pain patients using electroacupuncture. *American Journal of Chinese Medicine* 1989; 17: 85–87.

Berry H, Fernandes L, Bloom B, Clark RJ, Hamilton EB. Clinical study comparing acupuncture, physiotherapy, injection and oral anti-inflammatory therapy in shoulder-cuff lesions. *Curr Med Res Opin* 1980; 7: 121–126.

Bertolucci LE, DiDario B. Efficacy of a portable acustimulation device in controlling seasickness. *Aviation Space and Environmental Medicine* 1995; 66: 1155–1158.

Bhatt-Sanders D. Acupuncture for rheumatoid arthritis: an analysis of the literature. *Semin Arthritis Rheum* 1985; 14: 225–231.

Birch S, Jamison RN. Controlled trials of Japanese acupuncture for chronic myofascial neck pain: assessment of specific and nonspecific effects of treatment. *Clinical Journal of Pain* 1998; 14: 248–255.

Blom M, Dawidson I, Angmar Mansson B. The effect of acupuncture on salivary flow rates in patients with xerostomia. *Oral Surg Oral Med Oral Pathol* 1992; 73: 293–298.

Blom M, Dawidson I, Fernberg JO, Johnson G, Angmar-Mansson B. Acupuncture treatment of patients with radiation-induced xerostomia. *European Journal of Cancer Part B, Oral Oncology* 1996; 32B: 182–190.

Boureau F, Luu M, Kisielnicki E. Effects of transcutaneous nerve stimulation (TNS), electrotherapy (ET), electroacupuncture (EA) on chronic pain: a comparative study. *Pain* 1981; Suppl 1: S277 (abstract).

Brattberg G. Acupuncture therapy for tennis elbow. *Pain* 1983; 16: 285–288.

Brockhaus A, Elger CE. Hypalgesic efficacy of acupuncture on experimental pain in man. Comparison of laser acupuncture and needle acupuncture. *Pain* 1990; 43: 181–185.

Brown S, North D, Marvel MK, Fons R. Acupressure wrist bands to relieve nausea and vomiting in hospice patients: do they work? *American Journal of Hospice and Palliative Care* 1992; 9: 26–29.

Buguet A, Sartre M, Le KJ. Sleep pattern changes under nocturnal acupressure in healthy subjects. *Neurophysiologie Clinique* 1995; 25: 78–83.

Bullock ML, Culliton PD, Olander RT. Controlled trial of acupuncture for severe recidivist alcoholism. *Lancet* 1989; 1: 1435–1439.

Bullock ML, Umen AJ, Culliton PD, Olander RT. Acupuncture treatment of alcoholic recidivism: a pilot study. *Alcoholism* 1987; 11: 292–295.

Cahn AM, Carayon P, Hill C, Flamant R. Acupuncture in gastroscopy. *Lancet* 1978; 1: 182–183.

Camerlain M, Leung CY, Santerre A, et al. Double-blind evaluation of the effects of acupuncture in the treatment of rheumatoid arthritis of the knee. *Union Medicale Du Canada* 1981; 110: 1041–1044.

Cardini F, Marcolongo A. Moxibustion for correction of breech presentation: A clinical study with retrospective control. *Amer J Chin Med* 1993; 21: 133–138.

Cardini F, Weixin H. Moxibustion for correction of breech presentation: a randomized controlled trial. JAMA 1998; 280: 1580–1584.

Carlsson J, Augustinsson LE, Blomstrand C, Sullivan M. Health status in patients with tension headache treated with acupuncture or physiotherapy. *Headache* 1990; 30: 593–599.

Carlsson J, Fahlcrantz A, Augustinsson LE. Muscle tenderness in tension headache treated with acupuncture or physiotherapy. *Cephalalgia* 1990; 10: 131–141.

Carlsson J, Rosenhall U. Oculomotor disturbances in patients with tension headache treated with acupuncture or physiotherapy. *Cephalalgia* 1990; 10: 123–129.

Carlsson J, Wedel A, Carlsson GE, Blomstrand C. Tension headache and signs and symptoms of craniomandibular disorders treated with acupuncture or physiotherapy. *Pain Clinic* 1990; 3: 229–238.

Ceccherelli F, Altafini L, Lo Castro G, Avila A, Ambrosio F, Giron GP. Diode laser in cervical myofascial pain: a double-blind study versus placebo. *Clin J Pain* 1989; 5: 301–304.

Ceccherelli F, Ambrosio F, Adami MG, et al. Failure of high frequency auricular electrical stimulation to relieve postoperative pain after cholecystectomy. Results not improved by administration of aprotinin. *Deutsche Zeitschrift Für Akupunktur* 1985; 28: 87–92.

Chapman CR, Benedetti C, Colpitts YH, Gerlach R. Naloxone fails to reverse pain thresholds elevated by acupuncture: acupuncture analgesia reconsidered. *Pain* 1983; 16: 13–31.

Chapman CR, Wilson ME, Gehrig JD. Comparative effects of acupuncture and transcutaneous stimulation on the perception of painful dental stimuli. *Pain* 1976; 2: 265–283.

Chen L, Tang J, White PF, Sloninsky A, Wender RH, Naruse R, Kariger R. The effect of location of transcutaneous electrical nerve stimulation on postoperative opioid analgesic requirement: acupoint versus nonacupoint stimulation. *Anesthesia and Analgesia* 1998; 87: 1129–1134.

Cheng PT, Wong MK, Chang PL. A therapeutic trial of acupuncture in neurogenic bladder of spinal cord injured patients—a preliminary report. *Spinal Cord* 1998; 36: 476–480.

Cheng RSS, Pomeranz B. Electrotherapy of chronic musculoskeletal pain: Comparison of electroacupuncture and acupuncture-like transcutaneous electrical nerve stimulation. *Clinical Journal of Pain* 1986; 2: 143–149.

Chow OKW, So SY, Lam WK, Yu DYC, Yeung CY. Effect of acupuncture on exercise-induced asthma. *Lung* 1983; 161: 321–326.

Christensen BV, Juhl IU, Wilbek H et al. Acupuncture treatment of severe knee osteoarthrosis: A long term study. *Acta Anaesthesiol Scand* 1992; 36: 519–525.

Christensen BV, Juhl IU, Wilbek H, Bulow HH, Dreijer NC, Rasmussen HF. Acupuncture treatment of knee arthrosis. A long-term study. *Ugeskrift for Loeger* 1993; 155: 4007–4011.

Christensen PA, Noreng M, Andersen PE et al. Electroacupuncture and postoperative pain. *Brit J Anaesth* 1989; 62: 258–262.

Christensen PA, Laursen LC, Taudorf E, Srensen SC, Weeke B. Acupuncture and bronchial asthma. *Allergy* 1984; 39: 379–385.

Christensen PA, Noreng M, Andersen PE, Nielsen JW. Electroacupuncture and postoperative pain. *Brit J Anaesth* 1989; 62: 258–262.

Chu YC, Lin SM, Hsieh YC, Peng GC, Lin YH, Tsai SK, Lee TY. Effect of BL-10 (tianzhu), BL-11 (dazhu) and GB-34 (yanglinquan) acuplaster for prevention of vomiting after strabismus surgery in children. *Acta Anaesthesiologica Sinica* 1998; 36: 11–16.

Clavel F, Benhamou S, Company Huertas A, Flamant R. Helping people to stop smoking: randomised comparison of groups being treated with acupuncture and nicotine gum with control group. *Br Med J* [Clin Res] 1985; 291: 1538–1539.

Clavel-Chapelon F, Paoletti C, Benhamou S. A randomised 2 x 2 factorial design to evaluate different smoking cessation methods. *Revue Epidemiologie et de Sante Publique* 1992; 40: 187–190.

Clavel-Chapelon F, Paoletti C, Benhamou S. Smoking cessation rates 4 years after treatment by nicotine gum and acupuncture. *Prev Med* 1997; 26: 25–28.

Co LL, Schmitz TH, Havdala H, Reyes A, Westerman MP. Acupuncture: an evaluation in the painful crises of sickle cell anaemia. *Pain* 1979; 7: 181–185.

Coan RM, Wong G, Coan PL. The acupuncture treatment of neck pain: a randomized controlled study. *Am J Chin Med* 1981; 9: 326–332.

Coan RM, Wong G, Ku SL, et al. The acupuncture treatment of low back pain: a randomized controlled study. *Am J Chin Med* 1980; 8: 181–189.

Cottraux JA, Harf R, Boissel JP, Schbath J, Bouvard M, Gillet J. Smoking cessation with behavior therapy or acupuncture: a controlled study. *Behav Res Ther* 1983; 21(4): 417–424.

Cottraux J, Schbath J, Messy P, Mollard E, Juenet C, Collet L. Predictive value of MMPI scales on smoking cessation programs outcomes. *Acta Psychiatrica Belgica* 1986; 86: 463–469.

David J, Modi S, Aluko AA, Robertshaw C, Farebrother J. Chronic neck pain: a comparison of acupuncture treatment and physiotherapy. *British Journal of Rheumatology* 1998; 37: 1118–1122.

Davies A, Lewith G, Goddard J et al. The effect of acupuncture on nonallergic rhinitis: a controlled pilot study. *Altern Ther Health Med* 1998; 4: 70–74.

Dawson D, Lewith G, Machin D. The effects of acupuncture vs. placebo in the treatment of headache pain. *Pain* 1985; 21: 35–42.

DeAloysio D, Penacchioni P. Morning sickness control in early pregnancy by Neiguan point acupressure. *Obstet Gynecol* 1992; 80: 852–854.

Deluze C, Bosia L, Zirbs A et al. Electroacupuncture in fibromyalgia: results of a controlled trial. *Brit Med J* 1992; 305: 1249–1252.

Dias PL, Subramaniam S, Lionel ND. Effects of acupuncture in bronchial asthma: preliminary communication. *J R Soc Med* 1982; 75: 245–248.

Dickens W, Lewith G. A single-blind controlled and randomized clinical trial to evaluate the effect of acupuncture in the treatment of trapeziometacarpal osteoarthritis. *Complemen Med Res* 1989; 3: 5–8.

Doerr-Proske H, Wittchen HU. A muscle and vascular oriented relaxation program for the treatment of chronic migraine patients. A randomized clinical comparative study. *Zeitschrift Für Psychosomatische Medizin Und Psychoanalyse* 1985; 31: 247–266.

Doerr PH, Wittchen HU. A randomized clinical control group study on the effectiveness of a biobehavioral treatment program. *Zeitschrift Für Psychosomatische Medizin Und Psychoanalyse* 1985; 31: 247–266.

Dowson DI, Lewith GT, Machin D. The effects of acupuncture versus placebo in the treatment of headache. *Pain* 1985; 21: 35–42.

Dundee JW, Chestnutt WN, Ghaly RG, Lynas AG. Traditional Chinese acupuncture: a potentially useful antiemetic? *Br Med J* [Clin Res] 1986; 293: 583–584.

Dundee JW, Ghaly RG, Bill KM, Chestnutt WN, Fitzpatrick KT, Lynas AG. Effect of stimulation of the P6 antiemetic point on postoperative nausea and vomiting. *Br J Anaesth* 1989; 63:612–618.

Dundee JW, Ghaly RG, Fitzpatrick KTJ. Randomised comparison of the antiemetic effects of metoclopramide and electro-acupuncture in cancer chemotherapy. *British Journal of Clinical Pharmacology* 1988; 25: 678P–679P.

Dundee JW, Ghaly RG, Fitzpatrick KT, Abram WP, Lynch GA. Acupuncture prophylaxis of cancer chemotherapy-induced sickness. *J R Soc Med* 1989; 82: 268–271.

Dundee JW, McMillan C. Positive evidence for P6 acupuncture antiemesis. *Postgrad Med J* 1991; 67: 417–422.

Dundee JW, Sourial FB, Ghaly RG, Bell PF. P6 acupressure reduces morning sickness. *J R Soc Med* 1988; 81: 456–457.

Dundee JW, Yang J. Prolongation of the antiemetic effect of P6 acupuncture by acupressure in patients having cancer chemotherapy. *J Roy Soc Med* 1990; 83: 360–362.

Dunn PA, Rogers D, Halford K. Transcutaneous electrical nerve stimulation at acupuncture points in the induction of uterine contractions. *Obstet Gynecol* 1989; 73: 286–290.

Edelist G, Gross AE, Langer F. Treatment of low-back pain with acupuncture. *Can Anaesth Soc J* 1976; 23: 303–306.

Ehrlich D, Haber P. Influence of acupuncture on physical performance capacity and haemodynamic parameters. *Int J Sports Med* 1992; 13: 486–491.

El RM, Weston C. An investigation into the possible additive effects of acupuncture and autogenic relaxation in the management of chronic pain. *Acupuncture in Medicine* 1997; 15: 74–75.

Emery P, Lythgoe S. The effect of acupuncture on ankylosing spondylitis. *Br J Rheumatol* 1986; 25: 132–33.

Eriksson MB, Sjolund BH, Sundbarg G. Pain relief from peripheral conditioning stimulation in patients with chronic facial pain. *J Neurosurg* 1984; 61: 149–155.

Fargas-Babjak AM, Pomeranz B, Rooney PJ. Acupuncture-like stimulation with codetron for rehabilitation of patients with chronic pain syndrome and osteoarthritis. *Acupuncture and Electro-Therapeutic Research* 1992; 17: 95–105.

Fernandes L, Berry N, Clark RJ, Bloom B, Hamilton EB. Clinical study comparing acupuncture, physiotherapy, injection, and oral anti-inflammatory therapy in shoulder-cuff lesions. *Lancet* 1980; 1: 208–209.

Filshie J, Redman D. Acupuncture and malignant pain problems. *Eur J Surg Oncol* 1985; 11: 389–394.

Fox EJ, Melzack R. Transcutaneous electrical stimulation and acupuncture: comparison of treatment for low-back pain. *Pain* 1976; 2: 141–148.

Fung KP, Chow OK, So SY. Attenuation of exercise-induced asthma by acupuncture. *Lancet* 1986; 2: 1419–1422.

Furugard S, Hedin PJ, Eggertz A, Laurent C. Acupuncture worth trying in severe tinnitus. *Lakartidningen* 1998; 95: 1922–1928.

Gadsby JG, Franks A, Jarvis P, Dewhurst F. Acupuncture-like transcutaneous electrical nerve stimulation within palliative care: a pilot study. *Complementary Therapies in Medicine* 1997; 5: 13–18.

Gallacchi G, Muller W, Plattner GR. Akupunktur- und laserstrahlbehandlung beim zervikal- und lumbalsyndrom. *Schweiz Med Wochenschr* 1981; 111: 1360–1366.

Garvey TA, Marks MR, Wiesel SW. A prospective, randomized, double-blind evaluation of trigger-point injection therapy for low-back pain. *Spine* 1989; 14: 962–964.

Gaw AC, Chang LW, Shaw LC. Efficacy of acupuncture on osteoarthritic pain. A controlled, double-blind study. *N Engl J Med* 1975; 293: 375–378.

Geirsson G, Wang YH, Lindstrom S, Fall M. Traditional acupuncture and electrical stimulation of the posterior tibial nerve. A trial in chronic interstitial cystitis. *Scandinavian Journal of Urology and Nephrology* 1993; 27: 67–70.

Gerardi AU, Dominici S, Sapia F, et al. Reflexology in respiratory allergies. *Minerva Medica* 1983; 74: 2521–2531.

Gerhard I, Postneek F. Auricular acupuncture in the treatment of female infertility. *Gynecol Endocrinol* 1992; 6: 171–181.

Ghaly RB, Fitzpatrick KTJ, Dundee JW. Antiemetic studies with traditional Chinese acupuncture: a comparison of manual needling with electrical stimulation and commonly used antiemetics. *Anaesthesia* 1987; 42: 1108–1110.

Ghia JN, Mao W, Toomey TC, Gregg JM. Acupuncture and chronic pain mechanisms. *Pain* 1976; 2: 285–299.

Gilbey V, Meumann B. Auricular acupuncture for smoking withdrawal. *Am J Acupuncture* 1977; 5: 239–247.

Gillams J, Lewith GT, Machin D. Acupuncture and group therapy in stopping smoking. *Practitioner* 1984; 228: 341–344.

Godfrey CM, Morgan P. A controlled trial of the theory of acupuncture in musculoskeletal pain. *J Rheumatol* 1978; 5: 121–124.

Gosman-Hedstrom G, Claesson L, Klingenstierna U, Carlsson J, Olausson B, Frizell M, Fagerberg B, Blomstrand C. Effects of acupuncture treatment on daily life activities and quality of life: a controlled, prospective, and randomized study of acute stroke patients. *Stroke* 1998; 29: 2100–2108.

Grabow L. Controlled study of the analgetic effectivity of acupuncture. *Arzneimittel Forschung* 1994; 44: 554–558.

Gunn CC, Milbrandt WE, Little AS, Mason KE. Dry needling of muscle motor points for chronic low-back pain: a randomized clinical trial with long-term follow-up. *Spine* 1980; 5: 279–291.

Gunsberger M. Acupuncture in the treatment of sore throat symptomatology. *Am J Chin Med* 1973; 1: 337–340.

Hackett GI, Burke P, Harris I. An anti-smoking clinic in general practice. *Practitioner* 1984; 228: 1079–1082.

Hackett GI, Seddon D, Kaminski D. Electroacupuncture compared with paracetamol for acute low back pain. *Practitioner* 1988; 232: 163–164.

Haker E, Lundeberg T. Laser treatment applied to acupuncture points in lateral humeral epicondylalgia. A double-blind study. *Pain* 1990; 43: 243–247.

Haker EH, Lundeberg TC. Lateral epicondylalgia: report of noneffective mid-laser treatment. *Arch Phys Med Rehabil* 1991; 72: 984–988.

Hameroff SR, Crago BR, Blitt CD, Womble J, Kanel J. Comparison of bupivacaine, etidocaine, and saline for trigger-point therapy. *Anesth Analg* 1981; 60: 752–755.

Hansen PE, Hansen JH. Acupuncture treatment of chronic facial pain: a controlled cross-over trial. *Headache* 1983; 23: 66–69.

Hansen PE, Hansen JH. Acupuncture treatement of chronic facial pain. A double-blind crossover investigation. *Ugeskrift for Loeger* 1981; 143: 2885–2887.

Hansen PE, Hansen JH. Acupuncture treatment of chronic tension headache: a controlled cross-over trial. *Cephalalgia* 1985; 5: 137–142.

Hansen PE, Hansen JH. Acupuncture therapy for chronic tension headache. A controlled crossover study. *Ugeskrift for Loeger* 1984; 146: 649–652.

Hansen PE, Hansen JH, Bentzen O. Acupuncture treatment of chronic unilateral tinnitus: a double-blind cross-over trial. *Clin Otolaryngol* 1982; 7: 325–329.

Hansen PE, Hansen JH, Bentzen O. Acupuncture treatment of chronic unilateral tinnitus. A double-blind cross-over investigation. *Ugeskrift for Loeger* 1981; 143: 2888–2890.

Hao J, Zhao C, Cao S et al. Electric acupuncture treatment of peripheral nerve injury. *J Trad Chin Med* 1995; 15: 114–117.

He D, Berg JE, Hostmark AT. Effects of acupuncture on smoking cessation or reduction for motivated smokers. *Prev Med* 1997; 26: 208–214.

Helms JM. Acupuncture for the management of primary dysmenorrhea. *Obstet Gynecol* 1987; 69: 51–56.

Hesse J, Mogelvang B, Simonsen H. Acupuncture versus metoprolol in migraine prophylaxis: a randomized trial of trigger point inactivation. *J Internal Med* 1994; 235: 451–456.

Hirsch D, Leupold W. Placebo-controlled study on the effect of laser acupuncture in childhood asthma. *Atemwegs Und Lungenkrankheiten* 1994; 20: 701–705.

Ho CM, Hseu SS, Tsai SK, Lee TY. Effect of P-6 acupressure on prevention of nausea and vomiting after epidural morphine for post-cesarean section pain relief. *Acta Anaesthesiologica Scandinavica* 1996; 40: 372–375.

Ho RT, Jawan B, Fung ST, Cheung HK, Lee JH. Electro-acupuncture and postoperative emesis. *Anaesthesia* 1990; 45: 327–329.

Hu HH, Chung C, Liu TJ. A randomized controlled trial on the treatment for acute partial ischemic stroke with acupuncture. *Neurepidemiology* 1993; 12: 106–113.

Hu S, Stritzel R, Chandler A. P6 acupressure reduces symptoms of vection-induced motion sickness. *Avia Space Environ Med* 1995; 66: 631–634.

Hyde E. Acupressure therapy for morning sickness. A controlled clinical trial. *J Nurse Midwifery* 1989; 34: 171–178.

Jensen LB, Melsen B, Jensen SB. Effect of acupuncture on headache measured by reduction in number of attacks and use of drugs. *Scand J Dent Res* 1979; 87: 373–380.

Jerner B, Skogh M, Vahlquist A. A controlled trial of acupuncture in psoriasis: no convincing evidence. *Acta Derm Venerol* 1997; 77: 154–156.

Jobst K, Chen JH, McPherson K, et al. Controlled trial of acupuncture for disabling breathlessness. *Lancet* 1986; 2: 1416–1419.

Johansson A, Wenneberg B, Wagersten C et al. Acupuncture in treatment of facial muscular pain. *Acta Odontol Scand* 1991; 49: 153–158.

Johansson K, Lindgren I, Widner H et al. Can sensory stimulation improve the functional outcome in stroke patients? *Neurology* 1993; 43: 2189–2192.

Johansson V, Kosic S, Lindahl O. Effect of acupuncture in tension headache and brainstem reflexes. *Adv Pain Res* 1976; 1: 839–841.

Johnson MI, Kundu S, Ashton CH, Marsh VR, Tsai SK. The analgesic effects of acupuncture on experimental pain threshold and somatosensory evoked potentials in healthy volunteers. *Complementary Therapies in Medicine* 1996; 4: 219–225.

Joos S, Schott C, Zou H, Daniel V, Martin E. Acupuncture—immunological effects in treatment of allergic asthma. *Allergologie* 1997; 20: 63–68.

Junnila SYT. Acupuncture superior to piroxicam in the treatment of osteoarthritis. *Am J Acupuncture* 1982; 10: 341–346.

Junnila SYT. Acupuncture therapy for chronic pain. A randomised comparison between acupuncture and pseudoacupuncture with minimal peripheral stimulus. *Am J Acupuncture* 1982; 10: 259–262.

Junnila SYT. Intra-articular glycosaminoglycan vs acupuncture in the treatment of gonarthosis. *Acupunct Electrother Res* 1985; 10: 242 (abstract).

Kenyon JN, Knight CJ, Wells C. Randomised double-blind trial on the immediate effects of naloxone on classical Chinese acupuncture therapy for chronic pain. *Acupunct Electrother Res* 1983; 8: 17–24.

Kepes ER, Chen M, Schapira M. A critical evaluation of acupuncture in the treatment of chronic pain. *Adv Pain Res Ther* 1976; 1: 817–822.

Kho HG, Eijk RJ, Kapteijns WM, van Egmond J. Acupuncture and transcutaneous stimulation analgesia in comparison with moderate-dose fentanyl anaesthesia in major surgery. Clinical efficacy and influence on recovery and morbidity. *Anaesthesia* 1991; 46: 129–135.

Kho HG, Kloppenborg PW, van Egmond J. Effects of acupuncture and transcutaneous stimulation analgesia on plasma hormone levels during and after major abdominal surgery. *European Journal of Anaesthesiology* 1993; 10: 197–208.

Kho KH. The impact of acupuncture on pain in patients with reflex sympathetic dystrophy. *Pain Clinic* 1995; 8: 59–61.

Kjendahl A, Sallstrom S, Osten PE et al. A one year follow-up study on the effects of acupuncture in the treatment of stroke patients in the subacute stage: a randomized controlled trial. *Clin Rehabil* 1997; 11: 192–200.

Kleijnen J, ter Riet G, Knipschild P. Acupuncture and asthma: a review of controlled trials. *Thorax* 1991; 46: 799–802.

Kleinhenz J, Streitberg K et al. Randomised clinical trial comparing the effects of acupuncture and a newly designed placebo needle in rotator cuff tendinitis. *Pain* 1999; 83: 235–241.

Krause AW, Clelland JA, Knowles CJ, Jackson JR. Effects of unilateral and bilateral auricular transcutaneous electrical nerve stimulation on cutaneous pain threshold. *Phys Ther* 1987; 67: 507–511.

Kreczi T, Klingler D. A comparison of laser acupuncture versus placebo in radicular and pseudoradicular pain syndromes as recorded by subjective responses of patients. *Acupunct Electrother Res* 1986; 11: 207–216.

Krop J, Lewith GT, Gziut W, Radulescu C. A double-blind, randomized, controlled investigation of electrodermal testing in the diagnosis of allergies. *Journal of Alternative Complementary Medicine* 1997; 3: 241–248.

Lagrue G, Poupy JL, Grillot A, Ansquer JC. Antismoking acupuncture. Short-term results of a double-blind comparative study (letter). *Nouvelle Presse Medicale* 1980; 9: 966.

Laitinen J. Treatment of cervical syndrome by acupuncture. *Scand J Rehabil Med* 1975; 7: 114–117.

Laitinen J. Acupuncture and transcutaneous electric stimulation in the treatment of chronic sacrolumbalgia and ischialgia. *Am J Chin Med* 1976; 4: 169–175.

Lamontagne Y, Annable L, Gagnon MA. Acupuncture for smokers: lack of long-term therapeutic effect in a controlled study. *Can Med Assoc J* 1980; 122: 787–790.

Langley GB, Sheppeard H, Johnson M, Wigley RD. The analgesic effects of transcutaneous electrical nerve stimulation and placebo in chronic pain patients. A double-blind non-crossover comparison. *Rheumatology International* 1984; 4: 119–123.

Lao HH. A retrospective study on the use of acupuncture for the prevention of alcoholic recidivsm. *American Journal of Acupuncture* 1995; 23: 29–33.

Lao L, Bergman S, Hamilton GR, Langenberg P, Berman B. Evaluation of acupuncture for pain control after oral surgery: a placebo-controlled trial. *Archives of Otolaryngology—Head and Neck Surgery* 1999; 125: 567–572.

Lao L, Berman S, Langenberg P. et al. Efficacy of Chinese acupuncture on postoperative oral surgery pain. *Oral Surg Oral Med Oral Pathol Oral Radiol Endod* 1995; 79: 423–428.

Lee CK, Chien TJ, Hsu JC, Yang CY, Hsiao JM, Huang YR, Chang CL. The effect of acupuncture on the incidence of postextubation laryngospasm in children. *Anaesthesia* 1998; 53: 917–920.

Lee PK, Anderson TW, Modell JH, Saga SA. Treatment of chronic pain with acupuncture. JAMA 1975; 232: 1133–1135.

Lee YH, Lee WC, Chen MT, Huang JK, Chung C, Chang LS. Acupuncture in the treatment of renal colic. *J Urol* 1992; 147: 16–18.

Lehmann TR, Russell DW, Spratt KF. The impact of patients with nonorganic physical findings on a controlled trial of transcutaneous electrical nerve stimulation and electroacupuncture. *Spine* 1983; 8: 625–634.

Lehmann TR, Russell DW, Spratt KF, et al. Efficacy of electroacupuncture and TENS in the rehabilitation of chronic low-back pain patients. *Pain* 1986; 26: 277–290.

Lehmann V, Banzhaf E, Kunze E, Stube G, Theil G, Schilling C, Mobius M, Wenzel KP, Han D. Randomized clinically controlled study of the efficacy of acupuncture in comparison with electroacupuncture as well as drug therapy with propranolol in patients with recurrent migraine. *Deutsche Zeitschrift Für Akupunktur* 1991; 34: 27–30.

Lein DH, Jr., Clelland JA, Knowles CJ, Jackson JR. Comparison of effects of transcutaneous electrical nerve stimulation of auricular, somatic, and the combination of auricular and somatic acupuncture points on experimental pain threshold. *Phys Ther* 1989; 69: 671–678.

Lenhard L, Walte PME. Acupuncture in the prophylactic treatment of migraine headaches: pilot study. *N Z Med J* 1983; 96: 663–666.

Lewers D, Clelland JA, Jackson JR, Varner RE, Bergman J. Transcutaneous electrical nerve stimulation in the relief of primary dysmenorrhea. *Phys Ther* 1989; 69: 3–9.

Lewis IH, Pryn SJ, Reynolds PI, Pandit UA, Wilton NC. Effect of P6 acupressure on postoperative vomiting in children undergoing outpatient strabismus correction. *British Journal of Anaesthesia* 1991; 67: 73–78.

Lewith GT. How effective is acupuncture in the management of pain? *J R Coll Gen Pract* 1984; 34: 275–278.

Lewith GT, Field J, Machin D. Acupuncture compared with placebo in post-herpetic pain. *Pain* 1983; 17: 361–368.

Li CK, Nauck M, Loser C, Folsch UR, Creutzfeldt W. Acupuncture to alleviate pain during colonoscopy. *Deutsche Medizinische Wochenschrift* 1991; 116: 367–370.

Li J, Chenard JR, Marchand S, Charest J, Lavignolle B. Acupuncture points and trigger-points: reactivity to pressure and skin response in patients with chronic low-back pain. *Rheumatologie* 1994; 46: 11–19.

Lin JG, Ho SJ, Lin JC. Effect of acupuncture on cardiopulmonary function. *Chinese Medical Journal (Engl)* 1996; 109: 482–485.

Lipton DS, Brewington V, Smith M. Acupuncture for crack-cocaine detoxification: experimental evaluation of efficacy. *J Subst Abuse Treatment* 1994; 11: 2045–215.

List T. Acupuncture in the treatment of patients with craniomandibular disorders. Comparative, longitudinal and methodological studies. *Swedish Dental Journal Supplement* 1992; 87: 1-159: 1-159.

List T, Helkimo M. Acupuncture and occlusal splint therapy in the treatment of carniomandibular disorders, Part II. A one year follow-up study. *Acta Odontol Scand* 1992; 50: 375–385.

List T, Lundeberg T, Lundstrom et al. The effect of acupuncture in the treatment of patients with primary Sjögren's syndrome. A controlled study. *Acta Odontol Scand* 1998; 56: 95–99.

Loh L, Nathan PW, Schott GD, Zilkha KJ. Acupuncture versus medical treatment for migraine and muscle tension headaches. *J Neurol Neurosurg Psychiatry* 55 1984; 47: 333–337.

Longobardi AG, Clelland JA, Knowles CJ, Jackson JR. Effects of auricular transcutaneous electrical nerve stimulation on distal extremity pain: a pilot study. *Phys Ther* 1989; 69: 10–17.

Loy TT. Treatment of cervical spondylosis: electroacupuncture versus physiotherapy. *Med J Aust* 1983; 2: 32–34.

Lundeberg T. A comparative study of the pain alleviating effect of vibratory stimulation, transcutaneous electrical stimulation, electroacupuncture and placebo. *Am J Chin Med* 1984; 12: 72–79.

Lundeberg T, Bondesson L, Thomas M. Effect of acupuncture on experimentally induced itch. *British Journal of Dermatology* 1987; 117: 771–777.

Lundeberg T, Laurell G, Thomas M. Effect of acupuncture on sinus pain and experimentally induced pain. *Ear, Nose, and Throat Journal* 1988; 67: 565–566, 571, 572.

Lundeberg T, Hurtig T, Lundeberg S, Thomas M. Long-term results of acupuncture in chronic head and neck pain. *Pain Clinic* 1988; 2: 15–31.

Lundeberg T, Eriksson SV, Lundeberg S, Thomas M. Effect of acupuncture and naloxone in patients with osteoarthritis pain. A sham acupuncture controlled study. *Pain Clinic* 1991; 4: 155–161.

Luo H, Shen Y. A comparative study of the treatment of depression by electroacupuncture and amitriptyline. *Acupuncture* 1990; 1: 20–26.

Luu M, Maillard D, Pradalier A, Boureau F. Spirometric monitoring of the effects of puncturing thoracic pain points in asthmatic disease. *Respiration* 1985; 48: 340–345.

Lux G, Hagel J, Backer P, Backer G, Vogl R, Ruppin H, Domschke S, Domschke W. Acupuncture inhibits vagal gastric acid secretion stimulated by sham feeding in healthy subjects. *Gut* 1994; 35: 1026–1029.

Macdonald AJ, Macrae KD, Master BR, Rubin AP. Superficial acupuncture in the relief of chronic low-back pain. *Ann R Coll Surg Engl* 1983; 65: 44–46.

Machovec FJ, Man SC. Acupuncture and hypnosis compared: fifty-eight cases. *Am J Clin Hypn* 1978; 21: 45–47.

Man PL, Chen CH. Acupuncture for pain relief, a double-blind, self-controlled study. *Mich Med* 1974; 73: 15–8 passim.

Man PL, Chuang MY. Acupuncture in methadone withdrawal. *Int J Addict* 1980; 15: 921–926.

Man SC, Baragar FD. Preliminary clinical study of acupuncture in rheumatoid arthritis with painful knees. *Arthr Rheum* 1973; 16: 558–559 (abstract).

Man SC, Baragar FD. Preliminary clinical study of acupuncture in rheumatoid arthritis. *J Rheumatol* 1974; 1: 126–129.

Margolin A, Avants SK, Chang P et al. Acupuncture for the treatment of cocaine dependence in methadone-maintained patients. *Amer J Addict* 1993; 2: 194–201.

Mao W, Ghia JN, Scott DS, Duncan GH, Gregg JM. High versus low intensity acupuncture analgesia for treatment of chronic pain: effects on platelet serotonin. *Pain* 1980; 8: 331–342.

Marks NJ, Emery P, Onisiphorou C. A controlled trial of acupuncture in tinnitus. *J Laryngol Otol* 1984; 98: 1103–1109.

Martelete M, Fiori AM. Comparison of acupuncture and placebo in treatment of chronic shoulder pain. *Acupuncture and Electro-Therapeutic Research* 1985; 10: 183–193.

Martin GP, Waite PM. The efficacy of acupuncture as an aid to stopping smoking. *N Z Med J* 1981; 93: 421–423.

Martoudis S, Christofides K. Electroacupuncture for pain relief in labour. *Acupuncture in Med* 1990; 8: 51–53.

Mast R, Schoch T, Scharf HP. Acupuncture against postoperative pain after total knee replacement. A placebo-controlled trial on immediate effects. *Aktuelle Rheumatologie* 1995; 20: 131–134.

Matsumoto T, Levy B, Ambruso V. Clinical evaluation of acupuncture. *Am Surg* 1974; 40: 400–405.

Mazieres B, Frize B, Bayourthe L. Acupuncture treatment of chronic low-back pain: a short-term controlled trial. *Rev Rhum* 1981; 48: 447 (abstract).

McConaghy P, Bland D, Swales H. Acupuncture in the management of postoperative nausea and vomiting in patients receiving morphine via a patient-controlled analgesia system. *Acupuncture in Medicine* 1996; 14: 2–5.

McMillan AS, Nolan A, Kelly PJ. The efficacy of dry needling and procaine in the treatment of myofascial pain in the jaw muscles. *Journal of Orofacial Pain* 1997; 11: 307–314.

Melzack R, Katz J. Auriculotherapy fails to relieve chronic pain: a controlled crossover study. JAMA 1984; 251: 1041–1043.

Mendelson G, Kidson MA, Loh ST, Scott DF, Selwood TS, Kranz H. Acupuncture analgesia for chronic low-back pain. *Clin Exp Neurol* 1978; 15: 182–185.

Mendelson G, Selwood TS, Kranz H, Loh TM, Kidson MA, Scott DS. Acupuncture treatment of low-back pain: a double-blind placebo-controlled trial. *Am J Med* 1983; 74: 49–55.

Mendelson G, Selwood TS, Kranz H, Loh TS, Kidson MA, Scott DS. Acupuncture treatment of chronic back pain. A double-blind placebo-controlled trial. *Am J Med* 1983; 74: 49–55.

Molsberger A, Hille E. The analgesic effect of acupuncture in chronic tennis elbow pain. *Brit J Rheumatol* 1994; 33: 1162–1165.

Moore ME, Berk SN. Acupuncture for chronic shoulder pain. An experimental study with attention to the role of placebo and hypnotic susceptibility. *Ann Intern Med* 1976; 84: 381–384.

Myhal D, Lebel E, Leung CY, Camerlain M. Isotopic evaluation of the effects of acupuncture on the vascularisation of the knee with Tc-99m radioactive albumin. *Union Medicale Du Canada* 1981; 110: 1046–1048.

Naeser MA et al. Real versus sham laser acupuncture and microamps TENS to treat carpal tunnel syndrome and worksite wrist pain: pilot study. *Lasers and Surgical Medicine* 1996; (Supplement 8): 7.

Naeser MA, Alexander MP, Stiassny-Eder D et al. Real versus sham acupuncture in the treatment of paralysis in acute stroke patients: a CT scan lesion site study. *J Neuro Rehab* 1992; 6: 163–173.

Nepp J, Wedrich A, Akramian J, Ries E, Strenn K. The effect of acupuncture in conjunctivitis sicca. First results of a randomised double-blind study. *Spektrum Der Augenheilkunde* 1996; 10: 150–155.

Nepp J, Wedrich A, Akramian J, Derbolav A, Mudrich C, Ries E, Schauersberger J. Dry eye treatment with acupuncture. A prospective, randomized, double-masked study. *Advances in Experimental Medicine and Biology* 1998; 438: 1011–1016.

Newmeyer JA, Johnson G, Klot S. Acupuncture as a detoxification modality. *J Psychoactive Drugs* 1984; 16: 241–261.

Noling LB, Clelland JA, Jackson JR, Knowles CJ. Effect of transcutaneous electrical nerve stimulation at auricular points on experimental cutaneous pain threshold. *Phys Ther* 1988; 68: 328–332.

Oliveri AC, Clelland JA, Jackson J, Knowles C. Effects of auricular transcutaneous electrical nerve stimulation on experimental pain threshold. *Phys Ther* 1986; 66: 12–16.

Otto KC, Quinn C, Sung YF. Auricular acupuncture as an adjunctive treatment for cocaine addiction. A pilot study. *Am J Addict* 1998; 7: 164–170.

Parker LN, Mok MS. The use of acupuncture for smoking withdrawal. *Am J Acupuncture* 1977; 5: 363–366.

Parwatikar SD, Brown MS, Stern JA, et al. Acupuncture, hypnosis and experimental pain. 1. Study with volunteers. *Acupuncture and Electro-Therapeutic Research* 1978; 3: 161–190.

Peng A, Chua V, Karpe H. Smoking cessation utilizing acupuncture and the effect on carboxyhemoglobin. *Acupuncture* 1990; 1: 27–31.

Petrie JP, Hazelman BL. A controlled study of acupuncture in neck pain. *Br J Rheumatol* 1986; 25: 271–275.

Petrie J, Hazelman B. Credibility of placebo transcutaneous nerve stimulation and acupuncture. *American Journal of Acupuncture* 1985; 13: 69–71.

Petrie JP, Langley GB. Acupuncture in the treatment of chronic cervical pain: a pilot study. *Clin Exp Rheumatol* 1983; 1: 333–335.

Pintov S, Lahat E, Alstein M, Vogel Z, Burg J. Acupuncture and the opioid system: implications in management of migraine. *Neurology* 1997; 17: 129–133.

Podoshin L, Ben-David Y, Fradis M, Gerstel R, Felner H. Idiopathic subjective tinnitus treated by biofeedback, acupuncture and drug therapy. *Ear, Nose, and Throat Journal* 1991; 70: 284–289.

Raustia AM. Diagnosis and treatment of temporomandibular joint dysfunction. Advantages of computed tomography diagnosis. Stomatognathic treatment and acupuncture—a randomized trial. *Proceedings of the Finnish Dental Society* 1986; 82 Suppl 9–10: 1–41.

Raustia AM, Pohjola RT. Acupuncture compared with stomatognathic treatment for TMJ dysfunction. Part III: effect of treatment on mobility. *J Prosthet Dent* 1986; 56: 616–623.

Raustia AM, Pohjola RT, Virtanen KK. Acupuncture compared with stomatognathic treatment for TMJ dysfunction. Part I: a randomized study. *J Prosthet Dent* 1985; 54: 581–585.

Richards D, Marley J. Stimulation of auricular acupuncture points in weight loss. *Aust Fam Physician* 1998; 27: S73–77.

Richardson PH, Vincent CA. Acupuncture for the treatment of pain: a review of evaluative research. *Pain* 1986; 24:15–40.

Richter A, Herlitz J, Hjalmarson A. Effect of acupuncture in patients with angina pectoris. *Eur Heart J* 1991; 12: 175–178.

Rogvi-Hansen B, Perrild H, Christensen T, Detmar SE, Siersbaek-Nielsen K, Hansen JE. Acupuncture in the treatment of Graves' ophthalmopathy. A blinded randomized study. *Acta Endocrinologica* 1991; 124: 143–145.

Rutgers MJ, Van RLKJ, Osman PO. A small randomized comparative trial of acupuncture versus transcutaneous electrical neurostimulation in postherpetic neuralgia. *Pain Clinic* 1988; 2: 87–89.

Sallstrom S, Kjendahl A, Osten PE et al. Acupuncture in the treatment of stroke patients in the subacute stage: a randomized, controlled study. *Compl Ther Med* 1996; 4: 193–197.

Sallstrom S, Kjendahl A, Osten PE, Stanghelle JK, Borchgrevink CF. Acupuncture therapy in stroke during the subacute phase. A randomized controlled trial. *Tidsskrift For Den Norske Laegeforening* 1995; 115: 2884–2887.

Sanchez-Araujo M, Puchi A. Acupuncture enhances the efficacy of antibiotics treatment for canine otitis crises. *Acupunct Electrother Res* 1997; 22: 191–206.

Schwager KL, Baines DB, Meyer RJ. Acupuncture and postoperative vomiting in day-stay paediatric patients. *Anaesthesia and Intensive Care* 1996; 24: 674–677.

Shen AC, Whitehouse MJ, Powers TR. A pilot study of the effects of acupuncture in rheumatoid arthritis [abstract]. *Arthr Rheum* 1973; 16: 569–570.

Shlay JC, Chaloner K, Max MB et al. Acupuncture and Amitriptyline for Pain Due to HIV-Related Peripheral Neuropathy: A Randomized Controlled Trial. *J Amer Med Assoc* 1998; 280: 1590–1595.

Sodipo JOA. Transcutaneous electrial nerve stimulation (TENS) and acupuncture: comparison of therapy for low-back pain. *Pain* 1981; Suppl 1: S277 (abstract).

Spacek A, Huemer G, Grubhofer G, Lackner FX, Zwolfer W, Kress HG. The use of ear acupuncture (P29-PAD, Occiput) in the case of a drop in blood pressure following the administration of Theiopental. *Deutsche Zeitschrift Für Akupunktur* 1996; 39: 18–22.

Stacher G, Wancura I, Bauer P, Lahoda R, Schulze D. Effect of acupuncture of pain threshold and pain tolerance determined by electrical stimulation of the skin: a controlled study. *Am J Chin Med* 1975; 3: 143–149.

Steiner RP, Hay DL, Davis AW. Acupuncture therapy for the treatment of tobacco smoking addiction. *Am J Chin Med* 1982; 10: 107–121.

Steins A, Junger M, Rosch G, Mohrle M, Blum A, Lorenz F, Klyscz T, Hahn M. Efficiency of acupuncture in acral circulatory disturbances. *Phlebologie* 1996; 25: 139–143.

Steiss JE, White NA, Bowen JM. Electroacupuncture in the treatment of chronic lameness in horses and ponies: a controlled clinical trial. *Can J Vet Res* 1989; 53: 239–243.

Stewart D, Thomson J, Oswald I. Acupuncture analgesia: an experimental investigation. *Br Med J* 1977; 1: 67–70.

Strom H. Controlled triple-blind investigation of the effect of electro–ear acupuncture on movement and pain in the knee after meniscectomy. *Ugeskrift for Loeger* 1977; 139: 2326–2329.

Stux G. Migraine treatment with acupuncture. *Acupuncture* 1990; 1: 16–18.

Sung YF, Kutner MH, Cerine FC, Frederickson EL. Comparison of the effects of acupuncture and codeine on postoperative dental pain. *Anesth Analg* 1977; 56: 473–478.

Takeda W, Wessel J. Acupuncture for the treatment of pain of osteoarthritic knees. *Arthritis Care Research* 1994; 7: 118–122.

Takishima T, Mue S, Tamura G, Ishihara T, Watanabe K. The bronchodilating effect of acupuncture in patients with acute asthma. *Ann Allergy* 1982; 48: 44–49.

Tandon MK, Soh PF. Comparison of real and placebo acupuncture in histamine-induced asthma. A double-blind crossover study. *Chest* 1989; 96: 102–105.

Tandon MK, Soh PF, Wood AT. Acupuncture for bronchial asthma? A double-blind crossover study. *Med J Aust* 1991; 154: 409–412.

Tashkin DP, Bresler DE, Kroening RJ, Kerschner H, Katz RL, Coulson A. Comparison of real and simulated acupuncture and isoproterenol in methacholine-induced asthma. *Ann Allergy* 1977; 39: 379–387.

Tashkin DP, Kroening RJ, Bresler DE, Simmons M, Coulson AH, Kerschnar H. A controlled trial of real and simulated acupuncture in the management of chronic asthma. *J Allergy Clin Immunol* 1985; 76: 855–864.

Taub HA, Mitchell JN, Stuber FE, Eisenberg L, Beard MC, McCormack RK. Analgesia for operative dentistry: a comparison of acupuncture and placebo. *Oral Surg Oral Med Oral Pathol* 1979; 48: 205–210.

Tavola T, Gala C, Conte G, Invernizzi G. Traditional Chinese acupuncture in tension-type headache: a controlled study. *Pain* 1992; 48: 325–329.

Teng C, Liu T, Chang W. Effect of acupuncture and physical therapy in the management of cervical spondylosis. *Arch Phys Med Rehabil* 1973; 54: 601.

Ternov K, Nilsson M, Lofberg L. Acupuncture for pain relief during childbirth. *Acupunct Electrother Res* 1998; 23: 19–26.

Thomas M, Eriksson SV, Lundeberg T. A comparative study of diazepam and acupuncture in patients with osteoarthritis pain: a placebo controlled study. *Am J Chin Med* 1991; 19: 95–100.

Thomas M, Lundberg T. Importance of modes of acupuncture in the treatment of chronic nonciceptive low-back pain. *Acta Anaesthesiol Scand* 1994; 38: 63–69.

Thomas M, Lundeberg T, Bjork G, Lundstrom-Lindstedt V. Pain and discomfort in primary dysmenorrhea is reduced by preemptive acupuncture or low frequency TENS. *European Journal of Physical Medicine and Rehabilitation* 1995; 5: 71–76.

Tougas G, Yuan LY, Radamaker JW, Chiverton SG, Hunt RH. Effect of acupuncture on gastric acid secretion in healthy male volunteers. *Digestive Diseases and Sciences* 1992; 37: 1576–1582.

Toyama PM. Acupuncture induced mood changes reversed by the narcotic antagonist nalaxone. *J Holistic Med* 1981; 3: 46–52.

Toyama PM, Popell C, Evans J, Heyder C. Beta-endorphin and cortisol measurements following acupuncture and moxibustion. *J Holistic Med* 1982; 9: 58–67.

Uskok M, D'Aquila MG, Buscaglia G, Porro B, Mereto N, Gastaldo P, Launo C. Acupuncture versus diazepam as premedication in gynecological surgery. *Gazzetta Medica Italiana Archivio Per Le Scienze Mediche* 1995; 154: 97–100.

Vandevenne A, Rempp M, Burghard G, et al. Study of the specific contribution of acupuncture to tobacco detoxification. *Semaine Des Hopitaux* 1985; 61: 2155–2160.

Vilholm OJ, Moller K, Jorgensen K. Effect of traditional Chinese acupuncture on severe tinnitus: a double-blind, placebo-controlled, clinical investigation with open therapeutic control. *British Journal of Audiology* 1998; 32: 197–204.

Vincent CA. A controlled trial of the treatment of migraine by acupuncture. *Clin J Pain* 1989; 5: 305–312.

Vincent CA. The treatment of tension headache by acupuncture: a controlled single case design with time series analysis. *Journal of Psychosomatic Research* 1990; 34: 553–561.

Virsik K, Kristufek P, Bangha O, Urban S. The effect of acupuncture on pulmonary function in bronchial asthma. *Prog Respir Res* 1980; 14: 271–275.

Wang B, Tang J, White PF, Naruse R, Sloninsky A, Kariger R, Gold J, Wender RH. Effect of the intensity of transcutaneous acupoint electrical stimulation on the postoperative analgesic requirement. *Anesthesia and Analgesia* 1997; 85: 406–413.

Wang HH, Chang YH, Liu DM. A study in the effectiveness of acupuncture analgesia for cononscopic examination compared with conventional premedication. *Amer J Acupunct* 1992; 20: 217–221.

Warwick-Evans LA, Masters IJ, Redstone SB. A double-blind placebo controlled evaluation of acupressure in the treatment of motion sickness. *Aviation Space and Environmental Medicine* 1991; 62: 776–778.

Washburn AM, Fullilove RE, Fullilove MT, Keenan PA, McGee B, Morris KA, Sorensen JL, Clark WW. Acupuncture heroin detoxification: a single-blind clinical trial. *Journal of Substance Abuse Treatment* 1993; 10: 345–351.

Waylonis GW, Wilke S, O'Toole D, Waylonis DA, Waylonis DB. Chronic myofascial pain: management by low-output helium-neon laser therapy. *Arch Phys Med Rehabil* 1988; 69: 1017–1020.

Weightman WM, Zacharias M, Herbison P. Traditional Chinese acupuncture as an antiemetic. *Br Med J* [Clin Res] 1987; 295: 1379–1380.

Weinschutz TK, Niederberger U. Relevance of acupuncture in migraine therapy. *Nervenheilkunde* 1995; 14: 295–301.

Weintraub M, Petursson S, Schwartz M. Acupuncture in musculoskeletal pain: methodology and results in a double-blind controlled clinical trial. *Clin Pharmacol Ther* 1975; 248 (abstract).

Wells EA, Jackson R, Diaz OR, Stanton V, Saxon AJ, Krupski A. Acupuncture as an adjunct to methadone treatment services. *American Journal on Addictions* 1995; 4: 198–214.

Wen HL, Teo SW. Experience in the treatment of drug addiction by electroacupuncture. *Modern Med Asia* 1980; 15: 921–926.

Williams T, Mueller K, Cornwall MW. Effect of acupuncture-point stimulation on diastolic blood pressure in hypertensive subjects' a preliminary study. *Phys Ther* 1991; 71: 523–529.

White AR, Eddleston C, Hardie R, Resch KL, Ernst E. A pilot study of acupuncture for tension headache, using a novel placebo. *Acupuncture in Medicine* 1996; 14: 11–15.

Williamson L, Yudkin P, Livingstone R, Prasad K, Fuller A, Lawrence M. Hay fever treatment in general practice: a randomised controlled trial comparing standardised Western acupuncture with sham acupuncture. *Acupuncture in Medicine* 1996; 14: 6–10.

Winyuan W, Be L. Therapeutic effect of acupuncture at Zhonping point for periarthritis of the shoulder. *Acupuncture* 1990; 1: 13–15.

Wong AMK et al. Clinical trial of electrical acupuncture on hemophlegic stroke patients. *American Journal of Physical Medicine* 1999; 78: 117–122.

Worner TM, Zeller B, Schwarz H, Zwas F, Lyon D. Acupuncture fails to improve treatment outcome in alcoholics. *Drug and Alcohol Dependence* 1992; 30: 169–173.

Wu B, Zhou RX, Zhou MS. Effect of acupuncture on immunomodulation in patients with malignant tumors. *Chung-Kuo Chung Hsi I Chieh Ho Tsa Chih* 1996; 16: 139–141.

Wyon Y, Lindgren R, Hammar M, Lundeberg T. Acupuncture against climacteric disorders? Lower number of symptoms after menopause. *Lakartidningen* 1994; 91: 2318–2322.

Wyon Y, Lindgren R, Lundeberg T et al. Effects of acupuncture on climacteric vasomotor symptoms, quality of life, and urinary excretion of neutropeptides among postmenopausal women. *Menopause* 1995; 2: 3–12.

Xinsheng L, Hairui S. Clinical comparison of the acupuncture treatment of cerebral palsy with standard and 'special points' of the scalp. *American Journal of Acupuncture* 1994; 22: 215–219.

Yang LC, Jawan B, Chen CN, Ho RT, Chang KA, Lee JH. Comparison of P6 acupoint injection with 50% glucose in water and intravenous droperidol for prevention of vomiting after gynecological laparoscopy. *Acta Anaesthesiologica Scandinavica* 1993; 37: 192–194.

Yang X, Liu X, Juo H et al. Clinical observation on needling extrachannel points in treating mental depression. *J Trad Chin Med* 1994; 14: 14–18.

Yentis SM, Bissonnette B. Ineffectiveness of acupuncture and droperidol in preventing vomiting following strabismus repair in children. *Canadian Journal of Anaesthesia* 1992; 39: 151–154.

Ying YK, Lin JT, Robins J. Acupuncture for the induction of cervical dilatation in preparation for first-trimester abortion and its influence on HCG. *J Reprod Med* 1985; 30: 530–534.

Young MF, McCarthy PW. Effect of acupuncture stimulation of the auricular sympathetic point on evoked sudomotor response. *Journal of Alternative Complementary Medicine* 1998; 4: 29–38.

Yu DYC, Lee SP. Effect of acupuncture on bronchial asthma. *Clin Sci Molec Med* 1976; 51: 503–509.

Zamotrinsky A, Afanasiev S, Karpov RS, Cherniavsky A. Effects of electrostimulation of the vagus afferent endings in patients with coronary artery disease. *Coronary Artery Disease* 1997 8: 551–557.

Zhang AR, Pan ZW, Lou F. Effect of acupuncturing houxi and shenmen in treating cerebral traumatic dementia. *Chung Kuo Chung Hsi I Chieh Ho Tsa Chih* 1995; 15: 519–521.

APPENDIX F

THE FIVE PHASES
(*Wu Xing*)*

The theory of the Five Phases is an attempt to classify phenomena in terms of five quintessential processes, represented by the emblems Wood, Fire, Earth, Metal, and Water. Its place in Chinese medicine and other Chinese intellectual pursuits has been misunderstood ever since the first Occidentals tried to explain Chinese natural philosophy to the West over 300 years ago. During this century, the academic world has made some advances toward a better appreciation of the Five Phases theory.[1]

The Five Phases are not in any way ultimate constituents of matter. This misconception has long been embodied in the common mistranslation "Five Elements" and exemplifies the problems that arise from looking at things Chinese with a Western frame of reference. The Chinese term that we translate as "Five Phases" is *wu xing*. *Wu* is the number five, and *xing* means "walk" or "move," and, perhaps most pertinently, it implies a process. The *wu xing*, therefore, are five kinds of processes; hence the Five Phases, and not the Five Elements. The theory of Phases is a system of correspondences and patterns that subsume events and things, especially in relationship to their dynamics.

More specifically, each Phase is an emblem that denotes a category of related functions and qualities. The Phase called Wood is associated with

---

*This appendix was written in collaboration with Dan Bensky and the assistance of Kiiko Matsumoto.

active functions that are in a growing phase. Fire designates functions that have reached a maximal state of activity and are about to begin a decline or a resting period. Metal represents functions in a declining state. Water represents functions that have reached a maximal state of rest and are about to change the direction of their activity. Finally, Earth designates balance or neutrality; in a sense, Earth is a buffer between the other Phases. In the sense that the Phases correlate observable phenomena of human life into images derived from the macrocosm, they serve a similar function as that of elements in other medical systems.

In more concrete terms, the Five Phases can be used to describe the annual cycle in terms of biological growth and development. Wood corresponds to spring, Fire to summer, Metal to autumn, and Water to winter. And what of Earth? Earth may represent the transition between each season (and it is commonly used to represent "Indian summer"). These correlations, as diagramed in Figure 49, are known as the Mutual Production order of the Five Phases. They represent the way in which the Five Phases interact and arise out of one another in the typical yearly cycle. There are thirty-six mathematically possible orders in which the Five Phases can be arranged, but only a few of them are actually used either in medicine or in other disciplines.

FIGURE 49   *Mutual Production Order of the Five Phases*

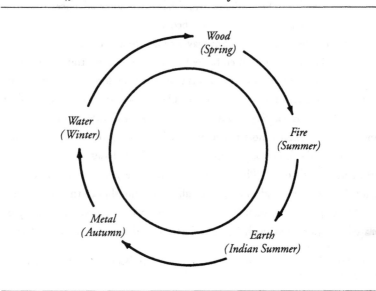

The application of the Five Phases to seasonable growth is only one example of how the system was used. In time, the five generic categories were used for classifying many more perceptions, from colors, sounds, odors, and taste sensations to emotions, animals, dynasties, the planets, and ultimately everything in the universe. (See Table 30.) Correlations were also made between the Phases and various Organs and anatomical regions, which is how the connection between the Phases and medicine came about.[2]

TABLE 30 *Five Phases Correspondences*

	WOOD	FIRE	EARTH	METAL	WATER
Direction	east	south	center	west	north
Color	blue-green	red	yellow	white	black
Climate	windy	hot	damp	dry	cold
Human Sound	shouting	laughing	singing	weeping	groaning
Emotion	anger	elation	pensive-ness	grief	fear
Taste	sour	bitter	sweet	pungent	salty
Yin Organ	Liver	Heart	Spleen	Lungs	Kidney
Yang Organ	Gall Bladder	Small Intestine	Stomach	Large Intestine	Bladder
Orifice	eyes	tongue	mouth	nose	ears
Tissue	tendons	blood vessels	flesh	skin	bones
Smell	goatish	burning	fragrant	rank	rotten
Spirit	Hun	Spirit	Yi	Po	will
Virtue	human kindness	propriety	faithful-ness	righteous-ness	wisdom

Before exploring the use of Five Phases theory in medicine, it is helpful to consider its history and relationship to Yin-Yang thinking. While Yin-Yang theory stretches back into China's remote antiquity, Five Phases theory was not documented until the fourth century B.C.E.[3] It is nevertheless reasonable to assume that a scheme as complex as the Five Phases theory did not emerge spontaneously. The framework must have been gestating for some time. Some intimation of the Five Phases can be found in many writings of the period from about 500 B.C.E. to 200 B.C.E., which was a time of great intellectual, political, and social ferment in China.[4] The Five Phases theory was first systematized by Zou Yen (approximately 350 B.C.E. to 270 B.C.E.) and his followers.[5] The original emphasis of the theory was as much political as it was scientific. The correct timing of rites and the succession of dynasties came to be interpreted through the dynamics of the Phases, which were then called the Five Virtues or Powers. As Joseph Needham comments, "there were intense and anxious debates about the proper color, musical notes and instruments, sacrifices, etc. [according to Five Phases], appropriate to a particular dynasty or emperor."[6]

The number five was important in the numerology of the period, particularly for classifications of Earthly things. Various other numbers, such as six, four, and three, turn up in early classification schemes for things pertaining to Heaven.[7] It is difficult to determine whether the importance of the number five led to Five Phases theory or the popularity of the Five Phases theory led to things being classified in fives.

During the third and fourth centuries B.C.E., the Five Phases theory and the Yin-Yang theory existed simultaneously and independently of each other.[8] For example, Lao Tzu and Chuang Tzu refer extensively to Yin and Yang but do not mention the Five Phases. Unlike other traditional cultures with systems of elemental correspondences (e.g., the Greek Four Elements or the Hindu Three Doshas), the Chinese thus had two systems of referents. It was not until the Han dynasty, a period of great eclecticism and synthesis, that the two systems began to merge in Chinese medicine. "The five elements [Phases] [which] had not been part of the most ancient Chinese medical speculations" were incorporated into the clinical tradition that culminated in the *Nei Jing*.[9] Certain parts of the *Nei Jing* refer to the Five Phases, while others do not. Yet other texts, such as the Discussion of Cold-Induced Disorders (the main early herbal text) and the biography of Bian Que in the *Shi Ji* or Historical Records,[10] make no mention whatsoever of Five Phases theory.[11] The Five Phases theory continued to undergo changes even after its incorporation into Chinese medicine. It is not until the Song dynasty (960–1279 C.E.) that the relationships between the Phases were commonly used to explain the etiology and processes of illness.[12]

Many attempts were made to fit the Five Phases neatly into the Yin-Yang structure. For example, Wood and Fire were considered the Yang Phases, being active in character, while Metal and Water, associated with quiescent functions, were the Yin Phases. Earth was the balance point between Yin and Yang. Yet, despite this apparently successful marriage between Five Phases and Yin-Yang theory, the two systems of correspondence frequently yielded different interpretations of health and disease.[13] For example, Five Phases theory might emphasize the following correspondences stated in the *Nei Jing*: The Liver opens into the eyes; the Kidney opens into the ears; the Heart opens into the tongue. Disorder in a particular orifice would necessarily be linked to its corresponding Organ. Yin-Yang theory, on the other hand, might emphasize the following quite different assertions of the *Nei Jing*: The pure Qi of all Organs is reflected in the eyes; all the Meridians meet in the ears; the tongue is connected to most of the Meridians. Yin-Yang theory would not necessarily see a link between a part and a part. Rather, all disharmonies of the eyes, ears, or tongue would be interpreted in terms of patterns. Thus, an eye disorder could be part of a Liver disharmony or perhaps a Lung, Kidney, or Spleen disharmony, depending on the configuration of other signs. The differences between these medical interpretations stem from the fact that Five Phases theory emphasizes one-to-one correspondences, while Yin-Yang theory emphasizes the need to understand the overall configuration upon which the part depends.

⊣ USE OF THE FIVE PHASES IN MEDICINE

At the bottom line, the Five Phases theory is a crucial emblem system used to discuss and represent clinical phenomena. In fact, one could have written this entire book from a Five Phases perspective. If this had been done then Earth would correspond to Spleen, Qi, Dampness, worry, Consciousness of Possibilities, and faithfulness; wood would correspond to Liver, Blood, wind, Non-Corporeal Soul, and human kindness; water would correspond to Kidneys, Essence, Cold, fear, and the Will; fire would correspond to Heart, warmth, elation, Heart Spirit, and propriety; and metal would correspond to Lungs, Fluids, dryness, Corporeal Soul, and righteousness. Much of what was presented would have fallen into place. Few practitioners would agree with these relationships, but in some situations the correspondence could be forced and be more metaphysical than practical.

To be valuable, the Five Phases theory requires flexibility and sensitivity. Distinguishing between useful and not useful correspondences can be difficult, and practitioners can disagree. For example, some practitioners are happy with such correspondence as those of plants and grains; others are not. Odors are excluded from many lists,[14] but a number of practitioners feel that they are clinically quite useful.[15] The correspondences that are in general use in medicine are listed in Table 30. The medically useful correspondences can be divided into two groups. There are those that make metaphysical sense in the Chinese mode of thought, or are construed to have associations outside the body (often forced associations). And there are correspondences derived not from metaphysical premises, but from the functions of the Organs or from empirical observation. The best example of the former is color: green for Wood (trees), red for Fire, yellow for Earth (the soil of northern China, where these correspondences originated, is yellow), white for Metal (silvery luster), and black for Water (the inky depths of the ocean). Similar explanations, however strained, are available for the seasons, climatic conditions, directions, tastes, and smells. An example of the latter type of correspondence is that between Metal and the nose. The nose has no actual relationship with Metal, and such a relationship was never posited by the ancient Chinese. The nose is, however, the opening most often affected by diseases of the Lungs, and in Chinese physiology the nasal tract is considered an extension of the Lungs. Because the Lungs are associated with Metal, the nose is also given that association. Similarly, the association of anger with the Liver is probably due to careful observation of people, rather than to any notion of the "woodenness" of becoming enraged. The distinctions between the two types of correspondence is important in explaining the dynamic behind the diagnostic use of the Five Phases theory, and also gives perspective on the whole system.

Chinese medicine has had to creatively adapt the Five Phases theory in order to fit it to actual medical experience. The physiology that grew out of Five Phases theory, for example, is not always identical with Eight Principal physiology. The Eight Principal tradition is based on empirical observation and is intimately connected to Yin-Yang theory, concentrating on the functions of the Organs and extrapolating their interrelationships from their functions. The Organs are thus the key to the system. Five Phases theory does not always agree with this understanding, and in that case, it is simply ignored.[16] For example, in Five Phases physiology, the Heart corresponds to Fire. Traditional

Chinese texts, however, consider the Kidneys (Life Gate Fire) to be the physiological basis for the Fire (Yang) of the other Organs. And so, the Five Phases theory's formal correspondence would be conveniently forgotten.

The Five Phases correspondence is often a convenient way to organize significant clinical reality. Let us take facial color correspondence, delineated in Table 30, as an example. A yellow complexion often appears in a Spleen disharmony (yellow and Spleen are both associated with Earth), and a darkish complexion often appears in a Kidney disharmony (black and Kidneys are associated with water). A red face, however, although it can be part of a Heart pattern, is just as likely to be part of the Heat pattern of any Organ. A white face can appear with Lung disharmonies, but can also be part of the Cold pattern of any Organ. A blue-green complexion, while often part of a Liver disharmony, might as easily be part of a Congealed Heart Blood pattern. The correspondences of climate work much the same way. Although it is true that the Spleen is especially sensitive to Dampness, the Kidney to Cold, the Lungs to Dryness, and the Liver to Wind, Dryness does not necessarily imply a Lung disharmony, for it can easily affect the Stomach, Intestines, or Heart. Coldness does not necessarily imply the Kidneys, because the Spleen, Lungs, and Heart can also be affected by Cold. And so on. The Five Phases correspondence can be helpful as a guide to clinical tendencies, but the test of veracity in Chinese medicine remains the pattern. Pattern thinking overrules all formal rules. The flexibility of Yin-Yang theory, including Five Phases, resides in its insistence that all correspondences finally depend on the configuration of a unique whole.

The Five Phases are often used to describe clinical processes and relationships and to help in the conceptualization of proper treatments. It is an explanatory theory and is not meant as a binding doctrine. For example, as has been shown (see Figure 49), the Five Phases can be used to describe the general processes that take place during the annual cycle. That sequence—the Mutual Production order of Wood, Fire, Earth, Metal, Water—describes normal generative functions. In the sequence, the producer is called the Mother and the produced, the Child (an example of the tendency toward concreteness in traditional Chinese thought). Some patterns of disharmony can be explained by reference to the Mutual Production order, especially patterns of Deficiency.

The Child of a Deficient Mother, for instance, becomes Deficient for want of proper nourishment. Conversely, when the child is Deficient, it may "steal the Qi" of the Mother, making it Deficient as well. If an Organ is Deficient, therefore, treatment can be affected by strengthening the Mother Organ. When there is an Excess in an Organ, the Child can be drained. The concept of treatment is important in acupuncture, but is seldom used in herbal medicine.[17]

Another sequence is known as the Mutual Checking or Mutual Control order. In this sequence, each Phase is said to check or control the succeeding Phase (see Figure 50). The Control order, like the Mutual Production order, describes naturally occurring phenomena, and it works to ensure that the Mutual Production order does not overgenerate and cause imbalances. A disharmony within the Control order might mean that an Organ is exerting Excess control over the Organ that it regulates. This would lead to a Deficiency in the regulated Organ. Or the Organ that should be regulated may become the regulator. Other situations can arise, but these two are the most likely. The former imbalance is known as an insulting cycle, and the latter as a humiliation cycle. Some common disharmonies of Five Phases patterns are summarized in Tables 31 and 32.[18] (Some of the examples may seem to contradict the presentation elsewhere in this book, or even to contradict Five Phases theory itself. In other words, one needs to have a sense of when to apply or not apply a rigid form of Five Phases.)

FIGURE 50   *Mutual Control Order of the Five Phases*

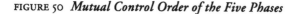

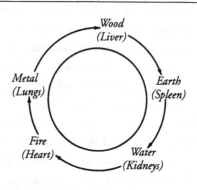

TABLE 31 *Disharmonies of the Mutual Production Cycle*

Description	Symptoms and Signs	Physiological Correlation
Wood not producing Fire		
Liver (Wood) Blood not nourishing Heart (Fire)	weakness; timidity; palpitations; poor memory; insomnia; thin or choppy pulse	general Deficient Blood pattern
Fire not producing Earth		
Heart (Fire) unable to warm Spleen (Earth)	aversion to cold; cold limbs; distended abdomen; diarrhea; edema	Kidney Yang unable to warm Spleen Yang
Earth not producing Metal		
Spleen (Earth) unable to nourish Lungs (Metal)	phlegm; cough; fatigue; empty pulse	Deficient Spleen producing Excess Mucus in Lungs (actually the reverse of the classic Five Phases relationship)
Metal not producing Water		
Lungs (Metal) not sending Water to Kidney (Water)	shortness of breath; thirst; scanty, dark urine; weak knees; sore lower back; other Deficient Yin	Deficient Kidney Yin
Water not producing Wood		
Kidney (Water) not nourishing Liver (Wood) Essence	tinnitius; low back pain; weak knees; vertigo; tremors; emaciation	Kidney Yin not nourishing Liver

TABLE 32 *Disharmonies of the Mutual Control Cycle*

DESCRIPTION	SYMPTOMS AND SIGNS	PHYSIOLOGICAL CORRELATION
Wood insults Earth		
Liver (Wood)Qi excessively Controls Spleen (Earth)	painful flanks; headache; distention; sore eyes; passing of gas (Excess Liver)with lack of appetite; diarrhea; lassitude (Deficient Spleen)	Liver Invading Spleen
Fire humiliated by-Metal		
Heart (Fire)Yang unable to control Lung (Metal) Fluids	frequent urination; palpitations; insomnia; shortness of breath	Deficient Heart Yang and Deficient Lung Qi
Earth's control of Wate not adjusted		
Spleen (Earth) insults Kidney (Water)	dry mouth and lips; thin, rapid pulse; constipation	Heat Pernicious Influence Injuring Yin (especially of Stomach)
Spleen (Earth) humiliated by Kidney (Water)	edema and other Deficient Kidney signs	Deficient Spleen Yang and Deficient Kidney Yang
Metal humiliated by Wood		
Lungs (Metal) unable to control Liver (Wood)	painful flanks; bitter taste in mouth; cough; irritability; wiry pulse	Liver Invading Lungs
Water humiliated by Fire		
Kidney (Water) unable to control Heart (Fire) Yang	spermatorrhea; lumbago; irritability; insomnia; red tongue; thin and rapid pulse	Deficient Kidney Yin and Deficient Heart Yin (also called "Heart and Kidney Unable to Communicate")

CRITICISM OF FIVE PHASES THEORY

The Five Phases theory has been the subject of criticism ever since its invention. The challenges to its veracity and practicality date as far back as Mohist contemporaries of Zou Yen (fourth century B.C.E.). For example, one comment on the Mutual Control order reads: "Quite apart (from any cycle) Fire naturally melts Metal, if there is enough Fire. Or Metal may pulverize a burning Fire to cinders, if there is enough Metal. Metal will store Water (but does not produce it). Fire attaches itself to Wood (but is not produced from it)."[19]

A few hundred years later, the great Han dynasty scientist and skeptic Wang Cong satirized the results of literal application of the Five Phases theory. Here are two short excerpts from his work:

The body of a man harbors the Qi of the Five Phases, and therefore (so it is said) he practices the Five Virtues, which are the Tao (Way) of the Phases. So long as he has the five inner Organs within his body, the Qi of the Five Phases are in order. Yet according to the theory, animals prey upon and destroy one another because they embody the several Qi of the Five Phases; therefore the body of a man with the five inner Organs within it ought to be the scene of internecine strife, and the heart of a man living a righteous life be lacerated with discord. But where is there any proof that the Phases do fight and harm each other, or that animals overcome one another in accordance with this?

The horse is connected with the sign wu *(Fire); the rat with the sign* zi *(Water). If Water really controls Fire, (it would be more convincing if) rats normally attacked horses and drove them away.*[20]

Despite such early criticism, the Five Phases theory became an important framework in Chinese medicine. One reason for this is that Chinese investigative study tends to be inductive only to a point and then proceeds with deductions based on the classics.[21] The Five Phases theory thus served as an orthodox reference for numerous speculative deductions.

Another major criticism, and a primary difficulty in the application of the Five Phases theory to medicine, is its lack of consistency. To fit the theory to reality, the referents of the Phases and the relationships between them have continually been changed. The results of such correction can be seen in Tables 31 and 32 on the clinical use of the Five Phases.

Such a problem exists in all traditional systems of elemental correspondence.[22] The original classical Greek formulation by Empedocles of Agrigentum (c. 504–433 B.C.E.) is a system in which the basic elements of fire, earth, water, and air were considered the ultimate constituents of matter and were associated with various other categories of four such as the four fundamental qualities and the four humors. All varieties and changes in the world were associated with different mixtures of the four elements. Figure 51 is a schematic representation of this theory.[23]

When they tried to apply this theory to empirical observations, however, the Greek natural philosophers and physicians had to change an element or add one, or just ignore the theory. Likewise, for the Chinese, Five Phase theory was interpreted in the framework of Yin and Yang: all rigidness and dogma was

FIGURE 51   *Greek System of the Four Elements*

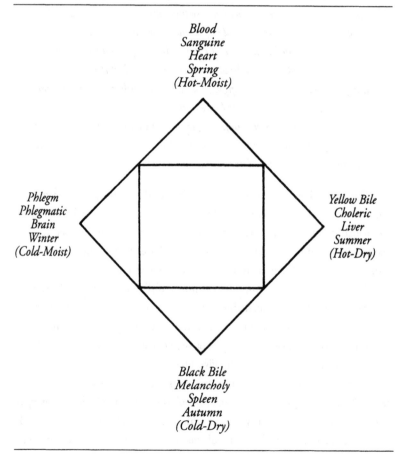

Blood
Sanguine
Heart
Spring
(Hot-Moist)

Phlegm
Phlegmatic
Brain
Winter
(Cold-Moist)

Yellow Bile
Choleric
Liver
Summer
(Hot-Dry)

Black Bile
Melancholy
Spleen
Autumn
(Cold-Dry)

subordinated to context and particularity. Some practitioners, especially in Korea, Japan, and parts of the West, have creatively emphasized the Five Phases Theory and made it the cornerstone of a rich and insightful clinical practice. And, just as important, all East Asian physicians recognize Five Phases as an important vocabulary in their semantic network, theoretical perspective, and clinical practice.

NOTES

1. While their approaches are too academic for the purpose of understanding the Five Phases in relationship to clinical medicine, both Joseph Needham in *Science and Civilization*, vol. 2, pp. 243–268, and Manfred Porkert in *Theoretical Foundations*, pp. 43–44, do an excellent job of explaining Five Phases theory.

2. In the early periods of Chinese history there were many Five Phases correspondence schemes altogether different from the one predominantly used in the *Nei Jing* and reflected in Table 30. Masao Maruyama, in a fascinating essay written in Japanese, describes several of these alternative schemes. For example, there is a compilation of philosophical theories prepared for the Prince of Huai-nan (known as the *Huai-nan-zi*) in the second century B.C.E., in which correspondences of Wood to the Spleen, Fire to the Lungs, Earth to the Heart, Metal to the Liver, and Water to the Kidneys appeared. The other correspondences are also different. The fact that various systems existed confirms the impression that Five Phases theory is a somewhat arbitrary and mechanical network of correspondences. See Masao Maruyama, *Studies of the Classics of Acupuncture Medicine* (*Shinkyu igaku no koten to kenkyu* [Osaka: Sogen Publishers, 1952]), pp. 15–25.

    Alternative and contradictory correspondences can be found even in the early medical texts. Perhaps they are remnants of prior schema or perhaps they recognize clinical realities. For example, in parts of the *Nei Jing*, fear corresponds to Deficient Liver Qi instead of to the Kidneys, and grief corresponds to Deficient Heart Qi instead of to the Lungs (*Su Wen*, sec. 2, chap. 8, p. 86). Another example is the three different correspondence schemas for the five tastes in *Su Wen*, chaps. 22 and 23, and *Ling Shu*, chap. 63.

    Such discrepancy in the formative period of philosophic speculative medical systems is universal. For example, the Hippocratic corpus has several versions of the four humors. In the *Nature of Man*, the later orthodox version appears: phlegm, blood, yellow bile, and black bile. In *Diseases IV*, they are phlegm, blood, bile, and water; while *Ancient Medicine* assumes an unlimited number of humors.

3. Needham, *Science and Civilization*, vol. 2, p. 242.

4. Jia De-dao, *Concise History* [95], p. 29.

5. Needham, *Science and Civilization*, vol. 2, p. 232.

6. Needham, *Grand Titration*, p. 231.

7. Jia De-dao, *Concise History*, pp. 29–30. For example, Lü's Spring and Autumn Annals (246–237 B.C.E.) mentions Four Phases, omitting Earth.

8. Fung Yu-lan, *History of Chinese Philosophy*, vol. I, p. 8; Chan, *Chinese Philosophy*, p. 224; Hans Agren, "Patterns of Tradition and Modernization in Contemporary Chinese Medicine," in *Medicine in Chinese Cultures: Comparative Studies of Health Care in Chinese and other Societies*, ed. by Arthur Kleinman et al. (Washington, D.C.: John E. Fogarty International Center, U.S. Dept. of HEW, NIH, 1975), p. 38.

9. Lu Gwei-djen and Joseph Needham, "Records of Diseases in Ancient China," *American Journal of Chinese Medicine 4*, no. 1 (1976): 12.

10. Dan Bensky, "The Biography of Bian Que in the *Shi Ji*," unpublished manuscript, University of Michigan, 1978, p. 2.

11. Recent archeological discoveries of pre–*Nei Jing* texts confirm the impression that Yin-Yang was originally a much more important part of Chinese medicine than the Five Phases theory. See "A Simple Introduction to Four Ancient Lost Medical Texts Found at the Tomb of Ma-wang," Medical History Text Research Group of the Academy of Traditional Medicine, *Wen Wu*, no. 6 (1975), pp. 16–19. The Five Phases are not mentioned in these ancient medical writings. See footnote 17.

12. Jia De-dao, *Concise History*, pp. 165–166.

13. Porkert, *Theoretical Foundations*, p. 118. Traditional Chinese thought has a general tendency to reconcile and harmonize different or even mutually exclusive ideas in an arbitrary syncretism. Contrary doctrines—for instance, Taoism and Confucianism—are asserted to be mutually complementary. Nakamura's discussion of this Chinese characteristic states: "What stands out in this sort of reasoning is a certain sort of utilitarianism and early compromise, with cold logical considerations completely abandoned." Hajime Nakamura, *Ways of Thinking of Eastern Peoples* (Honolulu: East-West Center Press, 1969), p. 291.

14. Nanjing Institute, *Introduction to Traditional Chinese Medicine* [50], p. 19; Shanghai Institute, *Foundations* [53], p. 28.

15. Often patients will spontaneously smell a particular odor or exude a particular odor when the corresponding Organ is involved.

16. Qin Bo-wei, Medical Lecture Notes [64], pp. 15–22.

17. Acupuncture points are selected primarily because of their effect on patterns or symptoms. Five Phases theory plays an important role in point selection only in relation to the Five Transporting (*wu-shu*) points on the extremities. Originally, and throughout history, these crucial points (individually known as well, gushing, transporting, transversing, and uniting: *jing, rong, shu, jing, he*) were defined by

their effect on patterns and symptoms (e.g., *Ling Shu*, sec. 1, chap. 1, p. 8; *Nan Jing*, "Difficulty 68," p. 148). The *Nei Jing* introduces a Five Phases connection with the Transporting points by mentioning that the well point of the Yang Meridians corresponds to Metal and the well point of the Yin Meridians corresponds to Wood (*Ling Shu*, sec. 1, chap. 2, pp. 14–28). No other point-Phase connection or therapeutic notion is mentioned in the *Nei Jing*. The *Nan Jing* completes a Five Phases connection with each of the Transporting points in "Difficulty 64" (p. 139), although no clear connection with point selection and therapeutics is made. (There are, however, some vague references in Difficulties 79 and 72.) Not until Gao Wu's famous text of 1529 C.E. is a precise connection made among Phase, Transporting point, and a therapeutic action of tonification or draining (Gao Wu, Gatherings from Eminent Acupuncturists [*Zhen-jiu Ju-ying*], [Shanghai: Shanghai Science and Technology Press, 1978], sec. 2, chap. 9, pp. 154–159). This particular method of Gao Wu's was only one of many he thought suitable for point selection, but nonetheless it became the basis of the rigid late-nineteenth-century Japanese *Nan Jing* school of acupuncture and therefore of the subsequent European emphasis on the Five Phases.

The *Nei Jing*, incidentally, mentions only one Transporting point (*fu-liu*, Kidney 7) as having a tonifying effect, and this mention is not in a Five Phases correspondence context (*Su Wen*, sec. 7, chap. 62, p. 338).

A second early source of this type of Five Phases usage in acupuncture is the famous "Song of Twelve Meridians, Mother-Child Points, and Tonification and Draining." This poem is later than Gao Wu's text and is reprinted in Selected Annotations of Acupuncture Songs and Odes (*Zhen-jiu Ge-fu Xuan-jie*) by Chen Bi-liu et al. (Hong Kong: China Medical Publishers, 1966 [reprint of 1959 Mainland edition]), pp. 213–226.

18. Tables 31 and 32 are based on Qin Bo-wei's discussion in Medical Lecture Notes, pp. 15–22. The chart includes examples of the Five Phases being used in sequences other than those described in the text. Such sequences result from the traditional attempt to make observable Organ disharmony fit into the Five Phases sequence, which is usually an attempt to make theory fit practice. There may also, however, be remnants of other Five Phases arrangements (see note 2). These different versions are explicit in early medical texts. For example, the Five Phases discussion in "Difficulty 75" of the *Nan Jing* indicates that to strengthen the Lungs it is necessary to strengthen the Kidneys instead of the Spleen. This reflects a version of the Five Phases that is different from the common one.

19. Quoted in Needham, *Science and Civilization*, vol. 2, pp. 259–260.

20. Ibid., pp. 265–266. Translation altered by author. Debate on Five Phases continues into modern times. For a discussion on the early-twentieth-century discussion,

see Bridie J. Andrews, *The Making of Modern Chinese Medicine, 1895–1937*, pp. 197–198.

21. Nakamura, *Ways of Thinking of Eastern Peoples*, p. 190.

22. To get a sense of the cultural, psychological, scientific, ideological, religious, and intellectual factors that are involved in a correspondence system, it is worth examining the transition from the Aristotelian system of Four Elements to the Paracelsian Three Elements (*tria prima:* salt, sulfur, and mercury) in sixteenth-century Europe. An interesting discussion appears in Allen G. Dobus, "The Medico-Chemical World of the Paracelsians," in *Changing Perspectives in the History of Science*, ed. by Mikuluas Teich and Robert Young (Dordrecht, Holland, and Boston: D. Reidel Pub. Co., 1973), pp. 88–92.

23. Figure 51 is adapted from Elson J. Garner, *History of Biology* (Minneapolis: Burgess Pub. Co., 1960, 1972), p. 31.

HISTORICAL BIBLIOGRAPHY: LINKS IN THE CHAIN OF TRANSMISSION

A complete list of Chinese medical writings can be found in Catalogue of China's Medical Books, Vols. I and II (*Zhong-guo Yi-xue Shu-mu*), edited by Gang and Hei [Taipei: Wenhai, 1971]. A much shorter version appears in Selected Explanations of Traditional Chinese Medical Terms [33], pp. 480–498. This annotated bibliography is a further condensation. Three versions of the *Nei Jing* are presented first; thereafter the titles are arranged in chronological order, by dynasty. Each entry includes an English translation or rendering of the Chinese title. The kind assistance of Dan Bensky in translating is gratefully acknowledged.

The Nei Jing

Inner Classic of the Yellow Emperor (*Huang-di Nei-jing* 黄帝内经). Includes the Simple Questions (*Su Wen* 素 问) and the Spiritual Axis (*Ling Shu* 灵 枢). The earliest book on Chinese medical theory, known in the tradition, this was probably compiled around 100 B.C.E., but the present version contains material of a much later date (see below). Many sources put the compilation date much earlier, but such dating has more to do with Chinese legend than with history. The *Su Wen* or Simple Questions deals mostly with theoretical concepts and medical cosmology, while the *Ling Shu* or Spiritual Axis is primarily concerned with acupuncture and moxibustion.

Inner Classic of the Yellow Emperor: Great Simplicity (*Huang-di Nei-jing Tai-su* 黄 帝 内 经 太 素), 605–617 c.e., edited by Yang Shang-shan. Of the thirty original chapters, twenty-three are extant. This is the earliest available edition of the *Nei Jing*. It is similar to the *Su Wen* but is without the *Su Wen's* additions.

Revised and Annotated Inner Classic of the Yellow Emperor: Simple Questions (*Chong-guang Bu-zhu Huang-di Nei-jing Su-wen* 重 广 补 注 黄 帝 内 经 素 问), 762 c.e., edited by Wang Bing-ci. This and a further amended edition by the Song-dynasty physician Lin Yi are the standard versions of the work. Wang Bing-ci reorganized the entire work and added at least seven chapters of his own.

Han Dynasty (206 b.c.e.–220 c.e.)

Before the second century c.e. Pharmacopoeia Classic of the Divine Husbandman (*Shen-nong Ben-cao Jing* 神 农 本 草 经). The original is long lost. The present text was compiled at a much later date. Describes 365 medicines and divides them into upper, middle, and lower classes, the highest promoting longevity and the lowest treating disease.

Second century c.e. Classic of Difficulties (*Nan Jing* 难 经). Consists of eighty-one questions and answers dealing with difficult portions of the *Nei Jing*.

c. 220 c.e. Discussion of Cold-Induced Disorders (*Shang-han Lun* 伤 寒 论), by Zhang Zhong-jing. Reorganized c. 300 by Wang Shu-he. Ten chapters, primarily concerned with the six stages of disease and diagnostic method in acute febrile diseases. This book is one of the clinical and practical foundations of traditional pharmaceutical medicine.

c. 220 C.E. Essential Prescriptions of the Golden Chest (*Jin-gui Yao-lue Fang Lun* 金匮要略方论), by Zhang Zhong-jing. The standard edition was put together in the early Song dynasty by Lin Yi. The subjects include miscellaneous internal diseases, women's disorders, emergencies, and dietary restrictions. This was originally one book, together with Discussion of Cold-Induced Disorders.

Jin Dynasty (265–420 c.e.)

280 C.E. Classic of the Pulse (*Mai Jing* 脉经), by Wang Shu-he. Description of twenty-four pulses and a discussion of their meaning in terms of Organs, Meridians, diseases, management, and prognosis.

282 C.E. Systematic Classic of Acupuncture, sometimes translated as ABC of Acupuncture (*Zhen-jiu Jia-yi Jing* 针灸甲乙经), by Huang-fu Mi. Discusses physiology, pathology, the Meridians, diagnosis, the points, and acupuncture treatment. It is a systematic presentation of material from the *Ling Shu* and other early, but now lost, texts.

c. 341 C.E. Emergency Prescriptions to Keep Up One's Sleeve (*Zhou-hou Bei-ji Fang* 肘后备急方), by Ge Hong. Simple prescriptions using easily accessible drugs for emergencies. Extensively revised in later dynasties.

Southern and Northern Dynasties (420–581 c.e.)

c. 495 C.E. Prescriptions Left by the Ghost of Liu Juan-zi (*Liu Juan-zi Gui-yi Fang* 刘涓子鬼遗方), Southern Qi dynasty, by Gong Qing-xuan. Earliest extant book on "external diseases." Primarily concerned with trauma, abscesses, rashes, and carbuncles. Includes discussion of antiseptic technique in minor surgery.

c. 536 C.E. Collection on Commentaries on the Pharmacopoeia Classic (*Ben-cao-jing Ji-zhu* 本草经集注), Liang dynasty, by Tao Hong-jing. The present text is actually a later compilation. The medicines are divided by type (mineral, plant, etc.).

Sui Dynasty (581–618 c.e.)

610 C.E. Discussion on the Origins of Symptoms in Illness (*Zhu-bing Yuan-hou Lun* 诸 病 源 候 论), by Chao Yuan-fang. Detailed descriptions of 1,720 illnesses under sixty-seven headings.

Tang Dynasty (618–907 c.e.)

652 C.E. Thousand Ducat Prescriptions (*Qian-jin Yao-fang* 千 金 要 方), by Sun Si-miao. A compilation of early Tang and previous works. Contents include important information on various specialties, acupuncture and moxibustion, and diet.

659 C.E. Newly Revised Pharmacopoeia (*Xin-xiu Ben-cao* 新 修 本 草), by Li Ji. All that is left of this book are fragments in Tang Shen-wei's Song-dynasty pharmacopoeia. (See Song-dynasty section.) Originally this was the National Pharmacopoeia with 844 entries detailing the type and flavor, area of origin, and use of the medicines. Illustrated.

682 C.E. Supplemental Wings to the Thousand Ducat Prescriptions (*Qian-jin Yi Fang* 千 金 翼 方), by Sun Si-miao. Important additions to the earlier Thousand Ducat Prescriptions, including pharmacology concerns, acupuncture, Cold-Induced disorders, gynecology, and pediatrics.

682 C.E. Subtleties of the Silver Sea (*Yin-hai Jing-wei* 银 海 精 微), by Sun Si-miao. Full exploration of various eye disorders and their treatment.

847 C.E. The Treasure Produced with Cessation of Menstruation (*Jing-xiao Chan-bao* 经 效 产 宝), by Zan Yin. Earliest extant book on obstetrics. Divided into three parts: pregnancy, labor and delivery, and postpartum.

Five Dynasties (907–960 c.e.)

752 C.E. Necessities of a Frontier Official (*Wai-tai Bi-yao* 外 台 秘 要), by Wang Tao. An important collection of medical knowledge from this period. Includes more than 6,000 prescriptions.

946 C.E. Secret Methods of Understanding Trauma and Rejoining Fractures (*Li-shang Xu-duan Mi-fang* 理 伤 续 断 秘 方), by Lin Dao-ren.

Earliest extant work on bone setting that deals with the subject both from a diagnostic and treatment perspective in great detail.

Song Dynasty (960–1279 c.e.)

992 c.e. Sagelike Prescriptions from the Taiping Era (*Taiping Sheng-hui Fang* 太 平 圣 惠 方), by Wang Huai-yin. A compilation of 16,834 subjects dealing primarily with textual and folk prescriptions to its time.

1026 c.e. The Illustrated Classic of Acupuncture Points as Found on the Bronze Model (*Tong-ren Shu-xue Zhen-jiu Tu Jing* 铜 人 输 穴 针 灸 图 经), by Wang Wei-yi. A description of the points listed in anatomical order on the Meridians.

1100 c.e. Discussion of Cold-Induced and General Illnesses (*Shang-han Zong-bing Lun* 伤 寒 总 病 论), by Pang An-shi. An expansion of the Discussion of Cold-Induced Disorders including such topics as summer diseases, epidemic diseases, pediatric and obstetrical Cold-Induced diseases, and rashes.

1107 c.e. Book That Revives Those with Cold-Induced or Similar Disorders (*Shang-han Lei-zheng Huo-ren Shu* 伤 寒 类 证 活 人 书), by Zhu Hong. Arranged in a question-and-answer format, with 101 questions. Explains the Discussion of Cold-Induced Disorders and the meaning of each formula with references and prescriptions from many other important texts.

1108 c.e. Historical and Precise Pharmacopoeial Index Arranged According to Pattern Group (*Jing-shi Zheng-lei Bei-ji Ben-cao* 经 史 证 类 备 急 本 妇), by Tang Shen-wei. Description of 1,558 medicines including use, Meridian entered, and preparation. Also included are 3,000 prescriptions. The work served as the base for many subsequent texts.

1114 c.e. Formulary of Pediatric Patterns and Medicines (*Xiao-er Yao-zheng Zhi-jue* 小 儿 药 证 直 决), by Qian Yi. Discussion of patterns, case histories, and prescriptions for children.

1117 c.e. General Record of Sagelike Benefit (*Sheng-ji Zong-lü* 圣 济 总 录), compiled by Imperial Medical College. A relatively complete record of contemporary medical knowledge.

1132 C.E. Prescriptions of Universal Benefit from My Own Practice (*Pu-ji Ben-shi Fang* 普济本事方), by Xu Shu-wei. A description of prescriptions and diagnostics, including those developed by the author.

1150 C.E. New Book for Infants (*You-you Xin-shu* 幼幼新书), by Liu Fang-ming. Includes discussion of etiology and diseases of the newborn.

1151 C.E. Professional and Popular Prescriptions from the Taiping Era (*Taiping Hui-min He-ji Ju-fang* 太平惠民和剂局方), by Chen Shi-wen. A contemporary formulary, with most prescriptions in powder or pill form.

1174 C.E. Discussion of Illnesses, Patterns, and Prescriptions Related to the Unification of the Three Etiologies (*San-yin Ji-yi Bing Zheng Fang Lun* 三因极一病证方论), by Chen Yen. An elaboration on the etiology scheme of the Essential Prescriptions of the Golden Chest, which deals with 180 illnesses.

1189 C.E. Formulary of the Pulse (*Mai Jue* 脉决), by Cui Jia-yen. Description of the pulses based on the classification scheme of the *Nan Jing*. Written in verse form for easy memorization.

1220 C.E. Classic of Nourishing Life with Acupuncture and Moxibustion (*Zhen-jiu Zi-sheng Jing* 针灸资生经), by Wang Shu-chuan. Has section on the location and use of the points as well as acupuncture treatments for various diseases. Based on earlier works and the author's clinical experience.

1237 C.E. Complete Book of Good Prescriptions for Women (*Fu-ren Da-quan Liang-fang* 妇人大全良方), by Chen Zi-ming. Discusses women's health problems under 260 headings. Appendixes of prescriptions and case histories

1241 C.E. Compass for Investigating Diseases (*Cha-bing Zhi-nan* 察病指南), by Shi Fa. Begins with a discussion of twenty-four pulses and their meanings. Also includes a description of the pulses of twenty-one disorders and a list of common obstetrical, gynecological, and pediatric pulses.

1253 C.E. Prescriptions Beneficial to Life (*Ji-sheng Fang* 济生方), by Yan Yong-huo. Practical explanations of 400 prescriptions.

Jin Tartar Dynasty (1115–1234 c.e.)

1186 C.E. Collection of Writings on the Mechanisms of Illnesses, Suitability of Qi, and the Safeguarding of Life as Discussed in the *Su Wen* (*Su-wen Bing-ji Qi-yi Bao-ming Ji* 素问病机气宜保命集), by Liu Wan-su. An exposition of many theoretical and practical medical issues.

1188 C.E. Standards of the Mysterious Inner Workings of the Origins of Illness as Discussed in the *Su Wen* (*Su-wen Xuan-ji Yuan-bing Shi* 素问玄机原病式), by Liu Wan-su. Discussions of the development of illness from the phase energetics section of the *Su Wen*. The use of cold treatments for Fire patterns is emphasized.

1228 C.E. Confucians' Duties to Their Parents (*Ru-men Shi-qin* 儒门事亲), by Zhang Cong-zheng. Promotes purgative treatment methods.

1231 C.E. Discussion of Dispelling Confusion Between External and Internal Injuries (*Nei Wai Shang Bian-huo Lun* 内外伤辨惑论), by Li Dong-yuan. A discussion of the differences between Externally and Internally generated disorders.

1249 C.E. Discussion of the Spleen and Stomach (*Pi-wei Lun* 脾胃论), by Li Dong-yuan. Based on his clinical experience, this book sets out Li's idea that the Spleen and Stomach are the most important Organs in health and disease. Many clinically useful concepts and prescriptions are included.

Yuan Dynasty (1271–1368 c.e.)

1335 C.E. Essential Meaning of External (Surgical) Diseases (*Wai-ke Jing-yi* 外科精义), by Qi De-zhi. A compendium and commentary of earlier physicians' ideas on diagnosis and treatment of swellings and carbuncles. Includes use of internal prescriptions for a systemic approach.

1341 C.E. Ao's Golden Mirror Reflections of Cold-Induced Disorders (*Ao-shi Shang-han Jin-jing Lu* 敖氏伤寒金镜录), by Dr. Ao. The first book devoted entirely to the tongue. An exhaustive description of thirty-six tongue types and their clinical significance. Illustrated.

1341 C.E. Elaboration of the Fourteen Meridians (*Shi-si Jing Fa-hui* 十 四 经 发 挥), by Hua Shou. Includes a discussion of Meridians, Extra Meridians, and special points.

1347 C.E. An Exhaustive Study of Excess (*Ge-zhi Yu Lun* 格 致 余 论), by Zhu Zhen-xiang. An elaboration of the notion that Yang is often in excess and Yin commonly insufficient.

1347 C.E. Secrets of the Cinnabar Creek Master (*Dan-xi Xin-fa* 丹 溪 心 法), by Zhu Zhen-xiang. The 100 topics in this book include Internally and Externally generated diseases, pediatrics, and obstetrics.

1361 C.E. The Meaning of the *Nan Jing* (*Nan-jing Ben-yi* 难 经 本 义), by Hua Shou. A collection of eleven commentaries on the *Nan Jing*, with corrections and emendations.

Ming Dynasty (1368–1644 c.e.)

1406 C.E. Prescriptions of Universal Benefit (*Pu-ji Fang* 普 济 方), by Zhu Xiao et al. The book with greatest number of prescriptions: 61,739 in all. Also has 239 illustrations.

1505 C.E. Collected Commentaries on the *Nan Jing* (*Nan-jing Ji-zhu* 难 经 集 注). Commentaries by Wang Jiu-si, Yang Xuan-cao, Ding De-yong, Wu Shu, and Yang Kang-hou emphasizing pulse diagnosis, Organ theory, and acupuncture.

1528 C.E. Essentials of the Mouth and Teeth (*Kou-chi Lei-yao* 口 齿 类 要), by Bi Ji. First, a discussion of the mouth and teeth, throat, and tongue; second, a discussion of the treatment of choking, bugs, and miscellaneous topics.

1529 C.E. Gatherings from Eminent Acupuncturists (*Zhen-jiu Ju-ying* 针 灸 聚 英), by Gao Wu. Acupuncture theory and practice along with formularies for beginners. A general work on acupuncture and moxibustion.

1529 C.E. Essentials for Correcting the Body (*Zheng-ti Lei-yao* 正 体 类 要), by Bi Ji. A detailed description of the symptoms, treatment, techniques, prescriptions, and instruments dealing with trauma.

c. 1540 C.E. Profound Pearl of the Red Water (*Chi-shui Xuan-zhu* 赤水玄珠), by Sun Dong-su. Primarily a discussion of internal medicine.

1549 C.E. Ordered Case Histories of Famous Physicians (*Ming-yi Lei An* 名医类案), by Jiang Quan. A collection of Ming and pre-Ming case histories.

1549 C.E. Elaboration of Pediatrics (*You-ke Fa-hui* 名医类案), by Wan Quan. A discussion of fetal, neonatal, and childhood illnesses.

1549 C.E. Secret Methods for Poxes and Rashes (*Dou-zhen Xin-Fa* 痘疹心法), by Wan Quan. Detailed descriptions of poxes and rashes including differential diagnosis of patterns.

1564 C.E. Pulse Studies of the Lakeside Master, also translated as the Pulse Studies of Li Shi-zhen (*Bin-hu Mai-xue* 濒湖脉学), by Li Shi-zhen. A description of twenty-seven pulse types in verse.

1565 C.E. Outline of Medicine (*Yi-xue Gang-mu* 医学纲目), by Lou Ying. A compilation of medical knowledge of the Jin Tartar–Yuan dynasty period.

1578 C.E. The Great Pharmacopoeia (*Ben-cao Gang-mu* 本草纲目), by Li Shi-zhen. The product of thirty years of work, this book describes the nature, flavor, use, region, preparation, shape, methods of cultivating and/or harvesting, and formulae of 1,892 medicines. Over 1,000 pages of illustrations and 1,000 prescriptions.

1601 C.E. Great Compendium of Acupuncture and Moxibustion (*Zhen-jiu Da-cheng* 针灸大成), by Yang Ji-zhou. A synthesis of the knowledge of acupuncture and moxibustion of the Ming and previous dynasties.

1617 C.E. Correct Lineage for External (Surgical) Diseases (*Wai-ke Zheng-zong* 外科正宗), by Chen Shi-gong. A description of the pathology, symptoms, diagnosis, management, and successful and unsuccessful case histories of over 100 patterns. Emphasizes oral treatment along with early surgery.

1624 C.E. Classic of Categories (*Lei Jing* 类经), by Zhang Jie-bing (Jing-yue). A reordering of the material in the *Nei Jing* by categories, along with commentary.

1624 C.E. Complete Works of Jing-yue (*Jing-yue Quan-shu* 景 岳 全 书), by Zhang Jie-bing. An important systematic presentation of theory, diagnosis, treatment methods, and discussion of various specialities.

1637 C.E. Essential Readings in Medicine (*Yi-zong Bi-du* 医 宗 必 读), by Li Zhong-zi. An introductory work including explanations of the pulses, pharmacopoeia, patterns, and medical theory with case histories.

1642 C.E. Discussion of Warm Epidemics (*Wen-yi Lun* 温 疫 论), by Wu You-xing. A preliminary discussion of Warm Diseases, their mode of infection, their progression in the body, and their differences from Cold-Induced disorders.

1642 C.E. Important Knowledge from the *Nei Jing* (*Nei-jing Zhi-yao* 内 经 知 要), by Li Zhong-zi. Material from the *Nei Jing* is divided into eight categories (lifestyle, Yin and Yang, various types of diagnoses, methodology of treatment, Meridians, etc.), and simple explanations are given.

Qing Dynasty (1644–1911 c.e.)

1658. Methods and Rules of Medicine (*Yi-men Fa-lu* 医 门 法 律), by Yu Chang. Presents miscellaneous disorders of the six Pernicious Influences from theoretical and practical perspectives.

1668. Mirror of the Tongue for Cold-Induced Disorders (*Shang-han She Jian* 伤 寒 舌 鉴), by Zhang Deng. Discussion of the tongue in Cold-Induced disorders, pregnancy, etc. With 120 illustrations.

1687. Medical Connection (*Yi Guan* 医 贯), by Zhao Xian-ke. Expounds the theory of the primary importance of the Kidney Yin and Yang.

1689. Discussion of Women's Disorders (*Nu-ke Jing Lun* 女 科 经 论), by Xiao Xun. A detailed description of women's disorders and their treatment.

1694. Concise Pharmacopoeia (*Ben-cao Bei-yao* 本 草 备 要), by Wang Ang. A clinical description of 460 commonly used medicines.

1723. The Four Examinations Pared Down to Their Essence (*Si-zhen Jue-wei* 四 诊 抉 微), by Lin Zhi-han. A compilation of previous works on examination techniques, with commentary.

1729. Collection of Pearls on Cold-Induced Disorders (*Shang-han Guan-zhu Ji* 伤寒贯珠集), by You Yi. A reorganization by treatment method of Discussion of Cold-Induced Disorders.

1742. Golden Mirror of Medicine (*Yi-zong Jin-jian* 医宗金鉴), edited by Wu Qian. A complete compilation of all aspects of Chinese medicine, including the major classics. Written in easily understandable form.

1746. Case Histories That Act as Clinical Compasses (*Ling-zheng Zhi-nan Yi-an* 临证指南医案), by Ye Tian-shi. Compilations and commentaries of the case histories of Ye Tian-shi.

c. 1746. Discussion of Warm Diseases (*Wen-re Lun* 温热论), by Ye Tian-shi. A discussion of the four stages of acute febrile diseases (*wei, qi, ying, xue*) by their developer.

1798. Refined Diagnosis of Warm Diseases (*Wen-bing Tiao-bian* 温病条辨), by Wu Ju-tong. An expansion of the work of Ye Tian-shi, dividing disease into Upper, Middle, and Lower Burners. Description of patterns such as Wind Fever, Fever Poison, Summer Fever, and Damp Fever.

1801. Field of Epidemic Raspy Throat Rash (*Yi-sha-cao* 疫痧草), by Chen Geng-dao. Devoted exclusively to Epidemic Raspy Throat Rash (analogue of scarlet fever).

1839. Ordering of Patterns and Deciding Treatments (*Lei-zheng Zhi-cai* 类证治裁), by Lin Pei-qin. A collection and systematic analysis of earlier concepts of pattern discernment and treatment methods.

1846. New Compilation of Tested Prescriptions (*Yan-fang Xin-bian* 验方新编), by Bao Yun-shao. A selection of simple prescriptions, arranged according to subject.

1885. Discussion of Blood Patterns (*Xue-zheng Lun* 血证论), by Tang Zong-hai. Describes the relationship between Qi and Blood as well as the mechanism and treatment of Blood disorders.

1897. Refined Diagnoses of White Throat (*Bai-hou Tian-bian* 白喉条辨), by Chen Bao-shan. Discusses the etiology, diagnosis by Meridian and pulse, prognosis, treatment, and prohibition for white throat (analogue of diphtheria).

APPENDIX H

SELECTED
BIBLIOGRAPHY

⊣ CHINESE SOURCES

As remarked in the Author's Note, this Chinese-language bibliography is idivided into eight sections to indicate subject matter or type of publication. In most of the sections, book entries are arranged alphabetically by author or editor. English translations, or renderings, of the titles are given first, followed by the romanization and the Chinese characters. The numbered book entries are keyed to citations in the notes.

Nei Jing and Nan Jing and Commentaries

1. Inner Classic of the Yellow Emperor: Simple Questions (*Huang-di Nei-Jing Su-wen* 黄帝内经素问). Beijing (Peking): People's Press, 1963. Cited as *Nei Jing* or *Su Wen*. This edition is the same as the revised and annotated one listed in Appendix I.

2. Classic of the Spiritual Axis with Vernacular Explanation (*Ling-shu-jing Bai-hua-jie* 灵枢经白·话解). Edited by Chen Bi-liu and Cheng Zhou-ren. Beijing: People's Hygiene Press, 1963. Cited as *Nei Jing* or *Ling Shu* (it is the second part of the *Nei Jing*).

3. Classic of Difficulties with Annotations (*Nan-jing Jiao-shi* 难 经 校 释). Edited by Nanjing Institute of Traditional Chinese Medicine. Beijing: People's Press, 1979. First appeared c. 200 C.E. Cited as *Nan Jing*.

4. Beijing Institute of Traditional Chinese Medicine, main ed. Explanations of the *Nei Jing* (*Nei-jing Shi-yi* 内 经 释 义). Shanghai: Science and Technology Press, 1964.

5. Chen Bi-liu, ed. Classic of Difficulties with Explanation in Vernacular Language (*Nan-jing Bai-hua-jie* 难 经 白 话 解). Beijing: People's Health Press, 1963. First appeared c. 200 C.E.

6. Gao Shi-zong. Genuine Explanation of the Yellow Emperor: Simple Questions (*Huang-di Su-wen Zhen-jie* 黄 帝 素 问 真 解). Beijing: Science and Technology Press, 1980. First appeared 1887 C.E.

7. Liu Wan-su. Standards of the Mysterious Inner Workings of the Origin of Illness as Discussed in the *Su Wen* (*Su-wen Xuan-ji Yuan-bing Shi* 素 问 玄 机 原 病 式). Beijing: People's Press, 1963. First appeared 1188 C.E.

8. Wang Jiu-si et al. Collected Commentaries on the *Nan Jing* (*Nan-jing Ji zhu* 难 经 集 注). Shanghai: Shanghai Commercial Press, 1955. First appeared 1505 C.E.

9. Yan Hong-chen and Gao Guang-zhen. Selections from the *Nei Jing* and *Nan Jing* with Elucidations (*Nei-nan-jing Xuan-shi* 内 难 经 选 释). Jilin (Kirin): People's Press, 1979.

10. Zhang Jie-bing. Classic of Categories (*Lei Jing* 类 经). Beijing: People's Health Press, 1957. First appeared 1624 C.E.

Other Classical Sources

11. Beijing Institute of Traditional Chinese Medicine, ed. Selected Readings in the Original Sources of Traditional Chinese Medicine (*Zhong-yi Yuan-zhu Xuan-du* 中 医 原 著 选 读). Beijing: People's Press, 1978.

12. Beijing, Nanjing, Shanghai, Guangzhou (Canton), and Chengdu Institutes of Traditional Chinese Medicine, eds. Lecture Notes on Selected Ideas and Case Histories of Famous Physicians of the Song, Yuan, Ming, and Qing Dynasties (*Zhong-yi Ming-jia Xue-shuo Ji Yi-an Xuan Jiang-yi: Song, Yuan, Ming, Qing* 中 医 名 家 学 说 及 医 案 选 讲 义: 宋，元，明 清). Beijing: People's Press, 1961.

13. Chao Yuan-fang. Discussion on the Origins of Symptoms in Illness (*Zhu-bing Yuan-hou Lun* 诸 病 源 候 论). Beijing: People's Health Press, 1955. First appeared 610 C.E.

14. Hua Shou. Elaboration of the Fourteen Meridians (*Shi-si Jing Fa-hui* 十 四 经 发 挥). Taipei: Whirlwind Press, 1980. First appeared 1341 C.E.

15. Huang-fu Mi. Systematic Classic of Acupuncture with Annotations (*Zhen-jiu Jia-yi Jing Jiao-shi* 针 灸 甲 乙 经 校 释). Annotations by Shandong Institute of Traditional Chinese Medicine. Beijing: People's Press, 1979. First appeared c. 282 C.E.

16. Li Shi-zhen. Pulse Studies of the Lakeside Master with Vernacular Explanation (*Bin-hu Mai-xue Bai-hua-jie* 濒 湖 脉 学 白 话 解). Edited and with commentary by Beijing Institute of Traditional Chinese Medicine, Fundamental Theory and Teaching Research Section. Beijing: People's Press, 1972. Text first appeared 1564 C.E. Cited as Pulse Studies.

17. Shanghai City Traditional Chinese Medical Archives Research Committee. Selections from Pulse Examination (*Mai-Zhen Xuan-yao* 脉 诊 选 要). Hong Kong: Commercial Press, 1970.

18. Sun Si-miao. Subtleties of the Silver Sea (*Yin-hai Jing-wei* 银 海 精 微). Beijing: People's Health Press, 1956. First appeared 682 C.E.

19. Sun Si-miao. Thousand Ducat Prescriptions (*Qian-jin Yao-fang* 千 金 要 方). Taipei: National Traditional Chinese Medical Research Bureau, 1965. First appeared 652 C.E.

20. Tang Zong-hai. Discussion of Blood Patterns (*Xue-zheng Lun* 血证论). Shanghai: People's Press, 1977. First appeared 1885 C.E.

21. Wang Shu-chuan. Classic of Nourishing Life with Acupuncture and Moxibustion (*Zhen-jiu Zi-sheng Jing* 针灸资生经). Taipei: Whirlwind Press, 1980. First appeared 1220 C.E.

22. Wang Shu-he. Classic of the Pulse (*Mai Jing* 脉经). Hong Kong: Taiping Book Publishers, 1961. First appeared c. 280 C.E.

23. Wu Ju-tong. Refined Diagnoses of Warm Diseases with Vernacular Explanation (*Wen-bing Tiao-bian Bai-hua-jie* 温病条辨白话解). Commentary by Zhejiang Institute of Traditional Chinese Medicine. Beijing: People's Health Press, 1963. Text first appeared 1798 C.E.

24. Wu Qian, main ed. Golden Mirror of Medicine (*Yi-zong Jin-jian* 医宗金鉴). 3 vols. Beijing: People's Health Press, 1972. First appeared 1742 C.E.

25. Wu You-xing. Discussion of Warm Epidemics with Notes and Commentary (*Wen-yi Lun Ping-zhu* 温疫论评注). Commentary by Zhejiang Province Traditional Medical Research Bureau. Beijing: People's Press, 1977. Text first appeared 1642 C.E.

26. Yang Ji-zhou. Great Compendium of Acupuncture and Moxibustion (*Zhen-jiu Da-cheng* 针灸大成). Beijing: People's Press, 1973. First appeared 1601 C.E.

27. Zhang Zhong-jing. Discussion on Cold-Induced Disorders with Clarifications (*Shang-han Lun Yu-yi* 伤寒论语译). Edited by Traditional Chinese Medical Research Institute. Beijing: People's Health Press, 1959, 1974. Text first appeared c. 220 C.E. Cited as Discussion.

28. Zhang Zhong-jing. Discussion on Cold-Induced Disorders with New Commentary (*Shang-han Lun Xin-zhu* 伤寒论新注). Commentary by Cheng Tan-an. Hong Kong: Shaohua Cultural Service Society, 1955. Main text first appeared c. 220 C.E.

29. Zhang Zhong-jing. Essential Prescriptions of the Golden Chest with Simple Commentary (*Jin-gui Yao-lue Qian-zhu* 金匮·要略浅注). Hong Kong: Taiping Book Publishers, 1970. Commentary by Chen Xiuyuan first appeared c. 1800 C.E. Text first appeared c. 200 C.E.

30. Zhang Jie-bing. Illustrated Wing to the Classic of Categories (*Lei-jing Tu-yi* 类经图翼). Beijing: People's Health Press, 1965. First published 1624 C.E.

Reference Books

31. Gansu Hygiene School. Explanation of Common Traditional Chinese Medical Terms (*Zhong-yi-xue Chang-yong Ming-ci Jie-shi* 中医学常用名词解释). Gansu: People's Press, 1975.

32. Jiangsu New Medical Institute. Encyclopedia of the Traditional Chinese Pharmacopoeia (*Zhong-yao Da-ci-dian* 中药大辞典). Shanghai: People's Press, 1977.

33. Traditional Chinese Medical Research Institute and Guangdong Institute of Traditional Chinese Medicine, eds. Selected Explanations of Traditional Chinese Medical Terms (*Zhong-yi Ming-ci Shu-yu Xuan-shi* 中医名词术语选释). Beijing: People's Press, 1973.

34. Traditional Chinese Medical Research Institute and Guangzhou (Canton) Institute of Traditional Chinese Medicine, main eds. Shanghai, Liaoning, Chengdu, Anhui, Hebei, Nanjing, Hunan, and Shanxi Institutes of Traditional Chinese Medicine, contributing eds. Concise Dictionary of Traditional Chinese Medicine (*Jian-ming Zhong-yi Ci-dian* 简明中医辞典). Hong Kong: Joint Publishing Company, 1979.

35. Wu Ke-qian. Dictionary of Sources of Illness (*Bing-yuan Ci-dian* 病源辞典). Hong Kong: Shiyong Publishers, 1965.

36. Xie Li-hang, ed. Traditional Chinese Medical Encyclopedia (*Zhong-guo Yi-xue Da-ci-dian* 中国医学大辞典), 4 vols. Hong Kong: Commercial Press, 1974. First published 1921.

Contemporary Introductory Texts Used to Train Traditional Physicians

37. Beijing Institute of Traditional Chinese Medicine. Foundations of Clinical Patterns in Traditional Chinese Medicine (*Zhong-yi Ling-zheng Ji-chu* 中医临证基础). Beijing: People's Press, 1975.

38. Beijing Institute of Traditional Chinese Medicine, main ed. Foundations of Traditional Chinese Medicine (*Zhong-yi-xue Ji-chu* 中医学基础). Shanghai: Science and Technology Press, 1978.

39. Beijing Traditional Chinese Medical Hospital Revolutionary Committee. Essentials of Distinguishing Patterns and Dispensing Treatment (*Bian-zhen Shi-zhi Gang-yao* 辨证施治纲要). Beijing: People's Press, 1974.

40. Chengdu Institute of Traditional Chinese Medicine. Internal Medicine and Pediatrics (*Nei-er-ke-xue* 内儿科学). Sichuan (Szechuan): People's Press, 1975.

41. Chengdu Institute of Traditional Chinese Medicine. Practical Traditional Chinese Medicine (*shi-yong Zhong-yi-xue* 实用中医学). Sichuan: People's Press, 1977.

42. Guangdong Institute of Traditional Chinese Medicine. Clinical Traditional Chinese Medicine: New Edition (*Zhong-yi Ling-chuang Xin-bian* 中医临床新编). Guangdong: People's Press, 1972.

43. Guangdong Institute of Traditional Chinese Medicine. Lecture Notes on Traditional Chinese Medical Diagnosis (*Zhong-yi Zhen-duan-xue Jiang-yi* 中医诊断学讲义). Shanghai: Science and Technology Press, 1964.

44. Guangdong Institute of Traditional Chinese Medicine. Traditional Chinese Internal Medicine (*Zhong-yi Nei-ke* 中医内科). Beijing: People's Press, 1976.

45. Hubei Institute of Traditional Chinese Medicine, main ed. Introduction to Traditional Chinese Medicine (*Zhong-yi-xue Gai-lun* 中医学概论). Shanghai: Science and Technology Press, 1978.

46. Jiangsu Institute of New Medicine. Traditional Chinese Medicine (*Zhong-yi-xue* 中医学). Jiangsu: People's Press, 1972.

47. Jiangsu Institute of New Medicine. Traditional Chinese Medicine Clinical Handbook of Common Illnesses (*Chang-jian Bing Zhong-yi Ling-chuang Shou-ce* 常见病中医临床手册). Beijing: People's Press, 1972.

48. Liaoning Institute of Traditional Chinese Medicine. Lecture Notes on Traditional Chinese Medicine (*Zhong-yi-xue Jiang-yi* 中医学讲义). Liaoning: People's Press, 1972.

49. Nanjing Institute of Traditional Chinese Medicine. Concise Traditional Chinese Internal Medicine (*Jian-ming Zhong-yi Nei-ke-xue* 简明中医内科学). Shanghai: Science and Technology Press, 1959.

50. Nanjing Institute of Traditional Chinese Medicine. Introduction to Traditional Chinese Medicine (*Zhong-yi-xue Gai-lun* 中医学概论). Beijing: People's Health Press, 1959.

51. Nanjing Institute of Traditional Chinese Medicine. Traditional Chinese Medical Ancillary Care (*Zhong-yi Hu-bing-xue* 中医护病学). Hong Kong: Shaohua Cultural Service Society, 1959.

52. Shanghai Institute of Traditional Chinese Medicine. Distinguishing Patterns and Dispensing Treatments (*Bian-zheng Shi-zhi* 辩证施治). Shanghai: People's Press, 1972.

53. Shanghai Institute of Traditional Chinese Medicine. Foundations of Traditional Chinese Medicine (*Zhong-yi-xue Ji-chu* 中 医 学 基 础). Hong Kong: Commercial Press, 1975.

54. Shanghai Institute of Traditional Chinese Medicine. Lecture Notes on Traditional Chinese Internal Medicine (*Zhong-yi Nei-ke-xue Jiang-yi* 中 医 内 科 学 讲 义). Shanghai: Science and Technology Press, 1964.

55. Tianjin City Traditional Chinese Medical Hospital. Traditional Chinese Internal Medicine (*Zhong-yi Nei-ke* 中 医 实 用 临 床 手 册). Tianjin: People's Press, 1974.

56. Tianjin Institute of Traditional Chinese Medicine. Practical Clinical Handbook of Traditional Chinese Medicine (*Zhong-yi Shi-yong Ling-chuang Shou-ce* 中 医 实 用 临 床 手 册). Hong Kong: Commercial Press, 1970.

57. Wuhan People's Liberation Army Health Committee. Concise Traditional Chinese Medicine (*Jian-ming Zhong-yi-xue* 简 明 中 医 学). Hubei: People's Press, 1972.

Contemporary Writings

58. Chen Yu-ming. Essentials of Pathology, Diagnosis, and Treatment (*Bing-li Yu Zhen-duan Zhi-liao Gang-yao* 病 理 与 诊 断 治 疗 纲 要). Ningxi: People's Press, 1973.

59. Fang Yao-zhong. Seven Lectures on the Study of Distinguishing Patterns and Treatments (*Bian-zheng Lun-zhi Yan-jiu Qi-jiang* 辩 证 论 治 研 究 七 讲). Beijing: People's Press, 1979.

60. Li Tiao-hua. Patterns and Treatment of the Kidneys and Kidney Illnesses (*Shen Yu Shen-bing De Zheng-zhi* 肾 与 肾 病 的 证 治). Hebei: People's Press, 1979.

61. Liu Guan-jun. Pulse Examination (*Mai-zhen* 脉 诊). Shanghai: Science and Technology Press, 1979.

62. Ma Ruo-shui. Theoretical Foundations of Traditional Chinese Medicine (*Zhong-yi Ji-chu Li-lun Zhi-shi* 中 医 基 础 理 论 知 识). Gui-yang: Guizhou People's Press, 1977.

63. Qin Bo-wei. Elementary Traditional Chinese Medicine (*Zhong-yi Ru-men* 中 医 入 门). Hong Kong: Taiping Book Publishers, 1971.

64. Qin Bo-wei. Medical Lecture Notes of Qian Zhai (*Qian Zhai Yi-xue Jiang-gao* 谦 斋 医 学 讲 稿). Shanghai: Science and Technology Press, 1964.

65. Qin Bo-wei et al. Traditional Chinese Medical References for Clinical Patterns (*Zhong-yi Ling-chuang Bei-yao* 中 医 临 证 备 要). Beijing: People's Press, 1973.

66. Ren Ying-qiu. Ten Lectures on the Study of Pulses in Traditional Chinese Medicine (*Zhong-yi Mai-xue Shi-jiang* 中 医 脉 学 十 讲). Hong Kong: Taiping Book Publishers, 1971.

67. Zhai Ming-yi. Clinical Foundations of Traditional Chinese Medicine (*Zhong-yi Ling-chuang Ji-chu* 中 医 临 床 基 础). Anyang: Henan People's Press, 1978.

Miscellaneous Sources

68. Anhui Institute of Traditional Chinese Medicine. Clinical Handbook of Traditional Chinese Medicine (*Zhong-yi Ling-chuang Shou-ce* 中 医 临 床 手 册). Anhui: People's Press, 1965.

69. Beijing Institute of Traditional Chinese Medicine, Diagnosis Research and Teaching Section. Traditional Chinese Tongue Examination (*Zhong-yi She-zhen* 中 医 舌 诊). Hong Kong: Commercial Press, 1970, 1973. This text and the one following seem to be modified editions.

70. Beijing Institute of Traditional Chinese Medicine, Fundamental Theory and Teaching Research Section. Traditional Chinese Tongue Examination (*Zhong-yi She-zhen* 中 医 舌 诊). Beijing: People's Press, 1960, 1980.

71. Chen Xin-qian, main ed. Pharmacology: New Edition (*Xin-bian Yao-wu-xue* 新编药物学). Beijing: People's Health Press, 1951, 1974.

72. Eleventh People's Hospital of the Shanghai Institute of Traditional Chinese Medicine, Research Committee on Hypertension. Theory and Treatment of Hypertension by Traditional Chinese Medicine (*Gao-xue-ya-bing De Zhong-yi-li-lun He Zhi-liao* 高血压病的中医理论和治疗). Hong Kong: Shiyong Publishers, 1971.

73. Guanganmen Hospital of the Traditional Chinese Medicine Research Institute. Collected Clinical Experiences of Zhu Ren-kang: Dermatology (*Zhu Ren-kang Ling-chuang Jing-yan-ji Pi-fu Wai-ke* 朱仁康临床经验集皮肤外科). Beijing: People's Press, 1979.

74. Guangdong Provincial Traditional Chinese Medicine Hospital, Department of Ophthalmology. Traditional Chinese Ophthalmology (*Zhong-yi Yan-ke* 中医眼科). Beijing: People's Press, 1975.

75. Guangzhou (Canton) Ministry of Health, Logistic Headquarters, Guangdong Dept. of Health, Hunan Province Dept. of Health, Guangxi Zhuang Autonomous Region Department of Health. Introduction to Traditional Chinese Medicine: New Edition (*Xin-bian Zhong-yi-xue Gai-yao* 新编中医学概要). Beijing: People's Press, 1974. Material for Western doctors to learn traditional Chinese medicine.

76. Hao Jin-kai, ed. Illustrative Charts of Extra Meridian Acupuncture Points (*Zhen-jiu Jing-wai-qi-xue Tu-pu* 针灸经外奇穴图谱), 2 vols. Shanxi: People's Press, 1974.

77. Huzhou Institute of Traditional Chinese Medicine. Traditional Chinese Gynecology (*Zhong-yi Fu-ke* 中医妇科). Beijing: People's Press, 1978.

78. Jinan City Health Dept. Revolutionary Committee, compilers and annotators. Clinical Cases of Wu Shao-huai (*Wu Shao-huai Yi-an* 吴少怀医案). Shandong: People's Press, 1978.

79. Luoyang Regional Revolutionary Health Commission, main ed. Internal Medicine: New Edition (*Xin-bian Nei-ke* 新编内科). Vols. 1 and 2. Henan: People's Press, 1978.

80. Nanjing Institute of Traditional Chinese Medicine. Lecture Notes on Warm Illnesses (*Wen-bing-xue Jiang-yi* 温病学讲义). Shanghai: Science and Technology Press, 1964.

81. Nanjing Institute of Traditional Chinese Medicine. Study of Warm Illnesses (*Wen-bing-xue* 温病学). Shanghai: Science and Technology Press, 1978.

82. Shanghai First Medical Hospital. Clinical Handbook of Antimicrobial Medicines (*Ling-chuang Kang-jun Yao-wu Shou-ce* 临床抗菌药物手册). Shanghai: People's Press, 1977.

83. Shanghai First Medical Hospital. Practical Internal Medicine (*Shi-yong Nei-ke-xue* 实用内科学). Beijing: People's Press, 1974.

84. Shanghai First Medical Hospital, Organ Research Committee. Studies on the Kidneys (*Shen De Yan-jiu* 肾的研究). Hong Kong: Zhonghua Publishers, 1970.

85. Shanghai Institute of Traditional Chinese Medicine. Acupuncture (*Zhen-jiu Xue* 针灸学). Beijing: People's Health Press, 1974.

86. Shanghai Institute of Traditional Chinese Medicine. Study of Acupuncture Points (*Zhen-jiu Shu-xue Xue* 针灸腧穴学). Hong Kong: Shaohua Cultural Service Society, 1964.

87. Shanghai Institute of Traditional Chinese Medicine. Study of Prescriptions (*Fang-ji-xue* 方剂学). Hong Kong: Commercial Press, 1975.

88. Shanghai Second Medical Hospital. Handbook of Internal Medicine (*Nei-ke Shou-ce* 内科手册). Beijing: People's Press, 1974.

89. Zhang Yao-qing and Chen Dao-long. Records of Clinical Patterns in Internal Medicine (*Nei-ke Ling-zheng Lü* 内科临证录). Shanghai: Science and Technology Press, Shanghai, 1978.

90. Zhejiang Provincial Committee for Trial Material for Western-Style Doctors Learning Traditional Chinese Medicine. Clinical Studies of Traditional Chinese Medicine (*Zhong-yi Ling-chuang-xue* 中医临床学). Zhejiang: People's Press, 1978. Cited as Clinical Studies.

91. Zhejiang Provincial Committee for Trial Material for Western-Style Doctors Learning Traditional Chinese Medicine. Foundations of Traditional Chinese Medicine (*Zhong-yi Ji-chu-xue* 中医基础学). Zhejiang: People's Press, 1972. Cited as Foundations.

92. Zhongshan Institute of Medicine. Clinical Use of Chinese Medicines (*Zhong-yao Ling-chuang Ying-yong* 中医临床应用). Guangdong: People's Press, 1975.

Sources on the History of Chinese Medicine

93. Beijing Institute of Traditional Chinese Medicine. Lecture Notes on the History of China's Medicine (*Zhong-guo Yi-xue Shi Jiang-yi* 中国医学史讲义). Shanghai: Science and Technology Press, 1964.

94. Chen Bang-xian. History of China's Medicine (*Zhong-guo Yi-xue Shi-lüe* 中国医学史). Shanghai: Shanghai Commercial Press, 1957, 1937.

95. Jia De-dao. Concise History of China's Medicine (*Zhong-guo Yi-xue Shi-lüe* 中国医学史略). Taiyuan: Shanxi People's Press, 1979.

Journals

Beijing Traditional Chinese Medicine (*Beijing Zhong-yi* 北京中医).

Chinese Journal of Internal Medicine (*Zhong-hua Nei-ke Za-zhi* 中华内科杂志). Cited as CJIM.

Fujian Traditional Chinese Medicine (*Fujian Zhong-yi-yao* 福 建 中 医 药).

Guangdong Traditional Chinese Medicine (*Guangdong Zhong-yi* 广 东 中 医).

Heilongjiang Traditional Chinese Medicine (*Heilongjiang Zhong-yi-yao* 黑 龙 江 中 医 药).

Harbin Traditional Chinese Medicine (*Ha-er-bin Zhong-yi* 哈 尔 滨 中 医).

Jiangsu Traditional Chinese Medicine (*Jiangsu Zhong-yi* 江 苏 中 医).

Journal of Traditional Chinese Medicine (*Zhong-yi-Za-zhi* 中 医 杂 志). Cited as JTCM.

New Traditional Chinese Medicine (*Xin Zhong-yi* 新 中 医).

Shanghai Journal of Traditional Chinese Medicine (*Shanghai Zhong-yi-yao Za -zhi* 上 海 中 医 药 杂 志). Cited as SJTCM.

Wen Wu (Cultural Objects; 文 物). Beijing.

Zhejiang Journal of Traditional Chinese Medicine (*Zhejiang Zhong-yi Za-zhi* 浙 江 中 医 杂 志).

ENGLISH-LANGUAGE SOURCES

Andrews, Bridie J. *The Making of Modern Chinese Medicine, 1895–1937.* Unpublished Ph.D. dissertation. Cambridge: University of Cambridge, 1996.

Barnes, Linda L. *Alternative Pursuits: A History of Chinese Healing Practices in the Context of American Religions and Medicines with an Ethnographic Focus on the City of Boston.* Unpublished Ph.D. dissertation. Cambridge: Harvard University, 1995.

Bates, Don (ed.). *Knowledge and the Scholarly Medical Traditions.* Cambridge: Cambridge University Press. 1995.

Bensoussan, Alan. *The Vital Meridian: A Modern Exploration of Acupuncture.* Melbourne, Australia: Churchill Livingstone, 1991.

Bensoussan, Alan, and Stephen P. Myers. *Toward a Safer Choice: The Practice of Traditional Chinese Medicine in Australia.* Campbelltown, NSW, Australia: University of Western Sydney, Macarthur, 1996.

Chan, Wing-tsit, trans. and comp. *A Source Book in Chinese Philosophy.* Princeton, NJ: Princeton University Press, Princeton Paperbacks, 1963. Cited as *Chinese Philosophy.*

Chiu, Martha Li. *Mind, Body, and Illness in a Chinese Medical Tradition.* Cambridge: Harvard University. Unpublished Ph.D. dissertation, 1986.

Dash, Vd. Bhagwan. *Ayurvedic Treatment for Common Diseases.* Delhi: Delhi Diary, 1979.

Department of Philosophy of Medicine and Science, comp. *Theories and Philosophies of Medicine.* New Delhi: Institute of History of Medicine and Medical Research, 1973.

Dwarkanath, C. *Introduction to Kayachikistsa.* Bombay: Popular Book Depot, 1959.

Ernst, Edzard, and Adrian White. *Acupuncture: A Scientific Appraisal.* Oxford: Butterworth-Heinemann, 1999.

Farquhar, Judith. *Knowing Practice: The Clinical Encounter of Chinese Medicine.* Boulder, CO: Westview Press, 1994.

Filshie, Jacqueline, and Adrian White. *Medical Acupuncture: A Western Scientific Approach.* Edinburgh: Churchill Livingstone, 1998.

Fung, Yu-lan. *A History of Chinese Philosophy.* 2 vols. Translated by Derk Bodde. Princeton, NJ: Princeton University Press, 1953, 1973.

Furth, Charlotte. *A Flourishing Yin: Gender in China's Medical History, 960–1665.* Berkeley: University of California Press, 1999.

Gruner, O. Cameron, ed. and trans. *The Canon of Medicine of Avicenna.* London: Luzac, 1930.

Hall, David L., and Ames, Roger T. *Anticipating China: Thinking Through the Narratives of Chinese and Western Culture.* Albany: State University of New York, 1995.

Hanson, Marta E. *Inventing a Tradition in Chinese Medicine: From Universal Canon to Local Medical Knowledge in South China in The Seventeenth to the Nineteenth Century.* (Ph. D. diss. University of Pennsylvania, 1997).

Harper, Donald J. *The "Wu Shih Erh Ping Fang": Translation and Prolegomena.* Berkeley: University of California. Unpublished Ph.D. dissertation, 1982.

Hsu, Elizabeth. *The Transmission of Chinese Medicine.* Cambridge: Cambridge University Press, 1999.

Jones, W. H. S., ed. and trans. *Hippocrates with an English Translation.* Vols. 1–4. Cambridge: Harvard University Press, 1931, 1952. Vol. 4 includes translations from *Heraceitis.* Cited as *Hippocrates.*

Jullien, François. *The Propensity of Things: Toward a History of Efficacy in China.* New York: Zone Books, 1995.

Kasulis, Thomas P. *Self as Body in Asian Theory and Practice.* Albany: State University of New York, 1993.

Keegan, David Joseph. *The "Huang-Ti Nei-Ching": The Structure of the Compilations; The Significance of the Structure.* Berkeley: University of California. Unpublished Ph.D. dissertation, 1986.

Kleinman, Arthur. *Writing at the Margin: Discourse Between Anthropology and Medicine.* Berkeley: University of California Press, 1995.

Kleinman, Arthur, et al., eds. *Medicine in Chinese Cultures: Comparative Studies of Health Care in Chinese and Other Societies.* Washington, DC: John E. Fogarty International Center, U.S. Dept. of HEW, NIH, 1975.

Kohn, Livia (ed.). *Taoist Meditation and Longevity Techniques.* Ann Arbor: Center for Chinese Studies, University of Michigan, 1989.

Kuriyama, Shigehisa. *The Expressiveness of the Body and the Divergence of Greek and Chinese Medicine.* New York: Zone Books, 1999.

Kuriyama, Shigehisa. *Varieties of Haptic Experience: A Comparative Study of Greek and Chinese Pulse Diagnosis.* Cambridge: Harvard University. Unpublished Ph.D. dissertation, 1986.

Leibowitz, J. O., and Shlomo Marcus, eds. *Moses Maimonides on the Causes of Symptoms.* Berkeley, CA: University of California Press, 1974.

Leslie, Charles, ed. *Asian Medical Systems.* Berkeley, CA: University of California Press, 1976.

Leslie, Charles, and Young, Alan (eds.). *Paths to Asian Medical Knowledge.* Berkeley: University of California Press, 1992.

Lloyd, G. E. R. *Adversaries and Authorities: Investigations into Ancient Greek and Chinese Science.* Cambridge: Cambridge University Press, 1996.

Maciocia, Giovanni. *The Foundations of Chinese Medicine.* Edinburgh: Churchill Livingstone, 1989.

Maciocia, Giovanni. *The Practice of Chinese Medicine.* Edinburgh: Churchill Livingstone, 1994.

May, Margaret Tallmadge, trans. *Galen on Usefulness of the Parts of the Body.* Ithaca, NY: Cornell University Press, 1968.

McKeon, Richard, ed. *The Basic Works of Aristotle.* New York: Random House, 1941.

Nakamura, Hajime. *Ways of Thinking of Eastern Peoples.* Edited by Philip P. Wiener. Honolulu: University Press of Hawaii, 1964, 1978.

Nakayama, Shigeru. Jerry Dusenbury (trans.). *Academic and Scientific Traditions in China, Japan, and the West.* Tokyo: University of Tokyo Press, 1984.

Needham, Joseph. *The Grand Titration: Science and Society in East and West.* London: George Allen & Unwin, 1969.

Needham, Joseph. *Science and Civilization in China.* Vol. 2. Cambridge: At the University Press, 1956.

Ozaki, Norman Takeshi. *Conceptual Changes in Japanese Medicine During the Tokugawa Period.* Cambridge: Harvard University. Unpublished Ph.D. dissertation, 1979.

Pomeranz, Bruce, and Stux, Gabriel (eds.). *Scientific Bases of Acupuncture.* New York: Springer-Verlag, 1989.

Porkert, Manfred. *The Theoretical Foundations of Chinese Medicine.* M.I.T. East Asian Science Series, Vol. 3. Cambridge, Mass.: M.I.T. Press, 1974.

Quinn, Joseph R., ed. *Medicine and Public Health in the People's Republic of China.* Washington, DC: John E. Fogarty International Center, U.S. Dept. of HEW, NIH, 1973.

Rosner, F., and S. Muntner, eds. and trans. *The Medical Aphorisms of Moses Maimonides,* 2 vols. New York: Bloch Publishing, 1971.

Sigerist, Henry E. *A History of Medicine,* 2 vols. New York: Oxford University Press, 1951, 1961.

Sivin, Nathan. *Chinese Alchemy: Preliminary Studies.* Cambridge: Harvard University Press, 1968.

Sivin, Nathan. *Traditional Medicine in Contemporary China.* Ann Arbor: Center of Chinese Studies, University of Michigan, 1987.

Temkin, Owsei. *Galenism: Rise and Decline of a Medical Philosophy.* Ithaca, NY: Cornell University Press, 1973.

Unschuld, Paul U. *Medicine in China: A History of Ideas.* Berkeley: University of California Press, 1985.

Unschuld, Paul U. *Nan-Ching: The Classic of Difficult Issues.* Berkeley: University of California Press, 1986.

Watson, James L., and Rawski, Evelyn S. (eds.). *Death Ritual in Late Imperial and Modern China.* Berkeley: University of California Press, 1988.

Zito, Angela, and Barlow, Tani E. (eds.). *Body, Subject & Power in China.* Chicago: University of Chicago Press, 1994.

INDEX

An italic *n* indicates a note number
(e.g., 31*n*32 refers to page 31, note 32).